T0348625

Genitourinary Emergencies

Editors

JOSHUA MOSKOVITZ
RYAN SPANGLER

EMERGENCY MEDICINE
CLINICS OF NORTH AMERICA

www.emed.theclinics.com

Consulting Editor
AMAL MATTU

November 2019 • Volume 37 • Number 4

ELSEVIER

1600 John F. Kennedy Boulevard ● Suite 1800 ● Philadelphia, Pennsylvania, 19103-2899

http://www.theclinics.com

EMERGENCY MEDICINE CLINICS OF NORTH AMERICA Volume 37, Number 4
November 2019 ISSN 0733-8627, ISBN-13: 978-0-323-70904-0

Editor: Colleen Dietzler
Developmental Editor: Casey Potter

Emergency Medicine Clinics of North America (ISSN 0733-8627) is published quarterly by Elsevier Inc., 360 Park Avenue South, New York, NY, 10010-1710. Months of issue are February, May, August, and November. Business and Editorial Offices: 1600 John F. Kennedy Boulevard, Suite 1800, Philadelphia, PA 19103-2899. Customer Service Office: 6277 Sea Harbor Drive, Orlando, FL 32887-4800. Periodicals postage paid at New York, NY, and additional mailing offices. Subscription prices are $100.00 per year (US students), $349.00 per year (US individuals), $679.00 per year (US institutions), $220.00 per year (international students), $462.00 per year (international individuals), $836.00 per year (international institutions), $220.00 per year (Canadian students), $411.00 per year (Canadian individuals), and $836.00 per year (Canadian institutions). International air speed delivery is included in all *Clinics'* subscription prices. All prices are subject to change without notice. **POSTMASTER:** Send address changes to *Emergency Medicine Clinics of North America*, Elsevier Periodicals Customer Service, 11830 Westline Industrial Drive, St. Louis, MO 63146. Customer Service (orders, claims, online, change of address): Elsevier Periodicals **Customer Service, 11830 Westline Industrial Drive, St. Louis, MO 63146. Tel: 1-800-654-2452 (U.S. and Canada); 314-453-7041 (outside U.S. and Canada). Fax: 314-453-5170. E-mail: journalscustomerservice-usa@elsevier.com (for print support);** **journalsonlinesupport-usa@elsevier.com (for online support)**.

Reprints. For copies of 100 or more of articles in this publication, please contact the Commercial Reprints Department, Elsevier Inc., 360 Park Avenue South, New York, NY 10010-1710. Tel.: 212-633-3874; Fax: 212-633-3820; E-mail: reprints@elsevier.com.

Emergency Medicine Clinics of North America is covered in *MEDLINE/PubMed (Index Medicus), Current Contents/Clinical Medicine, EMBASE/Excerpta Medica, BIOSIS, SciSearch, CINAHL, ISI/BIOMED,* and *Research Alert.*

Contributors

CONSULTING EDITOR

AMAL MATTU, MD
Professor and Vice Chair of Academic Affairs, Department of Emergency Medicine, University of Maryland School of Medicine, Baltimore, Maryland

EDITORS

JOSHUA MOSKOVITZ, MD, MBA, MPH
Associate Director of Operations of the Emergency Department, Department of Emergency Medicine, Jacobi Medical Center, Assistant Professor of Emergency Medicine, Albert Einstein College of Medicine, Bronx, New York; Adjunct Assistant Professor of Public Health, Hofstra School of Health and Human Services, Hempstead, New York

RYAN SPANGLER, MD
Clinical Assistant Professor, Assistant Director of Undergraduate Medical Education, Department of Emergency Medicine, University of Maryland School of Medicine, Baltimore, Maryland

AUTHORS

ANDREW BARBERA, MD
Department of Emergency Medicine, Jacobi/Montefiore/Einstein Emergency Medicine Residency Program, Site Director/Core Faculty, Jacobi Medical Center, Assistant Professor of Emergency Medicine, Albert Einstein College of Medicine, Bronx, New York

MICHAEL BILLET, MD
Assistant Professor, Department of Emergency Medicine, University of Maryland School of Medicine, Baltimore, Maryland

MOLLY M. BOURKE, DO
Resident, Jacobi/Montefiore Emergency Medicine Residency, Bronx, New York

ANDREW F. BRAGG, MD
Resident Physician, Department of Pediatrics, University of Rochester, Rochester, New York

MATTHEW J. COPPOLA, MD
Assistant Professor of Emergency Medicine, Donald and Barbara Zucker School of Medicine at Hofstra/Northwell, Hempstead, New York; North Shore University Hospital, Manhasset, New York

JILL CORBO, MD, RDMS
Associate Professor, Department of Emergency Medicine, Jacobi Medical Center, Bronx, New York

SARAH B. DUBBS, MD
Assistant Professor, Department of Emergency Medicine, University of Maryland School of Medicine, Baltimore, Maryland

TANVEER GAIBI, MD, FACEP
Clinical Assistant Professor of Emergency Medicine GWSM, Assistant Professor of Emergency Medicine, Virginia Commonwealth University, Chairman, Department of Emergency Medicine, Inova Fairfax Medical Center, Falls Church, Virginia

JOHN DAVID GATZ, MD
Clinical Instructor, Department of Emergency Medicine, University of Maryland School of Medicine, Baltimore, Maryland

ADITI GHATAK-ROY, MD
PGY-2 Resident, Department of Emergency Medicine, George Washington University, Washington, DC

KAMI M. HU, MD
Assistant Professor, Program Director, Combined Emergency/Internal/Critical Care Residency, University of Maryland, Baltimore, Maryland

JULIAN JAKUBOWSKI, DO
Core Faculty, Department of Emergency Medicine, Emergency Medicine Residency Marietta Memorial Hospital, Marietta, Ohio; Clinical Assistant Professor, The Ohio University Heritage College of Osteopathic Medicine, Athens, Ohio

MICHAEL P. JONES, MD
Vice Chair of Education/Residency Director, Associate Professor of Emergency Medicine, Albert Einstein College of Medicine, Jacobi and Montefiore Medical Centers, Bronx, New York

KATHRYN KOONS, MD
Resident, Jacobi/Montefiore Emergency Medicine Residency, Bronx, New York

NICOLE J. LEONARD, MD
Resident, Department of Emergency Medicine, Jacobi/Montefiore Emergency Medicine Residency, Bronx, New York

SARAH MAHONSKI, MD
Attending Physician, Heritage Valley Health System, Beaver, Pennsylvania

DENISE McCORMACK, MD, MPH
Assistant Professor, Department of Emergency Medicine, Albert Einstein College of Medicine, Jacobi Medical Center, Bronx, New York

KUMELACHEW MEKURIA, MD
Resident Physician, Department of Emergency Medicine, Albert Einstein College of Medicine, Jacobi and Montefiore Medical Centers, Bronx, New York

JOSHUA MOSKOVITZ, MD, MBA, MPH
Associate Director of Operations of the Emergency Department, Department of Emergency Medicine, Jacobi Medical Center, Assistant Professor of Emergency Medicine, Albert Einstein College of Medicine, Bronx, New York; Adjunct Assistant Professor of Public Health, Hofstra School of Health and Human Services, Hempstead, New York

JOSEPH OFFENBACHER, MD
Resident, Emergency Medicine, Jacobi/Montefiore/Einstein Emergency Medicine
Residency Program, Jacobi Medical Center, Bronx, New York

JOSHUA Z. SILVERBERG, MD
Assistant Professor of Emergency Medicine, Albert Einstein College of Medicine, Bronx,
New York

SARAH K. SOMMERKAMP, MD, RDMS
Assistant Professor, Department of Emergency Medicine, University of Maryland School
of Medicine, Baltimore, Maryland

RYAN SPANGLER, MD
Clinical Assistant Professor, Assistant Director of Undergraduate Medical Education,
Department of Emergency Medicine, University of Maryland School of Medicine,
Baltimore, Maryland

KATHLEEN STEPHANOS, MD
Senior Instructor of Clinical Emergency Medicine, Departments of Emergency Medicine
and Pediatrics, University of Rochester, Rochester, New York

SEMHAR Z. TEWELDE, MD
Assistant Professor, Department of Emergency Medicine, University of Maryland School
of Medicine, Baltimore, Maryland

JESSICA WANG, MD, RDMS
Department of Emergency Medicine, Jacobi Medical Center, Bronx, New York

GEORGE C. WILLIS, MD
Assistant Professor, Department of Emergency Medicine, University of Maryland School
of Medicine, Baltimore, Maryland

THOMAS ANDREW WINDSOR, MD
Assistant Professor, Department of Emergency Medicine, University of Maryland School
of Medicine, Baltimore, Maryland

JOSEPH OFFENBACHER, MD
Resident, Emergency Medicine, Bronx/Montefiore Einstein Emergency Residency Program, Jacobi Medical Center, Bronx, New York

JOSHUA Z. SILVERBERG, MD
Assistant Professor of Emergency Medicine, Albert Einstein College of Medicine, Bronx, New York

SAGAR K. SOMMERHALDER, MD, RDMS
Assistant Professor, Department of Emergency Medicine, University of Maryland School of Medicine, Baltimore, Maryland

RYAN SPANGLER, MD
Clinical Assistant Professor, Assistant Director of Undergraduate Medical Education, Department of Emergency Medicine, University of Maryland School of Medicine, Baltimore, Maryland

KATHLEEN STEPHANOS, MD
Senior Instructor of Pediatrics, Director, Departments of Emergency Medicine and Pediatrics, University of Rochester, Rochester, New York

BEMHAR Z. TEWELDE, MD
Assistant Professor, Department of Emergency Medicine, University of Maryland School of Medicine, Baltimore, Maryland

JESSICA WANG, MD, RDMS
Department of Emergency Medicine, Jacobi Medical Center, Bronx, New York

GEORGE D. WILLIS, MD
Assistant Professor, Department of Emergency Medicine, University of Maryland School of Medicine, Baltimore, Maryland

THOMAS ANDREW WINDSOR, MD
Assistant Professor, Department of Emergency Medicine, University of Maryland School of Medicine, Baltimore, Maryland

Contents

and complicated UTI are presented, as well as techniques for distinguishing them. The pathophysiology and clinical and laboratory diagnoses of UTI are described. Treatment of UTI is reviewed, with attention to bacteriuria and special populations, including pregnant, elderly/geriatric, and spinal cord injury patients.

The diagnosis and treatment of sexually transmitted infections is a crucial component of providing evidence-based care in the emergency department. Understanding how to make the diagnosis and implement effective treatment is essential to maintaining and improving public health. Providers should also be adept at giving care to sexual assault survivors and seeking out the expertise of specially trained professionals within networks known as SANE, SAFE, or SART. These networks are critical to providing standardized care to sexual assault patients. Prophylaxis remains a key element for the prevention of sexually transmitted infections in all patients who are considered high risk.

Pediatric patients pose a unique host of challenges to the emergency provider across all complaints and ages, but this is particularly notable in the genitourinary (GU) system. The pediatric GU system is different from that of the adult in its etiology of symptoms, complications, and treatments. Based on age, there are variations in the anatomy. These differences result in symptoms and diagnoses that must be managed differently. Although in many respects management is similar to GU emergency conditions in adults, there are, occasionally subtle, differences between the care of children and adults, which can greatly impact outcomes.

Hematuria is common; whether gross or microscopic, it is incumbent on emergency providers to consider life-threatening and benign processes when evaluating these patients. Most of the workup is driven by a focused history and physical, including laboratory studies and diagnostic imaging. The cause originates in the genitourinary tract and, as long as the patient remains stable, they can be discharged with close outpatient follow-up. The importance of this cannot be stressed enough because hematuria, especially in the elderly, frequently signals the presence of urologic malignancy. In addition, the workup occasionally yields a nongenitourinary tract cause, and these patients often require emergent management.

The emergency medicine provider sees a broad range of pathology involving the female genitourinary system on a daily basis. Must-not-miss diagnoses include pelvic inflammatory disease and ovarian torsion, as these diagnoses can have severe complications and affect future fertility. Although most patients with abnormal uterine bleeding are hemodynamically stable, it can present as a life-threatening emergency and providers should be adept at managing severe hemorrhage. Bartholin gland cysts are common complaints that often require procedural intervention. This article discusses these diagnoses and appropriate evaluation and management in the emergency department.

Emergency physicians rely on a multitude of different imaging modalities in the diagnosis of genitourinary emergencies. There are many considerations to be taken into account when deciding which imaging modality should be used first, as oftentimes several diagnostic tools can be used for the same pathologic condition. These factors include radiation exposure, sensitivity, specificity, age of patient, availability of resources, cost, and timeliness of completion. In this review, the strengths and weaknesses of different imaging tools in the evaluation of genitourinary emergencies are discussed.

Emergency medicine providers may encounter serious GU conditions that need rapid diagnosis and early intervention to avoid severe life- and limb-threatening complications. A fundamental knowledge of several key procedural interventions is incredibly important to optimal patient outcomes.

EMERGENCY MEDICINE
CLINICS OF NORTH AMERICA

SERIES OF RELATED INTEREST

Urologic Clinics
https://www.urologic.theclinics.com/

THE CLINICS ARE NOW AVAILABLE ONLINE!
Access your subscription at:
www.theclinics.com

EMERGENCY MEDICINE
CLINICS OF NORTH AMERICA

FORTHCOMING ISSUES

February 2020
Diagnostic Emergencies
Michael C. Bond and Amal Mattu, Editor

May 2020
Risk Management in Emergency Medicine
Lauren Nentwich and Jonathan Olshaker, Editors

August 2020
Emergency Department Operations and Administration
Josh Joseph and Kevin Klauer, Editors

RECENT ISSUES

August 2019
Critical Care in the Emergency Department
John Greenwood and Tiffany Murano, editors

May 2019
Obstetric and Gynecologic Emergencies
Joelle Borhart and Rebecca A. Bavolek, Editors

February 2019
Ear, Nose, and Throat Emergencies
Laura J. Bontempo and Jan Shoenberger, Editors

SERIES OF RELATED INTEREST

Urologic Clinics
https://www.urologic.theclinics.com

Foreword

Genitourinary Emergencies in Emergency Medicine

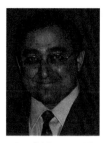

Amal Mattu, MD
Consulting Editor

I was recently talking to a colleague in emergency medicine about how he prioritizes his reading time, given how busy he is. He responded by stating that he focuses first on those organ systems that "make you die if they go bad." No surprise, he listed the cardiovascular system and neurologic system as his 2 main priorities when trying to keep up with the literature, and certain other organ systems, including the genitourinary (GU) system get only a passing glance with his limited time. At first, I thought this was quite a sensible method of time management. But then I started thinking about what happens when the GU system goes "bad."

Kidney failure can result in uremic encephalopathy, severe acidosis with cardiac dysfunction, hyperkalemia, and death. Ureteral stones cause, according to some patients, the worst pain they've ever experienced in their life. Bladder dysfunction leads to urinary abnormalities, including retention and eventually acute kidney injury. Mild urinary infections can lead to delirium in the elderly; and more severe infections are one of the most common causes of deadly sepsis. Testicular torsion leads to infertility and, commonly, litigation. Sexually transmitted infections can also lead to infertility, disseminated infections, and sepsis. It also bears noting that this organ system is responsible for mankind's ability to reproduce and carry on the species. Although cardiovascular and neurologic diseases receive far more attention in emergency medicine, there's no question that GU conditions are common and associated with significant morbidity and mortality in our patients.

In this issue of *Emergency Medicine Clinics of North America*, Guest Editors Drs Joshua Moskovitz and Ryan Spangler have assembled an outstanding group of authors to educate us on the importance of the GU system in emergency medicine. The authors discuss emergencies involving each anatomic structure from the kidneys to the genitals, including specific articles on renal colic, urinary retention, urinary and sexually transmitted infections, and hematuria. Special articles are added focusing

Emerg Med Clin N Am 37 (2019) xiii–xiv
https://doi.org/10.1016/j.emc.2019.08.002
0733-8627/19/© 2019 Published by Elsevier Inc.

on GU trauma and pediatric disorders, and they also separately discuss complications in the rapidly growing renal transplant population. Two final additional articles are provided on the special topics of imaging modalities in the GU system and also GU procedures.

This issue of *Emergency Medicine Clinics of North America* is an important addition to the emergency medicine literature. It is one of the only resources I've seen published in many years that focuses on the spectrum of GU emergencies in emergency medicine practice. It will certainly bring greater knowledge to an important but often neglected area of the emergency medicine, and help the reader truly understand what can happen when things "go bad." Our thanks to Drs Moskovitz and Spangler and the authors for their outstanding work!

Amal Mattu, MD
Department of Emergency Medicine
University of Maryland School of Medicine
110 South Paca Street
6th Floor, Suite 200
Baltimore, MD 21201, USA

E-mail address:
amalmattu@comcast.net

Preface

The Importance of Genitourinary Emergencies

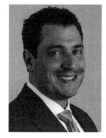
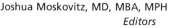
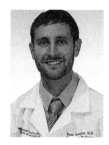

Joshua Moskovitz, MD, MBA, MPH   Ryan Spangler, MD

Editors

We hope you find this issue of Genitourinary Emergencies to be diverse with sufficient breadth and depth to help the pit doctor everywhere treat patients presenting with these complaints without angst or hesitation. We chose these articles to represent common presentations of genitourinary pathology that physicians in Emergency Departments everywhere may encounter. The majority of us treat these diseases each and every day, and we wanted to bring everyone up to speed on the latest and greatest in diagnosis, management, and intervention so we can all provide better quality care wherever we work to the patients we serve.

Joshua Moskovitz, MD, MBA, MPH
Department of Emergency Medicine
Jacobi Medical Center
Albert Einstein College of Medicine
1400 Pelham Parkway South
Building 6 Room 1B25
ED Administration Office
Bronx, NY 10461, USA

Hofstra School of Health and Human Services
Hempstead, NY 11549, USA

Emerg Med Clin N Am 37 (2019) xv–xvi
https://doi.org/10.1016/j.emc.2019.08.001
0733-8627/19/© 2019 Published by Elsevier Inc.

Ryan Spangler, MD
University of Maryland School of Medicine
Department of Emergency Medicine
110 South Paca Street
6th Floor, Suite 200
Baltimore, MD 21201, USA

E-mail addresses:
joshmoskovitz@gmail.com (J. Moskovitz)
rspangler@som.umaryland.edu (R. Spangler)

Penile Emergencies

Joseph Offenbacher, MD[a], Andrew Barbera, MD[b],*

KEYWORDS

- Penis • Penile emergency • Priapism • Paraphimosis • Phimosis • Balanitis
- Posthitis • Penile tourniquet syndrome

KEY POINTS

- Penile emergencies require prompt diagnosis and management to minimize organ dysfunction.
- Comprehension of the pathologic processes related to the unique anatomic structure and physiologic function of the penis is required for optimal treatment of penile emergencies and preservation of the organ function.
- Without prompt diagnosis and management, penile emergencies can lead to excretory or reproductive malfunction, penile loss, morbidity, or mortality.

INTRODUCTION

As an organ of central importance to both the urologic and reproductive systems, penile emergencies have the potential to lead to significant morbidity for patients. Although there is generally considered to be a defined set of pathologies affecting the penis in the acute setting, recognition and prompt diagnosis of these conditions often can be challenging for clinicians. Because of the organ's anatomy and physiology, failure or even moderate delays in identifying these acute conditions may result in permanent dysfunction and morbidity. In the broadest sense, penile emergencies can fall into 1 of 2 major categories: physiologic (relating to the venous outflow) or anatomic (relating to pathologies of the organ's complex tissue structure). Specific disease states include priapism, penile calciphylaxis, paraphimosis, phimosis, balanitis, posthitis, Peyronie disease, penile tourniquet syndrome.

PHYSIOLOGIC EMERGENCIES
Priapism

Priapism is defined as, "prolonged erection of the penis, generally lasting more than 4 hours, in the absence of sexual desire or stimulation."[1] The condition is generally

---

Disclosure Statement: The authors have no conflicts of interest or anything to disclose.
[a] Emergency Medicine, Jacobi//Montefiore/Einstein Emergency Medicine Residency Program, Jacobi Medical Center, 1400 Pelham Parkway South, Building 6, Suite 1B25, Bronx, NY 10461, USA; [b] Department of Emergency Medicine, Jacobi//Montefiore/Einstein Emergency Medicine Residency Program, Jacobi Medical Center, Albert Einstein College of Medicine, 1400 Pelham Parkway South, Building 6, Suite 1B25, Bronx, NY 10461, USA
* Corresponding author.
E-mail address: Barbera.Andrew@gmail.com

Emerg Med Clin N Am 37 (2019) 583–592
https://doi.org/10.1016/j.emc.2019.07.001
0733-8627/19/© 2019 Elsevier Inc. All rights reserved.

known to have 2 physiologic etiologies. The first, high-flow or nonischemic, is related to increased arterial flow to the penis. The second, commonly referred to as low-flow or ischemic priapism, is caused by an obstruction to venous outflow and subsequent engorgement.

Nonischemic, high-flow, priapism is not considered to be a urologic emergency, because penile tissue remains perfused by continued arterial supply and seldom requires emergent intervention. As described previously, this condition is caused by increased arterial flow to the organ, typically due to the development of traumatic fistulas between the artery and the cavernosum. This condition, although rare, is caused by blunt trauma to the perineum and penis with one such example being "straddle injury." Although this variant is often not painful, it is much less common than the ischemic subtype. Although not considered a true urologic emergency, if left untreated, it has been reported to lead to low-flow priapism states.[2]

Ischemic (low-flow) priapism is a painful urologic emergency necessitating emergent intervention. Caused by obstruction to venous outflow from the penis, this leads to venous engorgement and results in increased pressure and decreased arterial flow. The resulting inability to provide adequate flow of oxygenated blood to the organ leads to tissue necrosis and death. Ultimately, this condition can be thought of as an organ-specific type of compartment syndrome with permanent tissue death.[3] Ischemic priapism is known to have significant morbidity, often secondary to fibrosis of the penile tissue, with nearly one-third of treated patients suffering from fibrosis and permanent erectile dysfunction and subsequent infertility.[4]

Ischemic priapism is known to have several etiologies generally associated with either primary venous obstruction or secondary venous obstruction. Primary venous obstruction is related to either hematologic or vascular anatomic pathology, whereas secondary obstruction is related to failure of normal smooth muscle contraction within the spongy erectile tissue of the penis.[3] Secondary obstruction can have a number of different causes, including primary neurologic pathology, such as spinal cord injury or compression, and as a secondary sequalae to many different classes of medications.

Although hematologic diseases, primarily affecting red blood cells, contribute to the overall burden of disease incidence, it is well established that several hematologic pathologies place patients at increased risk for developing ischemic priapism. These conditions include sickle cell disease, leukemia, thalassemia, multiple myeloma, hemoglobin (Hb) Olmsted, parenteral hyperalimentation, hemodialysis, and glucose-6-phosphate dehydrogenase.[3] Taken together, these conditions contribute to blood hyperviscosity leading to impairment of flow and resulting in physiologic obstruction.

A subtype of this disorder, often seen in patients with sickle cell disease, is known as stuttering priapism. It is noted for leading to repeated episodes of priapism lasting less than 3 hours. In many cases, the condition resolves spontaneously without requiring further intervention. These patients do not require emergency intervention so long as the event does not last longer than approximately 3 hours.[5]

In addition to physiologic obstruction, mechanical obstruction of the venous outflow tracts has a known association with the development of priapism. These include several classes of pelvic malignancies, such as cancers to the penis, bladder, urethra, prostate, and rectum.[6] As tumor burdens begin to invade the venous outflow channels of the penis, risk of priapism becomes more acute. An additional significant etiology of mechanical obstruction to outflow of blood from the penis is related to trauma. This may include any significant injury to the pelvis, perineum, or penis, and is the result of blunt trauma to these regions.

In secondary venous obstruction, the primary mechanism by which medications lead to priapism is through their effect on smooth muscle contraction of the cavernous arteries and corporal bodies. This is generally a normal physiologic process through which erections can be attained. This process, however, requires subsequent contraction of the cavernous smooth muscle bodies to open the venous outflow tracts. Failure of normal smooth muscle contraction can lead to prolonged obstruction of venous outflow leading to hypoxia, acidosis, and cell death.

Medications that are known to be associated with this condition include drugs used for erectile dysfunction, antihypertensive agents (nitroglycerine, calcium channel blockers), alpha adrenergic antagonists, antipsychotic and antidepressant medications, recreational drugs (including cocaine, marijuana, and ethanol), and anticoagulants.[7] Other known agents include androgen hormones, immunosuppressants, and scorpion toxins.

Neurogenic causes of priapism include damage or disruption in both the central and peripheral nervous systems. Centrally these include damage to the brain, from vascular events or trauma, and to the spinal cord from trauma, iatrogenic anesthesia, disk disease, cauda equina syndrome, and central nervous system infections, such as neuro syphilis.[8,9] Peripherally, damage to peripheral pelvic nerves as sequelae of hip arthroplasty also have been shown to cause priapism.[10] Overall, these types of events have all been shown to lead to ischemic priapism by causing dysfunction of autonomic smooth muscle of the corpus cavernosum.

Regardless of its underlying cause, prolonged priapism, lasting roughly 4 hours, can lead to permanent dysfunction if not emergently treated. The proposed mechanism of the aforementioned time course relates to the onset of ischemia-induced cytokine release in the corpus cavernosum. This cytokine surge is thought to exacerbate smooth muscle necrosis, death, fibrosis, and dysfunction.[11]

In the emergency setting, rapid and accurate differentiation between ischemic and nonischemic priapism is essential to appropriately proceed with management. In this regard, there are several important signs and symptoms of ischemic priapism that should be noted.

A thorough medical history should be taken. Important features include painful, nontraumatic, erection. Patients with a past history of such events, as well as those with medical conditions, or those who use medications that are known to exacerbate the condition, should prompt a high level of clinical suspicion. Eliciting a thorough time course also can help in focusing the diagnosis. Patients with ischemic priapism often present immediately due to the early onset of pain. In contrast, patients with nonischemic priapism, which is typically not painful, present later in the course.

On physical examination, ischemic priapism often presents with a rigid penis and soft glans. In contrast, nonischemic priapism will typically present with a partial erection but a firm glans. The "peisis sign," whereby partial or complete resolution of the erection can be achieved by compression of the perineum, also is an important indicator of a nonischemic event.[1]

In addition to physical examination, a series of clinical tests can be performed to help achieve a diagnosis. These include analysis of blood aspiration from the corpora cavernosa as well as color duplex ultrasound of the penis and perineum looking for blood flow through the cavernosal arteries. In the case of ischemic priapism, aspirated blood tends to be dark in color and blood gas analysis will show pH of less than 7.25, Pao_2 less than 30 mm Hg, and Pco_2 greater than 60 mm Hg. This is in contrast to findings in nonischemic priapism, in which typically pH is greater than 7.3, Pao_2 is greater than 50 mm Hg, and Pco_2 is less than 40 mm Hg.[4]

Ischemic priapism is a true urologic emergency and, at least at the outset, should be managed in the emergency setting. Both medical and surgical management options are available in the acute setting. Oral terbutaline, a Beta-2-adrenergic agonist, at dose of 5 to 10 mg is often considered as an initial treatment to relax venous sinusoidal smooth muscle and enable increased venous outflow from the corpora.[12] If initial dose is ineffective, a second oral dose of again 5 to 10 mg can be used after 15 minutes.[13]

If this treatment does not show rapid (within 30 minutes) detumescence, there should be little hesitation in using more invasive options, such as corporal blood aspiration. This intervention can be associated with additional therapeutic adjuncts, such as saline irrigation and injection of alpha-adrenergic-agonists, such as dilute phenylephrine, with usual dose of 0.1 mg to 1 mg phenylephrine diluted into a 10-mL syringe with normal saline injecting 1 mL at a time.[7,14] As with most invasive penile procedures anesthesia via a penile block is recommended and is a procedure that can be done in the emergency setting.[15] In addition to direct management of the condition itself, efforts should be made to address the underlying cause of the priapism, as described previously. Patients whose condition does not respond to the aforementioned treatments would require a surgical shunt to prevent irreversible ischemia and tissue death[4] (Fig. 1).

Penile Calciphylaxis

Penile calciphylaxis is considered to be a rare disorder that can have both organ-specific and systemic morbidity and mortality.[1] Caused by calcification and fibrosis of the penile arteries, the most severe penile sequala of the disorder is gangrene of the organ. Despite its low incidence, penile calciphalix is often the result of underlying end-stage renal disease causing hyperparathyroidism.

The underlying pathophysiologic mechanism of the disorder often results in concurrent arterial calcification in the extremities, leading to systemic pathology. Calcification of the penile arteries can rapidly lead to ischemia, infection, and necrosis. Patients often can present in severe pain. The condition warrants emergent urologic evaluation for possible debridement and, in extreme cases, such as organ gangrene, amputation (penectomy).[16]

ANATOMIC EMERGENCIES
Paraphimosis

Paraphimosis is a pathologic process resulting from the anatomic structure of the distal foreskin in relation to the glans; specifically, where the foreskin in an uncircumcised male cannot be reduced distally to its usual anatomic position overlying the glans. This entrapment may result from inflammation of the foreskin in its retracted position leading to physiologic constriction of the penile shaft. This constriction may

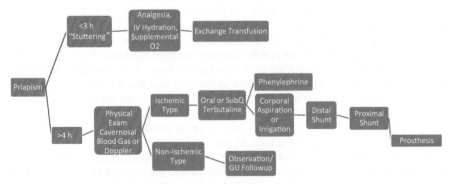

Fig. 1. Algorithm for priapism. GU, genitourinary; IV, intravenous; SQ, subcutaneous.

lead to obstruction of the venous outflow leading to glans edema and worsening penile shaft stricture. The constriction can become so severe that arterial blood supply may be compromised, leading to ischemia of the distal penile tissue. When this happens, tissue necrosis may ensue, leading to gangrene and death of the organ. There have been reports of such conditions leading to systemic sequela, such as necrotizing fasciitis.[17]

Diagnosis of the condition is based on history and physical examination. Paraphymosis is generally seen at the extremes of age in the very young and very old. It has been suggested that as men get older, a decreased frequency of erections can lead to less frequent dilation of the preputial orifice and increased risk of entrapment. In general, populations for whom genital hygiene presents a challenge are at significant risk for developing this condition.

In most cases, an inciting retraction of the foreskin has been known to contribute to the increased incidence of the condition. This has been known to occur during intercourse or medical examinations. Additional less common etiologies of paraphymosis include genital piercings, plasmodium falciparum, chancroid, lichen sclerosis, and contact dermatitis.[18]

Because of its ability to cause rapid gland necrosis, paraphymosis is considered a urologic emergency and must be managed immediately. This often can be accomplished in the emergency setting, and requires specialist intervention only if there is failure of manual reduction of foreskin or necrosis of tissue. Although many techniques exist, the overall goal of management is to reduce the glans back through the proximal foreskin. One method that is often described is the manual decompression of the swollen glans followed by reduction past the constricting band.[19]

Furthermore, several methods have been suggested for minimizing the edema of both the glans and the foreskin, which is ultimately essential for effective treatment. Reduction of the glans can be achieved through manual compression, ice packs, or wrapping the glans in compressive dressings. Reduction of the foreskin can be achieved through making micro-punctures in the foreskin, thereby releasing edematous fluid. Other methods for reducing foreskin edema include the invasive injection of hyaluronidase into the edematous foreskin, as well as the noninvasive, topical application of granulated sugar to the outside of the edematous structure.

If these emergent treatments should prove unsuccessful, surgical urologic management might be required to prevent tissue death. This can include dorsal slit procedures or circumcision (**Fig. 2**).

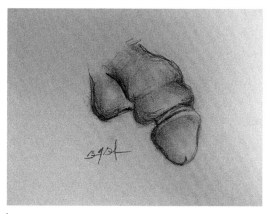

Fig. 2. Paraphimosis

Phimosis

Phimosis is a pathologic process also resulting from the anatomic structure of the distal foreskin in relation to the glans in uncircumcised male individuals. In this case, the foreskin cannot be retracted proximally over the glans. As with many penile conditions, the pathologic process varies slightly between the pediatric and adult patient. In newborns, this condition is considered normal and relates to the adherence of the epithelial layers of the glans and foreskin. It is not uncommon for the foreskin to not be fully retractable until age 3, and in some cases as late as adolescence. In adults, this condition is often caused by scaring and fibrosis of the distal prepuce.[20]

Although this condition is typically chronic and nonemergent, phimosis can become pathologic if it leads to urethral obstruction and chronic stone formation. In extreme cases of obstruction, surgical intervention with a slit procedure may be necessary. Severe cases of phimosis also may lead to balanitis and posthitis due to the similar anatomic etiologies of these related conditions (**Fig. 3**).

Balanitis/Posthitis/Balanoposthitis

Balanitis and posthitis are conditions of inflammation of the glans penis and foreskin, respectively. Often these conditions present together and are termed balanoposthitis. Uncircumcised men are at greater risk, as infection is a leading cause of developing this type of inflammation.

Patients often present with red, inflamed, and edematous tissue of the glans and foreskin. Discharge is also common. Depending on the underlying infectious etiology, papules and other penile lesions may be present. This is often seen secondary to candidiasis infections, which are known to be the most common cause of balanitis. These patients present with erythema, papules and "satellite lesions" to the foreskin and surrounding structures.

Candidiasis infections are commonly acquired through sexual intercourse with an infected partner. In addition, patients with comorbidities, such as diabetes mellitus, and poor hygiene are considered to be at increased risk for spontaneous infections. Patients presenting with spontaneous candidiasis balanitis should have a fingerstick glucose test, as this can be a presenting sign of new-onset diabetes. Those patients with known diabetes can present with candida balanitis as a presenting sign of uncontrolled hyperglycemia.[21] Patients presenting with evidence of balanitis secondary to candidiasis infection can be treated with topical

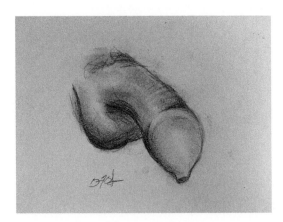

Fig. 3. Phimosis.

antifungals, such as clotrimazole cream 1% or miconazole cream 2% can be used twice daily for 2 weeks.[22] Those with underlying comorbidities or failure of topical treatment also may require oral antifungal therapy via a single 150-mg dose of fluconazole.[23]

In addition to candidiasis, other infectious conditions have been associated with the development of balanitis and posthitis. These include streptococcal and staphylococcal species. In addition, sexually transmitted infections, such as chlamydia and syphilis, are known etiologies. These conditions are managed by treating the underlying infectious condition with antibiotics. As a result, additional diagnostic evaluation with cultures and testing for sexually transmitted infections also may be appropriate to guide management.

Although balanitis and posthitis are typically not conditions of emergent acuity, they may have emergent sequalae if not properly managed. These include phimosis, cellulitis of the penile shaft, and abscess development. These conditions can be associated with high levels of morbidity and mortality, and should be recognized as possible consequences of failure to effectively manage the condition.

Although considerably less common, noninfectious etiologies of balanitis and posthitis must also be considered. These include contact dermatitis from condoms, spermicidals, and other substances that commonly come into contact with the penis.[24]

Noninfectious balanitis-specific conditions include lichen planus, which is clinically identified by itchy red and white plaques. It is typically treated with high-potency topical steroids. Balanitis xerotica obliterans is another glans-specific inflammatory condition. It is of unknown origin and causes chronic inflammation with possible pruritis and endarteritis.[25]

Peyronie Disease

Although not generally considered a penile emergency, Peyronie disease is a well described condition that can lead to significant morbidity, including erectile dysfunction, over time. It is a connective tissue disorder that is characterized by plaque and fibrotic collagen scar formation in the tunica albuginea.[26] Over time, these patients present with penile induration, palpable plaques, and an abnormal curvature of the erect penis.

Patients with this condition can present with pain and acute scar formation after penile trauma. Of note is that patients with this condition can present following very minor trauma, including microtrauma from intercourse. Patients are often not aware of the inciting event that led to their pain or scar formation. Management of these patients should focus on good, nonemergent, outpatient urologic follow-up for further treatment and possible surgical intervention.[27]

NONTRAUMATIC PENILE INJURY

The most common cause of nontraumatic but acute injuries to the penis are related to penile entrapment. In most cases, this condition results from circumferential entrapment of the organ leading to both venous and arterial compromise. This condition can be found, predominantly, in 2 distinct patient populations. In pediatrics, penile entrapment is most often accidental.

Penile tourniquet syndrome, although rare, if unrecognized can lead to progressive disease from edema to urethracutaneous fistula to severe consequences including tissue necrosis or amputation of the penis.[28] Penile tourniquet syndrome can be caused by any object that impedes blood flow and leads to penile strangulation and can occur at any age. However, it is recognized that infants are at higher risk, as they cannot communicate or localize to the pain or symptoms. In infants, penile tourniquet syndrome occurs usually between 2 and 6 months of age and the causative object is often hair from the mother. This time period coincides and is thought to be due to a process named "telogen effluvium," which is maternal post-partum hair loss that occurs 2 to 6 months postpartum and is due to reduced hormone production.[29,30] Infants who present with penile hair tourniquet syndrome often present with parental complaints of intractable crying or inconsolability. In these patients, it is especially important to expose their entire body and examine for hair tourniquets as part of the workup. Diagnosis of hair tourniquets is done by physical examination and very carefully, as patients may be uncooperative or the tourniquet can be masked by a skin fold[31] (**Fig. 4**).

In children and adults, although hair can still be the causative object, it is much less common, and children can present with a variety of household objects. Adolescents and adults commonly present with rings of different materials as the culprit object often used for sexual intent. Patients also may present in different disease stages, from minor pain and edema to penile necrosis, including adults who may feel stigmatized and delay medical evaluation. The first part of treatment is prompt diagnosis and, if possible, removal of strangulating object. If hair or thread tourniquet, it may be cut off with scissors, with care to ensure no second circumferential strands or hidden hair strands. If the object is of hard material and not easily cut, a technique previously described to take rings off of fingers can be used. Before any attempt at removal, local anesthesia should be applied to aid with patient tolerance and success of the procedure. Penile blocks are often all that is necessary to provide adequate anesthesia with minimal risk. After adequate anesthesia is achieved, a string can be passed beneath the ring and then bound tightly over the distal shaft of the penis to the glands to decrease edema. Then the proximal end of the string is lifted, allowing the ring to pass over the bound area of the penis. This procedure may be repeated as needed to affectively remove the object. Additional techniques, if this is unsuccessful, include aspiration of blood from the distal penis to decrease edema, the use of ring cutting devices, and, if needed, surgical debridement and removal in the operating room.[32] Of note, in children it is important to ensure that the penile tourniquet is not a form of parental punishment or abuse.

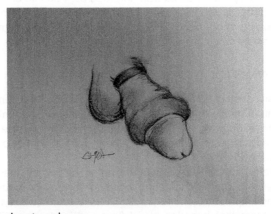

Fig. 4. Penile tourniquet syndrome.

SUMMARY

Penile emergencies most commonly result from pathologic processes related to the unique anatomic structure and physiologic function of the organ. As the organ itself is essential for excretory and reproductive function, its pathologies can lead to devastating morbidity and in some cases mortality. Even with prompt diagnosis and treatment, penile emergencies can lead to permanent organ dysfunction. Prompt diagnosis, management, and urologic consultation are essential for having the best chance of minimizing sequela of these conditions.

ACKNOWLEDGMENTS

Brian Barbera, illustrator of **Figs. 2–4**.

REFERENCES

1. Dubin J, Davis JE. Penile emergencies [review]. Emerg Med Clin North Am 2011; 29(3):485–99.
2. Carvajal A, Benavides JA. Combination high flow priapism with low flow priapism: case report. Sex Med 2018. https://doi.org/10.1016/j.esxm.2018.10.003.
3. Huang YC, Harraz AM, Shindel AW, et al. Evaluation and management of priapism: 2009 update. Nat Rev Urol 2009;6(5):262–71.
4. Burnett AL, Bivalacqua TJ. Priapism: current principles and practice [review]. Urol Clin North Am 2007;34(4):631–42, viii.
5. Muneer A, Minhas S, Arya M, et al. Stuttering priapism–a review of the therapeutic options [review]. Int J Clin Pract 2008;62(8):1265–70.
6. Persec Z, Persec J, Sovic T, et al. Penile metastases of rectal adenocarcinoma. J Visc Surg 2014;151(1):53–5.
7. Van Der Horst C, Stuebinger H, Seif C, et al. Priapism: etiology, pathophysiology and management. Int Braz J Urol 2003;29(5):391–400.
8. Hopkins A, Clarke C, Brindley G. Erections on walking as a symptom of spinal canal stenosis. J Neurol Neurosurg Psychiatry 1987;50(10):1371–4.
9. Munro D, Horne HW Jr, Paull DP. The effect of injury to the spinal cord and cauda equina on the sexual potency of men. N Engl J Med 1948;239(24):903–11.
10. Hishmeh S, DiMaio FR. Priapism as a complication after total hip arthroplasty: a case report and review of the literature [review]. Orthopedics 2008;31(4):397.
11. Bivalacqua TJ, Burnett AL. Priapism: new concepts in the pathophysiology and new treatment strategies [review]. Curr Urol Rep 2006;7(6):497–502.
12. Priyadarshi S. Oral terbutaline in the management of pharmacologically induced prolonged erection. Int J Impot Res 2004;16(5):424–6.
13. Vorobets D, Banyra O, Stroy A, et al. Our experience in the treatment of priapism. Cent European J Urol 2011;64(2):80–3.
14. Montague DK, Jarow J, Broderick GA, et al. Members of the erectile dysfunction guideline update panel; American Urological Association. American Urological Association guideline on the management of priapism. J Urol 2003;170(4 Pt 1): 1318–24.
15. Flores S, Herring AA. Ultrasound-guided dorsal penile nerve block for ED paraphimosis reduction. Am J Emerg Med 2015;33(6):863.e3-5.
16. Karpman E, Das S, Kurzrock E. Penile calciphylaxis: analysis of risk factors and mortality. J Urol 2003;169(6):2206–9.
17. Ahmed J, Mallick I. Paraphimosis leading to Fournier's gangrene. J Coll Physicians Surg Pak 2009;19(3):203–4.

18. Kessler CS, Bauml J. Non-traumatic urologic emergencies in men: a clinical review. West J Emerg Med 2009;10(4):281–7.
19. Choe JM. Paraphimosis: current treatment options. Am Fam Physician 2000;62: 2623–6.
20. McGregor TB, Pike JG, Leonard MP. Pathologic and physiologic phimosis: approach to the phimotic foreskin. Can Fam Physician 2007;53:445–8.
21. Kalra S, Chawla A. Diabetes and balanoposthitis. J Pak Med Assoc 2016;66(8): 1039–41.
22. Edwards SK. European guideline for the management of balanoposthitis. Int J STD AIDS 2001;12(Suppl 3):68–72.
23. Janik M, Heffernan M. Yeast infections: candidiasis and tinea (pityriasis) versicolor. In: Wolff K, Goldsmith LA, Katz SI, et al, editors. Fitzpatrick's dermatology in general medicine. 7th edition. New York: McGraw Hill; 2008. p. 1824–8.
24. Muratore L, Calogiuri G, Foti C, et al. Contact allergy to benzocaine in a condom. Contact Derm 2008;59:173–4.
25. Sakti D, Gurunadha HS, Tunuguntla R. Balanitis xerotica obliterans—a review. World J Urol 2000;18:382–7.
26. Ahuja SK, Sikka SC, Hellstrom WJ. Stimulation of collagen production in an in vitro model for Peyronie's disease. Int J Impot Res 1999;11(4):207–12.
27. Hellstrom W. Medical management of Peyronie's disease. J Androl 2009;30(4): 397–405.
28. Ozdamar MY, Zengin K, Tanik S, et al. The relationship between the localization and etiology in children's penile tourniquet syndrome: a case report and literature review. Pediatr Urol Case Rep 2014;1(3):16–20.
29. Harrison S, Sinclair R. Telogen effluvium. Clin Exp Dermatol 2002;27(5):389–95.
30. Hussin P, Mawardi M, Masran MS, et al. Hair tourniquet syndrome: revisited. G Chir 2015;36(5):219–21.
31. Hussain HM. A hair tourniquet resulting in strangulation and amputation of penis: case report and literature review. J Paediatr Child Health 2008;44(10):606–7.
32. Shukla P, Lal S, Shrivastava GP, et al. Penile incarceration with encircling metallic objects: a study of successful removal. J Clin Diagn Res 2014;8(6):NC01–5.

Acute Scrotal Emergencies

Molly M. Bourke, DO[a], Joshua Z. Silverberg, MD[b],*

KEYWORDS

- Scrotal emergencies • Testicular torsion • Fournier gangrene • Testicular trauma
- Scrotal ultrasonography

KEY POINTS

- Testicular torsion, Fournier gangrene, and testicular trauma are urologic emergencies.
- Testicular torsion is time sensitive with higher salvage rates under 6 hours.
- It is important to have a high index of suspicion for Fournier gangrene, because it has a high mortality rate.
- In the setting of trauma, testicular rupture and penetrating injuries through the dartos fascia require surgical exploration.

INTRODUCTION

Scrotal emergencies, however uncommon, can be life and fertility threatening. Testicular torsion, Fournier gangrene, and scrotal trauma are all considered emergent urologic conditions. These conditions need to be separated from the wide differential diagnoses presenting as acute scrotal pain to the emergency department.

Genitourinary complaints represent less than 1% of emergency department visits overall.[1] The more life-threatening and fertility-threatening diagnoses are less common than their more benign counterparts. The annual incidence of testicular torsion for boys under the age of 18 years is approximately 3.8 per 100,000.[2] A recent European study estimated the incidence of epididymitis to be 2.45 per 1000.[3]

Although these conditions are uncommon, it is important to diagnose and treat early. A review of pediatric malpractice claims in the emergency department from 2001 to 2015 demonstrated that male genital conditions were among the highest reported in malpractice suits, with misdiagnoses being the primary error.[4]

Diagnosis of testicular torsion is time sensitive. Testicular torsion has a greater than 90% salvage rate if surgery is performed within the first 6 hours of symptom onset. After 6 hours, there is a time-dependent increase in the rate of testicular atrophy and

Disclosure: M.M. Bourke has nothing to disclose. J.Z. Silverberg owns equity in Johnson and Johnson.
[a] Jacobi Montefiore Emergency Medicine Residency, 1400 Pelham Parkway South, Building 6, Suite 1B-25, Bronx, NY 10461, USA; [b] Albert Einstein College of Medicine, 1400 Pelham Parkway South, Building 6, Suite 1B-25, Bronx, NY 10461, USA
* Corresponding author.
E-mail address: joshua.silverberg@nychhc.org

Emerg Med Clin N Am 37 (2019) 593–610
https://doi.org/10.1016/j.emc.2019.07.002
0733-8627/19/© 2019 Elsevier Inc. All rights reserved.

orchiectomy.[5] It is important to establish the diagnosis early and advocate for definitive management with urology colleagues. Approximately 30% of cases of failed testicular salvage can be attributed to misdiagnosis and another 13% to delay in treatment after the diagnosis has been made.[6]

An acute scrotum is defined as acute pain of the scrotum. Pain is typically accompanied by local signs, such as swelling or tenderness, and/or generalized symptoms, such as vomiting or fever.[7] There is a large differential diagnosis for acute scrotal pain. True emergencies should be separated from urgencies. True urologic emergencies include testicular torsion, Fournier gangrene, and testicular trauma. Other abdominal emergencies to keep in mind that may present as scrotal pain include, but are not limited to, an incarcerated inguinal hernia, appendicitis, or referred pain from an abdominal aortic aneurysm.

Torsion should be differentiated from appendage torsion and epididymitis, whereas Fournier gangrene should be ruled out in infectious presentations of scrotal pain, including scrotal cellulitis and scrotal abscesses. In the setting of trauma, it is important to identify penetrating trauma and testicular rupture from simple testicular contusions. See **Box 1** for a full list of the differential diagnoses for acute scrotal pain.

PRESENTATION AND CAUSES

The presentation of an acute scrotum can be broken down into 4 subcategories: the painful swollen testicle, the painless swollen testicle, the erythematous testicle, and the traumatic testicle. Within each of these groups there is a diagnosis that cannot be missed.

However, not all scrotal emergencies present with pain in the genital area. It is important to rule out scrotal emergencies in patients presenting with lower abdominal pain. In a retrospective review of cases of testicular torsion, Progorelić and colleagues[9] investigated 9 cases of confirmed testicular torsion that presented with lower abdominal pain only. Of the 9 cases, 6 did not have an initial scrotal examination, which delayed diagnosis of testicular torsion, leading to orchiectomy in 5 of the 6 cases. The patient who was saved from orchiectomy was re-examined and underwent surgery within 5 hours. The other 5 cases did not receive a genitourinary examination or get definitive surgical intervention until after 18 hours (the range was from 18 to 72 hours). Of the 6 cases without a genitourinary examination, the first contact was with a general practitioner or an emergency physician.

The Painful Scrotum

Testicular torsion
Testicular torsion occurs when the spermatic cord twists causing venous congestion, decreased arterial blood flow and eventually ischemia of the testicle. There are 2 types of torsion: extravaginal and intravaginal. Extravaginal torsion occurs in the perinatal period, it occurs with twisting of the entire tunica vaginalis. It may present as a vanishing testicle or painless swollen hemiscrotum. Intravaginal torsion is the twisting inside the tunica vaginalis, occasionally as the result of a congenital bell clapper deformity. The deformity occurs when the testicle is not fully fused to the posterior scrotal wall. This results in the testicle being suspended horizontally, which predisposes it to torsion.[10] This deformity is estimated to be present in approximately 12% of men (**Fig. 1**).[11]

Testicular torsion can occur at any age, although it is most common at 2 peaks in life: during the first year of life and around puberty (12–18 years old).[2,12,13] Testicular torsion generally presents as acute onset scrotal pain with associated nausea or

Box 1
Differential diagnoses for acute scrotal pain

Ischemic
    Testicular torsion
    Torsion of the testicular appendage

Infectious
    Epididymitis
    Epididymo-orchitis
    Orchitis
    Scrotal cellulitis
    Scrotal abscess
    Fournier gangrene
    Hansen disease[a]
    Filariasis[b]

Traumatic
    Blunt:
        Testicular contusion
        Testicular rupture
    Penetrating
        Testicular rupture
    Hematocele
    Scrotal degloving

Inflammatory
    Henoch-Schonlein purpura

Idiopathic
    Idiopathic scrotal swelling

Oncologic
    Testicular tumors

Other
    Strangulated/incarcerated inguinal hernia
    Referred pain from abdominal pathology, for example, ruptured abdominal aortic aneurysm
    or nephrolithiasis

[a]Caused by *Mycobacterium leprae.*

[b]A parasitic disease caused by *Wuchereria bancrofti*, which manifests as lymphedema or a hydrocele often associated with epididymo-orchitis.[8]

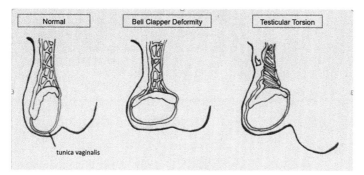

Fig. 1. Demonstration of normal testis, bell clapper deformity, and testicular torsion. (*Courtesy of* M. Bourke, DO, Bronx, NY.)

vomiting.[13] It can occur after minor trauma or during periods of testicular growth (ie, puberty); however, it usually occurs in the absence of a preceding event.[14] Fujita and colleagues[15] found there was an increased rate of onset during sleep. This is possibly owing to a unilateral cremasteric reflex or simply lower ambient temperatures, which have also been linked to an increased rate of torsion. It is important to keep in mind that intermittent torsion may also precede complete torsion.[16]

Testicular torsion can often be hard to differentiate from appendage torsion and epididymitis. There are 2 features of the clinical history that have been shown to increase the likelihood of diagnosis. Presence of nausea and/or vomiting and less than 24 hours since the onset of pain have both been proven to be associated with testicular torsion more often than the latter diagnosis.[13,17,18] One study demonstrated that, in patients with acute scrotal pain from testicular torsion, the presence of nausea and vomiting had a specificity of 93% and a sensitivity of 69%.[19] Thus, in the setting of acute scrotal pain, systemic symptoms of nausea and vomiting make testicular torsion more likely.

Appendage torsion

Appendage torsion, although not a scrotal emergency in itself, must be differentiated from testicular torsion. Appendage torsion is the twisting of a testicular or epididymal appendage, which is an embryologic remnant of the Mullerian ducts. Appendage torsion is usually seen in prepubertal boys 7 to 12 years old.[15] Onset is acute to subacute. It is often difficult to differentiate appendage torsion from testicular torsion based on history because both groups may have acute onset testicular pain and swelling. However, patients with appendage torsion are less likely to have systemic symptoms, including nausea or vomiting (**Fig. 2**).[19]

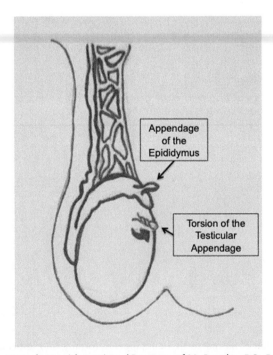

Fig. 2. Testicular appendage with torsion. (*Courtesy of* M. Bourke, DO, Bronx, NY.)

Epididymitis and orchitis

Like appendage torsion, epididymitis and orchitis may present similarly to testicular torsion. Epididymitis and orchitis are inflammation of the structures within the scrotum. Epididymitis is inflammation of the epididymis, whereas orchitis involves the testicle. The most common cause of both is bacterial infection.[7] The cause is generally broken down based on age group. In infants, epididymitis may be caused by sterile urine reflux secondary to a congenital anomaly.[18,20,21] In children, a post-viral infectious phenomenon is the most likely cause of the inflammation.[22,23] Therefore a careful history reviewing recent viral illness is important. In young boys under the age of 14, it is rare to have a bacterial cause.[22] In young men under 35 year old, the cause is most commonly sexually transmitted infection or complications from a sexually transmitted infection. In men over the age of 35 years, it is more commonly associated with benign prostatic hyperplasia. In the population of men who have sex with men, it is also important to consider *E. coli* or fungal infections.[7]

Epididymitis may present with hemiscrotal pain and swelling, similar to testicular torsion or appendage torsion. It may also present with associated symptoms of abdominal pain, nausea, or vomiting. However, epididymitis, unlike testicular or appendage torsion, is more likely to present with dysuria and micturition complaints.[18,20]

Isolated orchitis is rare; it typically presents as a progression of epididymitis.[24] When isolated, it is usually a result of a systemic viral infection (ie, Coxsackie virus, Epstein-Barr virus, varicella, or echovirus). Mumps is the most common viral cause of orchitis.[25] When the scrotum is involved, mumps presents as initial unilateral testicular involvement that later progresses to bilateral after 1 to 9 days.[25] When the causative organism is bacterial, it is almost always epididymo-orchitis.[24] Immunocompromised patients are also at risk of fungal infections.[7]

Inguinal hernia

In the differential diagnosis of painful scrotal swelling, it is important to consider an inguinal hernia. Inguinal hernias will not be further reviewed. It is mentioned here as a reminder that the presentation of acute scrotal pain and swelling can be caused by pathologic conditions of the abdomen.[7]

The Painless Swollen Scrotum

Hydrocele, varicocele, and spermatocele

Hydrocele is an accumulation of fluid around the testicle. It is the most common cause of painless scrotal swelling in children.[7] The swelling is often more prominent while awake, standing, or crying.

A varicocele is another cause of painless scrotal swelling. It most commonly occurs during puberty and on the left side due to a difference in venous drainage. A varicocele occurs when venous return from the scrotum is altered causing dilation of the spermatic cord veins, also known as the pampiniform plexus.

Finally, a spermatocele can also cause painless testicular swelling. This occurs when a sperm-filled cyst arises in the epididymis.

Testicular malignancy

Testicular malignancy is another cause of painless testicular swelling. However, this may be more easily distinguished from the above diagnoses on physical examination. It usually presents as an asymptomatic testicular mass. However, in rare cases, a mass may present with pain caused by acute bleeding within a tumor.[7]

The Erythematous Scrotum

Idiopathic scrotal edema
Idiopathic scrotal edema is a rare, self-limiting cause of an acute scrotum. It occurs between the ages of 3 to 9 years. It is defined as swelling of the scrotal skin without swelling of the deeper tissues. It is an important diagnosis to be aware of, because it needs to be differentiated from more malignant causes of scrotal edema and pain.[26,27]

Scrotal abscess and Fournier gangrene
Scrotal infections can range from mild cellulitis to a surgical emergency, such as Fournier gangrene. Patients can develop superficial or deep infections. A scrotal abscess and cellulitis are examples of superficial infections. Scrotal abscesses are derived from simple hair follicles and only involve the scrotal wall. Deep infections involve deeper structures, such as the testes or epididymis. Fournier gangrene is a rapidly progressive polymicrobial necrotizing fasciitis of the perineal, perianal, or genital areas.[7] The national incidence of Fournier gangrene is 1.6 per 100,000. Immunocompromised patients, particularly patients with a history of diabetes or alcohol abuse, are at higher risk for acquiring Fournier gangrene.[28] Previous studies had reported a mortality rate averaging between 20% and 40%; however, Sorensen and Krieger[29] reviewed the State Inpatient Database for the years of 2001 and 2004 and found a lower mortality rate of 7.5%. The mortality rate improves in hospitals treating more than 1 case of Fournier gangrene a year.[29] The most important predictors of mortality are age more than 60 years or complications during treatment, such as need for mechanical ventilation or red blood cell transfusion.[30]

The Traumatic Scrotum

Testicular trauma
Isolated urologic trauma is relatively uncommon. It is more commonly found in patients with multiple traumatic injuries.[31] Approximately 10% of all abdominal traumas also have a genitourinary injury.[31]

Traumatic injuries to the scrotum include blunt injuries, penetrating injuries, burns, bites, and scrotal avulsions. Blunt traumatic injuries may include scrotal hematoma, hematocele, testicular contusion, and complete testicular rupture. Scrotal hematocele occurs when the tunica vaginalis fills with blood, whereas disruption of the tunica albuginea is considered to be a ruptured testicle.[31] Testicular rupture and penetrating injuries are true scrotal emergencies requiring surgical management.

Testicular trauma commonly occurs playing sports or during motor vehicle accidents. Injury is more likely in motor vehicle accidents involving 2-wheeled vehicles.[32] Testicular dislocation is rare, but may occur with straddle injuries associated with motorcycle accidents.[33,34] Half of all blunt testicular injuries occur while playing sports.[34] Patients may present several days after blunt injury with symptoms similar to epididymitis. Traumatic epididymitis is a self-limiting inflammatory reaction after blunt trauma.

Strangulation injuries, that is, entrapment in a zipper, are another source of testicular trauma. According to the textbook *Urology* by Campbell and Walsh, [35] zipper injuries more often occur in "impatient boys or intoxicated men." String, hair, or rubber bands can also cause strangulation injuries. In these cases, Campbell and Walsh recommend keeping child abuse on the differential.

PHYSICAL EXAMINATION

In all cases of scrotal pain or lower abdominal pain in boys or men, a thorough genitourinary examination should be performed to assess for scrotal swelling, tenderness to palpation, location of tenderness, vascular swelling, discoloration, erythema, drainage, or warmth.

The Painful Scrotum

Testicular torsion

There are several physical examination findings that increase the likelihood of testicular torsion being the source of the painful scrotum. Multiple studies found that an abnormal cremasteric reflex and high position of the testicle were more commonly found in patients with testicular torsion.[13,17,18] The cremasteric reflex is defined as ipsilateral elevation of the testicle after stroking of the medial thigh. If absent, torsion may be more likely; however, if present, this by no means rules out torsion. The reflex can be absent in a significant percentage of normal men, as well as in those with upper and lower motor neuron disorders, spinal cord injuries, or nerve injuries after hernia repair.[36] Absence of the cremasteric reflex has been shown to have a negative predictive value of 98%, meaning if the reflex is present, torsion is less likely.[19] Another helpful physical examination finding is anterior rotation of the epididymis, which was found to have a 98% specificity in testicular torsion.[19] Elevation of the testicle and transverse location of the testicle also had high negative predictive values of 95%.[19] Beni-Israel and colleagues[17] found that high position of the testes had an odds ratio of 58.8 in cases of testicular torsion. When testicular torsion is suspected, a wide-based gait may be seen, because patients try to avoid leg contact with the tender scrotum.[13]

In perinatal torsion, it is possible that the contralateral side may also be torsed, without evidence or abnormal findings on clinical examination.[37]

Combination of history and physical examination can help narrow the diagnosis as well as differentiate between testicular torsion, torsion appendage, and epididymitis.

Appendage torsion

On examination, isolated superior pole tenderness has a strong correlation with torsion of the testicular appendage.[18] Patients may also have the blue dot sign, which is visualization of the infarcted appendage through the scrotal skin appearing as a blue dot. This sign is pathognomonic for appendage torsion[18,38] (see **Table 1** for comparison with testicular torsion and epididymitis).

Table 1
Comparing testicular torsion, epididymitis, and appendage torsion

History	Testicular Torsion	Epididymitis	Appendage Torsion
Age	Neonates, adolescents	Adolescents, young adults	Prepubertal
Pain onset	Acute	Gradual, progressive	Acute to subacute
Associated symptoms	N/V	Dysuria	
Physical examination		Fever	
Cremasteric reflex	Absent	Present or absent	Present or absent
Testicle	Testicular swelling, progressive to diffuse hemiscrotal involvement High riding, transverse alignment	Epididymal swelling progressing to diffuse hemiscrotal involvement Normal position	Head of the affected testicle or epididymis; normal position

Epididymitis and orchitis

On normal physical examination, the epididymis is found at the posterior-lateral aspect of the testicle. When palpated it feels soft and fleshy, similar to an earlobe. In epididymitis, the epididymis may be tender on palpation.[18] Patients may not have testicular tenderness. The provider should also check for Prehn sign, which is relief of pain in the lateral recumbent position or with scrotal elevation. If orchitis is present, patients will have more testicular involvement, with increased testicular swelling and tenderness. Testicles should have a normal position in both disease processes[18] (see **Table 1** for comparison with testicular torsion and appendage torsion).

Painless Scrotal Swelling

Hydrocele, varicocele, and spermatocele

Hydrocele may be more prominent while awake, standing, or crying. It presents as posterior swelling behind the testicle. An otoscope can be used to shine light through the scrotal wall. A fluid-filled scrotum will allow light to shine through, whereas a thickened scrotal wall or enlarged testicle will not transilluminate.[7]

Varicoceles are often palpable on the posterior superior portion of the testes; often described as a "bag of worms."

Finally, a spermatocele may feel like a painless cyst on the testicle. All painless masses should be differentiated from testicular malignancy.

Testicular malignancy

Testicular malignancy generally presents as a firm nontender mass on examination.

The Erythematous Scrotum

Idiopathic scrotal edema

Idiopathic scrotal edema generally presents as unilateral or bilateral scrotal swelling, erythema, and pain. It should be differentiated from scrotal abscess and deeper infections.[26,27]

Scrotal abscess and Fournier gangrene

Differentiating a scrotal abscess or cellulitis from Fournier gangrene may be difficult on first visualization. Patients may have overlying erythema or swelling. Crepitus and ecchymosis are common features in Fournier gangrene.[39] Patients may also present with purulent discharge from the perineum or with fever.[39] It is important to remember that fever may not always be present. Oguz and colleagues[39] found that only 42% of patients had fever on first presentation.

The Traumatic Scrotum

Testicular trauma

Scrotal trauma often presents with scrotal pain and swelling. Patients may have scrotal discoloration or a tender, firm scrotal mass that fails to transilluminate. This could indicate a hematocele.[7] An empty hemiscrotum in the setting of trauma is suggestive of testicular dislocation.[7] In a patient with scrotal trauma, external signs may not correlate with internal injury. There should be high suspicion of testicular injury with any open wounds to the scrotum.[40]

DIAGNOSIS

Aside from clinical diagnosis, ultrasonography is the diagnostic modality of choice for the presentation of acute scrotal pain.[41] In general, ultrasonography is performed by a radiologist or ultrasonography technician; however, bedside ultrasonography by an emergency physician can also aid in diagnosis.[42]

Emergency physicians can accurately diagnose patients presenting with acute scrotal pain using bedside ultrasonography. In 1 study, emergency physicians were able to differentiate between surgical emergencies, such as testicular torsion, and other less-urgent conditions. In this study, the emergency physicians' ultrasonography findings agreed with confirmatory testing in all but 1 case. The 1 case that was identified as an epididymal mass by the emergency physician turned out to be epididymitis.[42]

The Painful Scrotum: Testicular Torsion, Appendage Torsion, Epididymitis, and Orchitis

In the presentation of an acute painful scrotum, testicular torsion must be identified. It is imperative to rule out testicular torsion in a timely manner. In general, laboratory work and urinalysis are not helpful in the diagnosis of testicular torsion but may help with ruling in epididymitis. Ultrasonography is the diagnostic modality of choice when evaluating a painful scrotum.[43] According to the American College of Radiology, color Doppler ultrasonography is the primary modality to evaluate patients with acute scrotal pain.[41] Ultrasonography findings consistent with testicular torsion include absent or diminished intratesticular blood flow in the symptomatic testicle when compared with the asymptomatic testicle, or evidence of spermatic cord torsion with a "whirlpool or snail sign."[44] One study from 2010 found that overall sensitivity, specificity, positive predictive value, and negative predictive value for color Doppler ultrasonography in testicular torsion diagnosis were 96.8%, 97.9%, 92.1%, and 99.1%, respectively.[43] Other more recent studies from 2013, found a sensitivity of 100% with a lower specificity of 97.9% to 75.2%.[44,45] Overall the studies agree in the sense that ultrasonography is a good rule out test despite occasional false negatives. False-positives can also occur, especially in infants and young boys who have normally reduced blood flow.[46] As many as 50% of boys younger than 8 years old do not show intratesticular flow.[47] This is the reason that it is important to compare both testicles in 1 view.

Comparison of flow between both testicles is an important step in assessing for torsion. Imaging the spermatic cord to find a kink in the cord is more sensitive than color Doppler alone in adults and children[48–51] (**Box 2**).[52–54]

More recently, researchers have been looking at a clinical scoring system to help diagnosis of testicular torsion.[55] The Testicular Workup for Ischemia and Suspected Torsion (TWIST) score may help guide younger clinicians to the diagnosis of testicular torsion.[56] In a validation study using the TWIST score among pediatric emergency physicians, a high TWIST score of 7 had a 100% specificity and 100% positive predictive value for testicular torsion (**Box 3**).[57,58]

When there is high suspicion for testicular torsion given the history and physical presentation, ultrasonography should not delay surgical consultation or exploration, because ultrasonography is not 100% sensitive. If ultrasonography shows Doppler flow and there is still high suspicion for torsion, the patient should undergo surgical exploration, because that is the definitive diagnostic modality.[59]

Epididymitis and appendage torsion may be hard to differentiate on ultrasonography. Epididymitis generally appears with increased or normal color Doppler flow with an enlarged epididymis and sometimes a reactive hydrocele. Appendage torsion will appear to have normal flow, with an area of hyperechoic material near the superior portion of the testicle.[47] Urinalysis may show pyuria in the setting of epididymitis.

Box 2
Bedside ultrasonography of the scrotum

Positioning the patient: Use a sheet or towel under the scrotum to support the testicles. Have the patient hold the penis or position it superior laterally. Cover the penis for more privacy.[53]

Transducer: Use a linear high-frequency 6- to 15-MHz probe. Start the examination by asking where it hurts.
1. First obtain a midline transverse view with both testicles, also known as the saddle view, with the indicator to the right of the patient. Look for decreased flow in the symptomatic testicle compared with the asymptomatic side.
   • Take transverse static color Doppler images of both testicles
   • Take a color Doppler clip to demonstrate flow
2. Scan each testicle in the long axis (longitudinal plane) with the indicator to the head of the patient. The epididymis should be on the left of the screen and the testicle on the right.
3. Rotate the probe 90° with the indicator to the right of the patient for the transverse plane. Scan through the entire testicle. Make sure to scan both testicles.
4. Scan the spermatic cord in the longitudinal plane. Follow the cord from the testicle to the inguinal canal. Image the spermatic cord in the longitudinal and transverse planes; again, repeating on both sides. Look for the whirlpool or snail sign.

Data from Bandarkar AN, Blask AR. Testicular torsion with preserved flow: key sonographic features and value-added approach to diagnosis. Pediatr Radiol. 2018 May;48(5):735-744. https://doi.org/10.1007/s00247-018-4093-0. Epub 2018 Feb 21 and Blaivas. M. O.J. Ma, J. Mateer (Eds.). Emergency ultrasound. New York, NY: McGraw-Hill 2002: 221-228

The Painless Scrotal Swelling: Hydrocele, Varicocele, and Spermatocele; Testicular Malignancy

Differentiating painless scrotal swelling is primarily clinical. However, ultrasonography can help confirm the diagnosis by identifying fluid-filled, vascular, or solid structures (**Figs. 3** and **4, Table 2**).

The Erythematous Scrotum: Idiopathic Scrotal Edema, Scrotal Abscess, and Fournier Gangrene

It is important to differentiate scrotal edema and scrotal abscesses from the life-threatening Fournier gangrene. Idiopathic scrotal edema can be identified with ultrasonography. It is often seen as a hyperemic thickened scrotal wall around the testicle, described as the fountain sign.[61] A scrotal abscess may look like a fluid-filled structure within the scrotal wall.

Box 3
TWIST score (testicular workup for ischemia and suspected torsion)

History and Physical Presentation	Points
Testicular swelling	2
Hard testicle	2
Absent cremasteric reflex	1
Nausea or vomiting	1
High-riding testicle	1

High risk = 7 points.
   100% sensitive and specific for testicular torsion.

Data from Refs.[56–58]

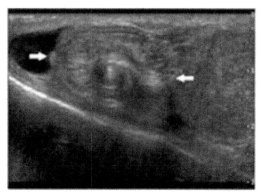

Fig. 3. The arrows indicate the Whirlpool sign on this gray scale ultrasonogram of the spermatic cord. (*From* Vijayaraghavan SB. Sonographic differential diagnosis of acute scrotum: real-time whirlpool sign, a key sign of torsion. *J Ultrasound Med.* 2006 May;25(5):563-74.)

The diagnosis of Fournier gangrene is primarily clinical.[62] However, advanced imaging can be helpful if the diagnosis is not clear clinically. A computed tomography (CT) scan can play an important role in evaluating the extent of disease for surgical planning.[63] CT findings may include fascial thickening, fluid collections, fat stranding, or subcutaneous emphysema.[63] Ultrasonography may also be used in the early diagnosis of Fournier gangrene.[53] On gray-scale ultrasograms, the scrotal wall appears with multiple echogenic foci and areas of shadowing representing gas.[53]

The Traumatic Scrotum: Testicular Trauma

Testicular rupture and penetrating injuries to the scrotum are both surgical emergencies. Although testicular rupture is rare, it is crucial to rule it out. Ultrasonography can

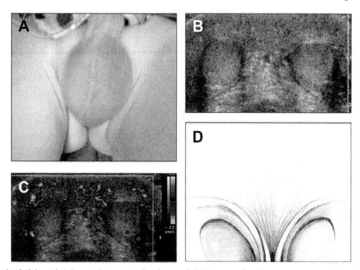

Fig. 4. (*A*) Child with idiopathic scrotal edema. (*B*) Gray-scale ultrasonogram of testicles with scrotal edema. (*C*) Transverse color Doppler image of both testicles showing increased blood flow in the peritesticular scrotal soft tissues, resembling a colored fountain due to intense hyperemia. (*D*) Representation of ultrasonography findings. (*From* Geiger J, Epelman M, Darge K. The fountain sign: a novel color Doppler sonographic finding for the diagnosis of acute idiopathic scrotal edema. *Journal of Ultrasound in Medicine.* 2010;29(8):1233–1237.)

Table 2 Scrotal ultrasonography findings	
	Ultrasonography Findings
Testicular torsion	Absent or decreased flow in testicle, kink in spermatic cord (whirlpool, snail, or spiral sign)
Appendage torsion	Normal flow of the testicle with a hyperechoic area near the superior pole
Epididymitis	Increased or normal blood flow of testicle, sometimes a reactive hydrocele, enlarged epididymis with increased flow[47,60]
Scrotal edema	Thickening of the scrotal wall, hypervascularity of the scrotum with normal appearance of the testicle and epididymis, ie, Fountain sign[61]
Fournier gangrene	Multiple echogenic foci (representing gas) with areas of dirty shadowing may be identified within the scrotal wall
Varicocele	Single vein diameter above 3 mm and/or more than 1 mm increase in diameter during the Valsalva maneuver or prominence of venous plexus[47]
Hydrocele	Fluid collection separating the 2 layers of the tunica vaginalis[60]
Testicular fracture	Hypoechoic, linear stripe without disruption of the tunica albuginea[60]
Testicular rupture	Disruption of the homogeneous echogenic tunica albuginea[47]

demonstrate disruption of the tunica albuginea with 100% sensitivity; however, it only has a 65% to 93.5% specificity.[64,65] Most other scrotal trauma is clinically diagnosed. Surgical exploration should be considered in all patients with clinical suspicion of penetration of the dartos fascia.[66]

TREATMENT AND MANAGEMENT
The Painful Scrotum: Testicular Torsion, Appendage Torsion, Epididymitis, and Orchitis

As mentioned in the Introduction, testicular torsion is time sensitive. Manual detorsion can be attempted before surgical intervention but should not delay surgical intervention.[67] Trials of manual detorsion have been found to decrease ischemia time.[68] Even if the testicle is manually detorsed, surgery is still required. Surgical exploration is the definitive management for testicular torsion.

Before performing manual detorsion, it must be explained that the procedure is painful but, if successful, it will alleviate the pain. Analgesic medication, local analgesia injection (ie, local lidocaine), or procedural sedation should be administered.

Stand at the foot of the bed or to the right of the patient. Holding the testicle between the thumb and index finger, rotate it in an outward direction (like opening a book) from medial to lateral. The initial attempt should be with one and a half full rotations (540°). Relief of pain is a positive end point. You can also reassess with bedside ultrasonography. If the pain worsened with detorsion in the medial to lateral rotation, detorse in the lateral to medial direction, because a third of testicular torsions occur with medial to lateral rotation.[67]

After manual detorsion, patients still require emergent surgical intervention. The urologist will expose the scrotum in the operating room and examine the testicle for viability after detorsion of the spermatic cord. If viable, the testicle is sutured into the inner scrotal lining (also known as an orchiopexy). The noninvolved testicle is also sutured into the lining to prevent torsion. If the testicle is found to be nonviable, the patient will undergo unilateral orchiectomy.[69]

One exception to emergent surgical intervention is in the neonatal population. Because it is nearly impossible to ascertain when the torsion occurred, the testicle is considered not salvageable. Most surgeons take the neonates to the operating room on a semi-elective basis, usually several months later to decrease the risk of anesthesia.[37]

Transferring a patient with testicular torsion to a tertiary pediatric facility after diagnosis delays definitive management and threatens testicular viability. Urologists at the initial facility should correct testicular torsion when possible.[70]

Epididymitis treatment is based on age at presentation. For patients under the age of 14 years, treatment varies. If urine cultures are positive, some clinicians cover for urinary bacteria, whereas others conservatively manage without antibiotics. There should be follow-up with a pediatric urologist for evaluation of congenital genitourinary anomalies.[71]

For sexually active patients over the age of 14 years and younger than 35 years, antibiotics are the mainstay of therapy. According to the Centers for Disease Control and Prevention, treatment should cover gonorrhea and chlamydia. The preferred treatment is ceftriaxone 250 mg intramuscularly plus doxycycline 100 mg daily for 10 days. If the patient practices anal penetration, use fluoroquinolone instead of doxycycline. The Centers for Disease Control and Prevention suggest levofloxacin 500 mg daily for 10 days or ofloxacin 300 mg twice daily for 10 days.[72]

For patients more than 35 years of age, single coverage with fluoroquinolone is appropriate.[72]

Adjuvants, including bed rest, ice, scrotal elevation, and nonsteroidal anti-inflammatory drugs (NSAIDs), can be helpful for symptom relief. Treatment of epididymo-orchitis is the same as described above. Isolated orchitis management is determined by the cause of the orchitis (which is not discussed in this article). If the patient seems to be suffering from toxicity, they may require admission; otherwise patients can have urologic follow-up in 5 to 7 days.[7]

Finally, management of appendage torsion solely consists of symptom relief. The same adjuvants used to treat epididymitis can be used with appendage torsion. The pain usually resides when the appendage degenerates in 1 to 2 weeks. It can recur depending on the number of appendages and their positions.[73]

The Painless Scrotal Swelling: Hydrocele, Varicocele, Spermatocele, or Testicular Malignancy

After diagnosis of a hydrocele, varicocele, or spermatocele, the management is primarily with nonemergent urologic follow-up. With pediatric patients, the parents can be counseled that most hydroceles resolve by 18 to 24 months of age.[7] With suspected testicular malignancy, the emergency clinician can start the work up with laboratory tests, including α-fetoprotein and β-human chorionic gonadotropin. These patients will need urgent urologic follow-up or even consultation while in the emergency department.[7]

The Erythematous Scrotum: Idiopathic Scrotal Edema, Scrotal Abscess, and Fournier Gangrene

Idiopathic scrotal edema is self-limiting. Episodes resolve in 1 to 4 days with symptom management: scrotal elevation, rest, and NSAIDs.[61,74] Scrotal abscesses can be treated similarly to abscesses on other areas of the body with drainage and antibiotic treatment. Depending on abscess location and clinical picture, surgical consultation may be necessary.

Fournier gangrene needs aggressive antibiotic therapy and surgical debridement. Like testicular torsion, Fournier gangrene is a true surgical emergency. Broad-spectrum antibiotics are recommended, but specific coverage for Fournier varies.[75] Most articles, primarily case reviews and retrospective data, recommend broad-spectrum antibiotics[63,75] The Infectious Diseases Society of America guidelines from 2014 recommend empirical coverage with piperacillin/tazobactam and vanco-mycin.[76] Ultimately, these patients need wide surgical debridement.[77] Surgery is the definitive treatment. There is mixed evidence on hyperbaric oxygen as adjuvant ther-apy; most evidence comes from small retrospective studies or case reports, but they demonstrate some benefit or decreased mortality.[78,79] All patients should be admitted to an intensive care unit because of the high mortality risk.

The Traumatic Scrotum: Testicular Trauma

Minor testicular trauma, such as contusions or zipper injuries, are managed conserva-tively with supportive care (ice, NSAIDs, scrotal support, and elevation), whereas ma-jor trauma is typically managed surgically.

If there is suspicion of testicular rupture, the American Urologic Association recom-mends scrotal exploration. Early exploration is associated with higher rates of testic-ular salvage.[80] For penetrating injuries, surgical exploration is also recommended.[81] More than half of all penetrating scrotal injuries have testicular involvement.[66]

For zipper injuries, there are several options for management. One technique is to use mineral oil. After local anesthesia, the clinician can use mineral oil on the zipper and surrounding skin to gently untangle the zipper from the skin.[82] The clinician may also try using a wire cutter or bone-cutting pliers. Cut the diamond (or the median bar) of the zipper, which will cause the zipper to fall apart, freeing the skin.[83]

SUMMARY

Although scrotal emergencies are rare within the emergency department, they can be life and fertility threatening. It is important to differentiate the surgical emergencies (testicular torsion, Fournier gangrene, and testicular trauma) from the less-urgent di-agnoses of acute scrotal pain. Among the wide differential, it is imperative that the emergency physician identify the more concerning causes early to save lives and pre-serve fertility.

REFERENCES

1. Lewis AG, Bukowski TP, Jarvis PD, et al. Evaluation of acute scrotum in the emer-gency department. J Pediatr Surg 1995;30:277–82.
2. Zhao LC, Lautz TB, Meeks JJ, et al. Pediatric testicular torsion epidemiology us-ing a national database: incidence, risk of orchiectomy and possible measures toward improving the quality of care. J Urol 2011;186(5):2009–13.
3. Street EJ, Justice ED, Kopa Z, et al. The 2016 European guideline on the man-agement of epididymo-orchitis. Int J STD AIDS 2017;28(8):744–9.
4. Glerum KM, Selbst SM, Parikh PD, et al. Pediatric malpractice claims in the emer-gency department and urgent care settings from 2001 to 2015. Pediatr Emerg Care 2018. https://doi.org/10.1097/PEC.0000000000001602.
5. Visser AJ, Heyns CF. Testicular function after torsion of the spermatic cord. BJU Int 2003;92(3):200–3.
6. Bayne AP, Madden-Fuentes RJ, Jones EA, et al. Factors associated with delayed treatment of acute testicular torsion—do demographics or interhospital transfer matter? J Urol 2010;184(4 Suppl):1743–7.

7. Davis JE. Male genital problems. In: Tintinalli JE, editor. Tintinalli's emergency medicine: a comprehensive study guide. 8th edition. New York: McGraw-Hill; 2016. p. 601–9.

8. Vashisht D, Oberoi B, Venugopal R, et al. Acute scrotum: Hansen's disease versus filariasis. Int J Mycobacteriol 2018;7(2):195–7.

9. Pogorelić Z, Mrklić I, Jurić I. Do not forget to include testicular torsion in differential diagnosis of lower acute abdominal pain in young males. J Pediatr Urol 2013; 9(6):1161–5.

10. Favorito LA, Cavalcante AG, Costa WS. Anatomic aspects of epididymis and tunica vaginalis in patients with testicular torsion. Int Braz J Urol 2004;30(5): 420–4.

11. Caesar RE, Kaplan GW. Incidence of the bell-clapper deformity in an autopsy series. Urology 1994;44(1):114–6.

12. Pogorelic Z, Mustapi K, Juki M, et al. Management of acute scrotum in children: a 25-year single center experience on 558 pediatric patients. Can J Urol 2016; 23(6):8594–601.

13. Boettcher M, Bergholz R, Krebs TF, et al. Clinical predictors of testicular torsion in children. Urology 2012;79:670.

14. Seng YJ, Moissinac K. Trauma induced testicular torsion: a reminder for the unwary. J Accid Emerg Med 2000;17(5):381–2.

15. Fujita N, Tambo M, Okegawa T, et al. Distinguishing testicular torsion from torsion of the appendix testis by clinical features and signs in patients with acute scrotum. Res Rep Urol 2017;9:169–74.

16. Eaton SH, Cendron MA, Estrada CR, et al. Intermittent testicular torsion: diagnostic features and management outcomes. J Urol 2005;174(4 Pt 2):1532–5.

17. Beni-Israel T, Goldman M, Bar Chaim S, et al. Clinical predictors for testicular torsion as seen in the pediatric ED. Am J Emerg Med 2010;28(7):786–9.

18. Kadish HA, Bolte RG. A retrospective review of pediatric patients with epididymitis, testicular torsion, and torsion of testicular appendages. Pediatrics 1988; 102(1 Pt 1):73–6.

19. Ciftci AO, Senocak ME, Tanyel FC, et al. Clinical predictors for differential diagnosis of acute scrotum. Eur J Pediatr Surg 2004;14(5):333–8.

20. Redshaw JD, Tran TL, Wallis C, et al. Epididymitis: a 21 year retrospective review of boys presenting to an outpatient urology clinic. J Urol 2014;192(4):1203–7.

21. Siegel A, Snyder H, Duckett JW. Epididymitis in infants and boys: underlying urogenital anomalies and efficacy of imaging modalities. J Urol 1987;138:1100–3.

22. Gkentzis A, Lee L. The aetiology and current management of prepubertal epididymitis. Ann R Coll Surg Engl 2014;96(3):181–3.

23. Somekh E, Gorenstein A, Serour F. Acute epididymitis in boys: evidence of a postinfectious etiology. J Urol 2004;171(1):391–4.

24. Trojian TH, Lishnak TS, Heiman D. Epididymitis and orchitis: an overview. Am Fam Physician 2009;79(7):583–7.

25. Masarani M, Wazait H, Dinneen M. Mumps orchitis. J R Soc Med 2006;99(11): 573–5.

26. Breen M, Murphy K, Chow J, et al. Acute idiopathic scrotal edema. Case Rep Urol 2013;2013:829345.

27. Qvist O. Swelling of the scrotum in infants and children, and non-specific epididymitis: a study of 158 cases. Acta Chir Scand 1956;110(5):417–21.

28. Yılmazlar T, Işık Ö, Öztürk E, et al. Fournier's gangrene: review of 120 patients and predictors of mortality. Ulus Travma Acil Cerrahi Derg 2014;20(5):333–7.

29. Sorensen MD, Krieger JN. Fournier's gangrene: epidemiology and outcomes in the general US population. Urol Int 2016;97:249–59.

30. Roghmann F, von Bodman C, Löppenberg B, et al. Is there a need for the Fournier's gangrene severity index? Comparison of scoring systems for outcome prediction in patients with Fournier's gangrene. BJU Int 2012;110(9):1359–65.

31. Morey AF, Brandes S, Dugi DD, et al. Urotrauma: AUA guideline. J Urol 2014; 192(2):327–35.

32. Paparel P, N'Diaye A, Laumon B, et al. The epidemiology of trauma of the genitourinary system after traffic accidents: analysis of a register of over 43,000 victims. BJU Int 2006;97:338–41.

33. Bhatt S, Dogra VS. Role of US in testicular and scrotal trauma. Radiographics 2008;28(6):1617–29.

34. Naseer A, King D, Lee H, et al. Testicular dislocation: the importance of scrotal examination in a trauma patient. Ann R Coll Surg Engl 2012;94(2):109–10.

35. Morey AF, Zhao LC. Genital and lower urinary tract trauma. In: Wein AJ, Kavoussi LR, Partin AW, et al, editors. Campbell-walsh urology. 11th edition. Philadelphia: Elsevier; 2016. chap 101.

36. Schwarz GM, Hirtler L. The cremasteric reflex and its muscle—a paragon of ongoing scientific discussion: a systematic review. Clin Anat 2017;30(4):498–507.

37. Yerkes EB, Robertson FM, Gitlin J, et al. Management of perinatal torsion: today, tomorrow, or never? J Urol 2005;174(4 Pt 2):1579–82.

38. Yang C Jr, Song B, Liu X, et al. Acute scrotum in children: an 18-year retrospective study. Pediatr Emerg Care 2011;27(4):270–4.

39. Oguz A, Gümüş M, Turkoglu A, et al. Fournier's gangrene: a summary of 10 years of clinical experience. Int Surg 2015;100(5):934–41.

40. Ramchandani P, Buckler PM. Review: imaging of genitourinary trauma. AJR Am J Roentgenol 2009;192(6):1514–23.

41. Remer EM, Casalino DD, Arellano RS, et al. ACR appropriateness criteria ® acute onset of scrotal pain—without trauma, without antecedent mass. Ultrasound Q 2012;28:47–51.

42. Blaivas M, Sierzenski P, Lambert M. Emergency evaluation of patients presenting with acute scrotum using bedside ultrasonography. Acad Emerg Med 2001; 8(1):90–3.

43. Waldert M, Klatte T, Schmidbauer J, et al. Color Doppler sonography reliably identifies testicular torsion in boys. Urology 2010;75:1170–4.

44. Altinkilic B, Pilatz A, Weidner W. Detection of normal intratesticular perfusion using color coded duplex sonography obviates need for scrotal exploration in patients with suspected testicular torsion. J Urol 2013;189:1853–8.

45. Liang T, Metcalfe P, Sevcik W, et al. Retrospective review of diagnosis and treatment in children presenting to the pediatric department with acute scrotum. AJR Am J Roentgenol 2013;200(5):444–9.

46. Sung EK, Setty BN, Castro-Aragon I. Sonography of the pediatric scrotum: emphasis on the Ts–torsion, trauma, and tumors. AJR Am J Roentgenol 2012; 198(5):996–1003.

47. Dudea SM, Ciurea A, Chiorean A, et al. Doppler applications in testicular and scrotal disease. Med Ultrason 2010;12:43–51.

48. Kalfa N, Veyrac C, Baud C, et al. Ultrasonography of the spermatic cord in children with testicular torsion: impact on the surgical strategy. J Urol 2004;172: 1692–5.

49. Hao JW, Du GH, Ding DG, et al. Value of spermatic cord sonography in the early diagnosis and treatment of testicular torsion. Zhonghua Nan Ke Xue 2012;18(5): 419–21 [in Chinese].

50. Baud C, Veyrac C, Couture A, et al. Spiral twist of the spermatic cord: a reliable sign of testicular torsion. Pediatr Radiol 1998;28:950–4.

51. McDowall J, Adam A, Gerber L, et al. The ultrasonographic "whirlpool sign" in testicular torsion: valuable tool or waste of valuable time? A systematic review and meta-analysis. Emerg Radiol 2018;25(3):281–92.

52. Bandarkar AN, Blask AR. Testicular torsion with preserved flow: key sonographic features and value-added approach to diagnosis. Pediatr Radiol 2018;48(5): 735–44.

53. McAdams CR, Del Gaizo AJ. The utility of scrotal ultrasonography in the emergent setting: beyond epididymitis versus torsion. Emerg Radiol 2018;25(4): 341–8.

54. Blaivas M, Ma OJ, Mateer J, editors. Emergency ultrasound. New York: McGraw-Hill; 2002. p. 221–8.

55. Barbosa JA, Tiseo BC, Barayan GA, et al. Development and initial validation of a scoring system to diagnose testicular torsion in children. J Urol 2013;189: 1859–64.

56. Sheth KR, Keays M, Grimsby GM, et al. Diagnosing testicular torsion before urological consultation and imaging: validation of the TWIST score. J Urol 2016; 195(6):1870–6.

57. Manohar CS, Gupta A, Keshavamurthy R, et al. Evaluation of testicular workup for ischemia and suspected torsion score in patients presenting with acute scrotum. Urol Ann 2018;10(1):20–3.

58. Frohlich LC, Paydar-Darian N, Cilento BG Jr, et al. Prospective validation of clinical score for males presenting with an acute scrotum. Acad Emerg Med 2017;24: 1474–82.

59. Stehr M, Boehm R. Critical validation of colour Doppler ultrasound in diagnosis of acute scrotum in children. Eur J Pediatr Surg 2003;13:386–92.

60. Kühn AL, Scortegagna E, Nowitzki KM, et al. Ultrasonography of the scrotum in adults. Ultrasonography 2016;35(3):180–97.

61. Geiger J, Epelman M, Darge K. The fountain sign: a novel color Doppler sonographic finding for the diagnosis of acute idiopathic scrotal edema. J Ultrasound Med 2010;29(8):1233–7.

62. Eke N. Fournier's gangrene: a review of 1726 cases. Br J Surg 2000;87(6): 718–28.

63. Chennamsetty A, Khourdaji I, Burks F, et al. Contemporary diagnosis and management of Fournier's gangrene. Ther Adv Urol 2015;7(4):203–15.

64. Guichard G, El Ammari J, Del Coro C, et al. Accuracy of ultrasonography in diagnosis of testicular rupture after blunt scrotal trauma. Urology 2008;71:52–6.

65. Buckley JC, McAninch JW. Use of ultrasonography for the diagnosis of testicular injuries in blunt scrotal trauma. J Urol 2006;175:175–8.

66. Phonsombat S, Master VA, McAninch JW. Penetrating external genital trauma: a 30-year single institution experience. J Urol 2008;180:192.

67. Sessions AE, Rabinowitz R, Hulbert WC, et al. Testicular torsion: direction, degree, duration and disinformation. J Urol 2003;169:663–5.

68. Demirbas A, Demir DO, Ersoy E, et al. Should manual detorsion be a routine part of treatment in testicular torsion? BMC Urol 2017;17(1):84.

69. Palmer LS, Palmer JS. Management of abnormalities of the external genitalia in boys. In: Wein AJ, Kavoussi LR, Partin AW, et al, editors. Campbell-walsh urology. 11th edition. Philadelphia: Elsevier; 2016. p. 3368–98, chap 146.

70. Preece J, Ching C, Yackey K, et al. Indicators and outcomes of transfer to tertiary pediatric hospitals for patients with testicular torsion. J Pediatr Urol 2017; 13(4):388.

71. Gkentzis A, Lee L. The aetiology and current management of prepubertal epididymitis. Ann R Coll Surg Engl 2014;96(3):181–3.

72. Workowski KA, Bolan GA. Sexually transmitted diseases treatment guidelines. MMWR Recomm Rep 2015;64:82–4.

73. Skoglund RW, McRoberts JW, Ragde H. Torsion of testicular appendages: presentation of 43 new cases and a collective review. J Urol 1970;104(4):598–600.

74. Lee A, Park SJ, Lee HK, et al. Acute idiopathic scrotal edema: ultrasonographic findings at an emergency unit. Eur Radiol 2009;19(8):2075–80.

75. Lin WT, Chao CM, Lin HL, et al. Emergence of antibiotic-resistant bacteria in patients with Fournier gangrene. Surg Infect (Larchmt) 2015;16(2):165–8.

76. Stevens DL, Bisno AL, Chambers HF, et al. Practice guidelines for the diagnosis and management of skin and soft tissue infections: 2014 update by the Infectious Diseases Society of America. Clin Infect Dis 2014;59(2):10–52.

77. Shyam DC, Rapsang AG. Fournier's gangrene. Surgeon 2013;11(4):222–32.

78. Mindrup SR, Kealey GP, Fallon B. Hyperbaric oxygen for the treatment of Fournier's gangrene. J Urol 2005;173(6):1975–7.

79. Li C, Zhou X, Liu L-F, et al. Hyperbaric oxygen therapy as an adjuvant therapy for comprehensive treatment of Fournier's gangrene. Urol Int 2015;94(4):453–8.

80. Cass AS, Luxenberg M. Testicular injuries. Urology 1991;37:528.

81. Morey AF, Brandes S, Dugi DD, et al. Urotrauma: AUA guideline. J Urol 2014; 192(2):327–35.

82. Kanegaye JT, Schonfeld N. Penile zipper entrapment: a simple and less threatening approach using mineral oil. Pediatr Emerg Care 1993;9:90–1.

83. Flowerdew R, Fishman IJ, Churchill BM. Management of penile zipper injury. J Urol 1977;117(5):671.

Emergency Diagnosis and Management of Genitourinary Trauma

Matthew J. Coppola, MD[a,b,*], Joshua Moskovitz, MD, MBA, MPH[c,d]

KEYWORDS

- Genitourinary trauma • Kidney injury • Ureteral injury • Bladder injury
- Bladder rupture • Penile injury

KEY POINTS

- Injury to the genitourinary tract (GU) often occurs in the setting of concomitant injury to multiple abdominopelvic organs. Misdiagnosis or delay in diagnosis of GU injury can lead to significant downstream morbidity.
- The presence of gross (visible) hematuria in the trauma patient is highly suggestive of underlying GU injury when present; however, its absence does not rule out GU tract injury.
- Intravenous contrast-enhanced computed tomography (CT) remains the imaging modality of choice for diagnosing renal trauma in stable blunt and penetrating trauma patients and to screen for other GU injury.
- Bladder and urethral injury can be particularly challenging to diagnose in the acute phase of trauma. CT cystography is required to accurately diagnose bladder injury, whereas retrograde urethrography is required to diagnose urethral injury.

INTRODUCTION

Injury to the genitourinary (GU) tract is rarely life-threatening in the acute phase of trauma and is often prioritized until after the diagnosis and management of other abdominopelvic injuries are completed. Up to 10% of all trauma cases will involve injuries to the GU tract. Most GU injury occurs by blunt trauma, with the kidneys being the most commonly injured GU organ, followed by the urethra and bladder.[1] GU trauma is rarely encountered in isolation; rather it is seen associated with injury to

Disclosure Statement: No commercial or financial conflicts of interest to disclose.
[a] Donald and Barbara Zucker School of Medicine at Hofstra/Northwell, 500 Hofstra University, Hempstead, NY 11549, USA; [b] North Shore University Hospital, 300 Community Drive, Manhasset, NY 11030, USA; [c] Albert Einstein College of Medicine, 1300 Morris Park Avenue, Bronx, NY 10461, USA; [d] Hofstra School of Health Sciences and Human Services, Hempstead, NY, USA
* Corresponding author. North Shore University Hospital, 300 Community Drive, Manhasset, NY 11030, USA.
E-mail address: mcoppola2@northwell.edu

Emerg Med Clin N Am 37 (2019) 611–635
https://doi.org/10.1016/j.emc.2019.07.003
0733-8627/19/© 2019 Elsevier Inc. All rights reserved.

other solid organs in both blunt and penetrating abdominal trauma. Trauma patients with GU tract injuries experience higher overall morbidity and mortality than those without GU injury.[2]

Although immediately life-threatening traumatic injuries are addressed first, it is important to consider concomitant GU injury because misdiagnosis, or delay in diagnosis, can lead to significant downstream morbidity for the trauma patient. Major long-term consequences of missed GU injury include sepsis, intraabdominal abscess, erectile dysfunction, incontinence, urethral strictures, fistulas, chronic kidney disease, and hypertension, to name a few.[3] The biggest pitfall in the management of GU trauma for emergency practitioners is failing to consider the potential for GU injury in the polytrauma patient. This review emphasizes when to suspect, how to effectively diagnose, and how to efficiently manage specific GU traumatic emergencies.

RENAL TRAUMA
Epidemiology

The kidney is the most commonly injured organ of the GU system despite its relatively protected retroperitoneal position. Renal trauma is involved in 1% to 3% of all trauma patients,[1,4] however rarely is seen as an isolated injury. Concomitant traumatic injuries are identified in 80% to 95% cases of renal injury.[4]

Blunt trauma is the most common mechanism by which the kidney is injured in trauma, accounting for 70% to 95% of renal trauma cases. Approximately 60% to 70% of blunt renal trauma cases occur in motor vehicle collisions (MVC) in adults.[4] The remainder of blunt renal trauma in adults has been attributed to falls, sports injuries, and pedestrian accidents. In the pediatric population, fewer MVCs (~30%) were responsible for blunt renal injury, whereas falls and pedestrian accidents were more often seen.[5]

Penetrating renal trauma is generally seen more in underdeveloped areas and urban centers. Most penetrating injury to the kidney occurs by firearms (80%–90%) and stab wounds in civilian settings. Multiorgan injury is seen in the vast majority (94%) of cases of penetrating renal trauma.[6] Compared with blunt renal trauma, a penetrating mechanism very often leads to higher severity injury to the kidney.

Anatomic Considerations

The kidney is a retroperitoneal organ covered by fat and Gerota fascia, which may shield it to some degree against blunt traumatic injury. Anchored in place only by the renal pelvis and without other reliable attachment points, the kidney is particularly vulnerable to injury by rapid deceleration forces as opposed to direct trauma. A spectrum of renal parenchymal injury occurs from deceleration forces, including contusions, hematomas, and lacerations. Injury to the renal vascular supply also can occur in blunt renal trauma.[4]

The kidney is the most commonly injured organ in children and adolescents. This greater susceptibility to injury is explained by the larger relative size of the kidneys, weaker Gerota fascia, less ossified ribs, and less developed paraspinal and abdominal musculature.[7]

Kidneys with anatomic pathologic condition (hydronephrosis, cysts, tumors, abnormal kidney position) are especially susceptible to blunt traumatic injury. The force needed to injure kidneys with preexisting renal lesions (PERL) can be trivial compared with anatomically normal kidneys. PERLs have been involved in blunt renal trauma cases in as much as 4% to 19% of adult patients and 12% to 35% of pediatric patients.[8] Most cases of PERL are identified incidentally after imaging of the trauma patient. In cases of known PERL and blunt trauma, a lower threshold for advanced imaging should be observed given higher overall susceptibility and severity of renal injury.

History and Physical Examination

Ascertaining the mechanism of trauma in stable patients is crucial in the initial steps of evaluating for the possibility of renal injury. Rapid deceleration or acceleration poses a high risk for potential renal trauma. Motor vehicle accidents or a fall from significant height would be common examples of rapid deceleration or acceleration mechanism injuries leading to kidney injury. A history of a direct blow to the flank or back is particularly suggestive of the possibility of isolated renal trauma. For penetrating injuries, the size of the weapon or projectile and entry trajectory may provide clues to possible associated renal injury. Penetrating wounds to the upper abdomen and lower chest should raise suspicion for renal involvement and liberal advanced imaging should be pursued.

A patient history of preexisting abnormal kidneys is helpful to obtain because the force required to injure these kidneys is much less. The threshold to obtain imaging to investigate for renal trauma in these cases should be much lower, as discussed earlier.[4] A history of a solitary kidney or significant baseline renal dysfunction provides additional reinforcement as to the importance of avoiding nephrectomy after renal trauma if at all possible.

Examination findings suggestive of renal trauma include flank or left upper-quadrant tenderness or ecchymosis. Chest wall tenderness, especially in the lower rib cage, may signify rib fractures and associated renal injury. Unfortunately, it is not uncommon for there to be no specific examination findings at all in cases of renal trauma. Thus, a high index of suspicion for renal trauma must be maintained based on the mechanism of injury and, if present, the knowledge of preexisting structurally abnormal kidneys. **Table 1** summarizes the important history and examination findings seen in renal trauma.

Diagnostic Studies

A urinalysis (UA) should be performed on all patients with blunt abdominal trauma to screen for gross (visible) hematuria. The presence of gross hematuria is highly suggestive of underlying kidney injury; however, the absence of gross hematuria does not rule it out. Gross hematuria was present only 65% of the time in cases of renal trauma, in 1 study.[9] Gross hematuria is even less commonly seen in penetrating renal trauma.

Intravenous (IV) contrast-enhanced multidetector computed tomography (CT) remains the gold standard in the diagnosis of blunt and penetrating renal trauma in the hemodynamically stable patient. CT imaging is more sensitive and specific for renal and GU trauma than ultrasound (US) and intravenous pyelography (IVP) and can rapidly identify associated abdominal and pelvic injuries.[10] Delayed excretory contrast phase (5–10 minutes after contrast administration) images allow for detection and further characterization of collecting system leaks and renal vascular injuries. Many trauma CT protocols screening for thoracoabdominal injury in polytrauma patients do not routinely include delayed phase contrast images and are at risk for missing injuries to the renal vasculature, collecting system, pelvis, and ureter. Thus, if high suspicion for renal or ureteral trauma is present, delayed excretory contrast phase images should be obtained after conventional "trauma CT protocol images"

Table 1
Kidney injury scale: 2018 revision

AAST Grade	AIS Severity	Imaging Criteria (CT Findings)	Pathologic Criteria
I	2	• Subcapsular hematoma and/or parenchymal contusion without laceration	• Subcapsular hematoma or parenchymal contusion without parenchymal laceration
II	2	• Perirenal hematoma confined to Gerota fascia • Renal parenchymal laceration ≤1-cm depth without urinary extravasation	• Perirenal hematoma confined to Gerota fascia • Renal parenchymal laceration ≤1-cm depth without urinary extravasation
III	3	• Renal parenchymal laceration >1-cm depth without collecting system rupture or urinary extravasation • Any injury in the presence of a kidney vascular injury or active bleeding contained within Gerota fascia	• Renal parenchymal laceration >1-cm depth without collecting system rupture or urinary extravasation
IV	4	• Parenchymal laceration extending into urinary collecting system with urinary extravasation • Renal pelvis laceration and/or complete ureteropelvic disruption • Segmental renal vein or artery injury • Active bleeding beyond Gerota fascia into the retroperitoneum or peritoneum • Segmental or complete kidney infarction(s) due to vessel thrombosis without active bleeding	• Parenchymal laceration extending into urinary collecting system • Renal pelvis laceration and/or complete ureteropelvic disruption • Segmental renal vein or artery injury • Segmental or complete kidney infarction(s) due to vessel thrombosis without active bleeding

(continued on next page)

AAST Grade	AIS Severity	Imaging Criteria (CT Findings)	Pathologic Criteria
Table 1 *(continued)*			
V	5	• Main renal artery or vein laceration or avulsion of hilum • Devascularized kidney with active bleeding • Shattered kidney with loss of identifiable parenchymal renal anatomy	• Main renal artery or vein laceration or avulsion of hilum • Devascularized kidney • Shattered kidney with loss of identifiable parenchymal renal anatomy

Vascular injury is defined as a pseudoaneurysm or arteriovenous fistula and appears as a focal collection of vascular contrast that decreases in attenuation with delayed imaging. Active bleeding from a vascular injury presents as vascular contrast, focal or diffuse, that increases in size or attenuation in delayed phase. Vascular thrombosis can lead to organ infarction.
Grade based on highest grade assessment made on imaging, at operation or on pathologic specimen.
More than 1 grade of kidney injury may be present and should be classified by the higher grade of injury.
Advance 1 grade for bilateral injuries up to Grade III.
Abbreviations: AIS, abbreviated Injury scale.
Adapted from Kozar RA, Crandall M, Shanmuganathan K, et al. Organ injury scaling 2018 update: Spleen, liver, and kidney. *J Trauma Acute Care Surg.* 2018;85(6):1119-1122.

have been completed.[10] **Fig. 1** depicts a renal laceration identified on IV contrast-enhanced CT.

IVP has been replaced by contrast-enhanced CT for the diagnosis of renal trauma except for patients too unstable to undergo CT imaging. IVP is used intraoperatively to confirm renal function in the contralateral uninjured kidney.

US is not adequately sensitive in ruling out renal injury in the trauma patient.[7] US is useful in evaluating for intraperitoneal free fluid when used in the Focused Assessment by Sonography in Trauma. Unfortunately, retroperitoneal free fluid, which may indicate renal injury, is often not appreciated on US. There may be an emerging role, however, for serial US assessments of known renal injury.

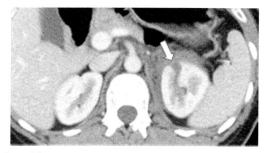

Fig. 1. CT image of renal laceration. IV contrast-enhanced CT demonstrating grade III renal laceration. The laceration extends into the renal medulla, and there is associated perinephric hematoma (*arrow*). (*From* Dane B, Baxter AB, Bernstein MP. Imaging Genitourinary Trauma. Radiol Clin North Am. 2017;55(2):321-335; with permission.)

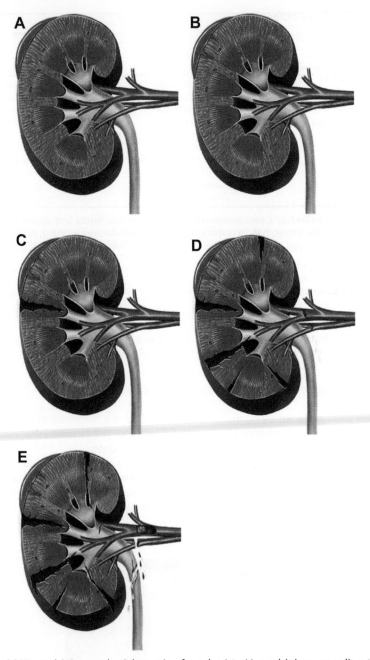

Fig. 2. AAST renal injury scale. Schematic of grades I to V renal injury according to AAST scale. (*A*) Grade I: subcapsular hematoma. (*B*) Grade II: laceration less than 1 cm, hematoma confined to perirenal space. (*C*) Grade III: laceration greater than 1 cm involving renal medulla. (*D*) Grade IV: laceration involving collecting system and vascular structures. (*E*) Grade V: hilum avulsed, "shattered kidney." (*From* Chong ST, Cherry-Bukowiec JR, Willatt JM, Kielar AZ. Renal trauma: imaging evaluation and implications for clinical management. *Abdom Radiol (NY)*. 2016;41(8):1565-1579; with permission.)

Renal Injury Classification

Renal trauma is classified most commonly according to the American Association for the Surgery of Trauma (AAST) grading system (**Fig. 2**, see **Table 1**). The system is an anatomically based injury grading scale based on the injury pattern seen at time of surgery. Grade I to III injuries involve renal parenchymal injury, whereas the more severe grade IV and V injuries involve collecting system and vascular injury. Higher-grade AAST scores were found to be associated with a higher need for nephrectomy, dialysis, and mortality in blunt renal trauma.[11,12]

Management

Most renal trauma is managed nonoperatively with close observation, bed rest, serial laboratory monitoring, and minimally invasive procedures, such as angioembolization or ureteral stenting if deterioration is identified. Recent studies indicate that 84% to 95% of renal trauma has been managed nonoperatively; failure and subsequent intervention occur only 2% to 5% of the time.[13] The detailed approach to management of renal trauma is guided by injury mechanism (blunt vs penetrating), hemodynamic stability and AAST injury grade.

Grade I and II blunt renal injuries are exclusively managed nonoperatively with no reported need for nephrectomy in recent study. Grade III blunt injuries have become

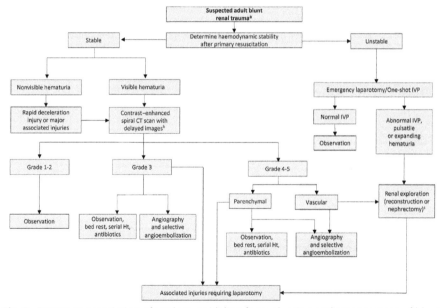

Fig. 3. European Association of Urology guideline for evaluation and management of blunt renal trauma. Ht, hematocrit. CT, computed tomography; Ht, haematocrit; IVP, intravenous pyelography. [a] Suspected renal trauma results from reported mechanism of injury and physical examination. [b] Renal imaging: CT scans are the gold standard for evaluating blunt and penetrating renal injuries in stable patients. In settings where CT is not available, the urologist should rely on other imaging modalities (IVP, angiography, radiographic scintigraphy, MRI). [c] Renal exploration: Although renal salvage is a primary goal for the urologist, decisions concerning the viability of the organ and the type of reconstruction are made during the operation. (*From* Kitrey ND., Djakovic N, Hallscheidt P, et al. Urological Trauma. EAU Urogenital Trauma Guidelines. Available at: https://uroweb.org/guideline/urological-trauma/. Accessed July 10, 2019. Reprinted with permission of the European Association of Urology.)

nonoperatively managed as well with the increasing role of selective angioembolization when deterioration occurs during a period of observation.[4]

Grade IV and V blunt renal injuries that are hemodynamically stable are suitable for nonoperative management with selective angioembolization. A success rate of 82% for nonoperative management of grade IV and V injuries has been recently reported.[14] **Fig. 3** summarizes the proposed evaluation and treatment algorithm for blunt and penetrating renal trauma according to the European Association of Urology.

Penetrating renal trauma traditionally had been an absolute indication for operative management; however, significant success has been seen recently with nonoperative management in stable patients. Nonetheless, higher-grade injury and penetrating mechanism remain the strongest predictors for nephrectomy in renal trauma.

Prophylactic antibiotics are considered in some instances of renal trauma in an attempt to avoid potential downstream urinary tract infection (UTI) and perinephric abscess formation. There is minimal evidence, however, to support routine administration of antibiotics in renal trauma. High-risk features that are thought to increase the risk of UTI and perinephric abscess formation include devitalized kidney segments, immunosuppression, or concomitant bowel or pancreatic injury.[15,16] Routine IV antibiotic administration in cases of patients with these high-risk features for 48 to 72 hours followed by 5 days of oral antibiotics has been proposed by some experts, regardless of injury grade. In the absence of these risk factors, routine antibiotic prophylaxis is considered in grade IV and V renal injuries.[15] Suggested antibiotic regimens include first-generation cephalosporins, ciprofloxacin, or ampicillin with gentamicin. The addition of metronidazole for gastrointestinal microbes is generally recommended when concomitant bowel injury is present (**Box 1**).

Box 1
Key points in renal trauma

History

- Gross hematuria
- Rapid deceleration or acceleration injury (MVC most common)
- Preexisting abnormal kidney anatomy (hydronephrosis, cysts, tumor) predisposes to renal injury

Examination

- Flank or back ecchymosis
- Chest wall tenderness or deformity in lower rib cage

Diagnostics

- UA: gross hematuria not reliably present (seen ~60% of the time)
- *IV contrast-enhanced CT* gold standard for diagnosis
  - *Delayed excretory contrast phase* (5–10 minutes after initial contrast administration) should be performed to rule out collecting system injury

Management

- Shift in management recently to favor nonoperative management with selective angioembolization in stable patients (see **Fig. 3**)
- Consider antibiotic prophylaxis:
  - In presence of risk factors (ischemic renal segments, bowel or pancreatic injury, immunosuppression) or fevers regardless of injury grade
  - Grade IV and V renal injury

URETERAL TRAUMA
Epidemiology

Ureteral trauma is very rare, accounting for less than 1% of all GU traumatic injury.[1] Most ureteral injury occurs by an iatrogenic mechanism, occurring during gynecology, urogynecologic, urologic, and other pelvic surgeries. Noniatrogenic ureteral injury occurs mostly during penetrating trauma from gunshot wounds. Blunt trauma resulting in ureteral injury is much less common than penetrating trauma. MVCs account for most incidences of blunt ureteral trauma.[1,17]

Anatomic Considerations

The ureter is a retroperitoneal structure that is divided into 3 segments based on location relative to other abdominal and pelvic structures. The segments are classified as the proximal, middle, and pelvic (distal) ureter. The pelvic ureter is the most commonly injured segment of the ureter and courses from the level of the iliac vessels to the bladder.[18] The close proximity of the ureter to numerous abdominopelvic structures explains its susceptibility to injury during various surgical procedures. In penetrating and blunt trauma, the proximal and middle ureter are injured most commonly and are thought to occur not by direct transection, but rather by injury to the surrounding blood supply to the ureter.

History and Physical Examination

Specific clinical indicators of ureteral injury are often not present, leading to misdiagnosis or a delay in diagnosis in up to 80% of cases of iatrogenic trauma to the ureter.[19] A recent history of gynecologic, urologic, or colorectal surgery coupled with worsening flank or abdominal pain, gross hematuria, prolonged ileus, or fevers should raise suspicion for possible iatrogenic ureteral injury.[19,20] Noniatrogenic ureteral trauma should be considered in cases of penetrating trauma or rapid deceleration injuries, especially when concurrent renal injury has already been confirmed.

Classic examination findings suggestive of ureteral injury are often not present, but secondary signs, such as prolonged ileus or persistently elevated surgical drain output, can be potential clues to ureteral injury.

Diagnostic Studies

As is the case with renal trauma, gross hematuria is not a reliable indicator of ureteral injury and is seen, at times, in only 40% of ureteral injury cases.[21] An elevation in serum blood urea nitrogen (BUN) and creatinine after a surgical procedure known to be associated with a high risk of ureteral injury should prompt consideration of ureteral injury.

The diagnostic imaging modality of choice in diagnosing suspected ureteral injury is contrast-enhanced CT with delayed renal excretory phase images in the stable trauma patient.[21] As discussed previously, typical portal venous phase "trauma protocol" CT images should be acquired first to identify all potential abdominopelvic injuries. It has been reported that up to 80% of ureteral injuries can be missed on initial portal venous phase CT images and may only be detected on delayed renal excretory imaging.[22] Retrograde pyelography is largely considered to be the most accurate modality in identifying ureteral injury, however is not often feasible in the initial assessment of potentially unstable trauma patients.[21]

Management

The management of ureteral injury is influenced heavily by whether its identification is early or delayed. If ureteral injury is identified immediately, which most often occurs intraoperatively during gynecologic, urogynecologic, or colorectal procedures, surgical repair over a stent is largely preferred. In cases of delayed diagnosis or the unstable trauma patient requiring attention to other abdominal or pelvic injury, urinary diversion away from the damaged ureter is favored most commonly with percutaneous nephrostomy placement. Urinomas or abscesses that may be present are often drained percutaneously. Reconstruction of the ureter is typically performed in a delayed fashion weeks to months later[23] (**Box 2**).

Box 2
Key points in ureteral trauma

History

- Recent gynecologic, colorectal, or urologic surgery (iatrogenic ureteral trauma most common)
- Flank or abdominal pain
- Gross hematuria
- Fevers
- Prolonged postoperative ileus

Examination

- Ileus
- Increasing or persistent surgical drain output (suggestive of urinary leak)

Diagnostics

- UA: gross hematuria not reliably present (seen ~40% of the time)
- *IV contrast-enhanced CT with delayed excretory phase* images is preferred imaging modality for diagnosis
- *Retrograde pyelography* most accurate for diagnosis but often not feasible as initial diagnostic step

Management

- Early identification: primary repair intraoperatively
- Late identification or unstable: urinary diversion with percutaneous nephrostomy and drainage of urinoma or abscess followed by delayed reconstruction of ureter

---

BLADDER TRAUMA
Epidemiology

Bladder injury in trauma is relatively uncommon given the protection the bony pelvis provides to the organ. It has been estimated that 1.6% of blunt abdominal trauma cases involve injury to bladder.[1] Blunt trauma accounts for most bladder injury (50%–86%). MVC followed by pedestrian versus vehicle accidents account for most blunt injuries to the bladder. Gunshot wounds account for most instances of penetrating trauma to the bladder.

Special attention should be taken in cases of confirmed pelvic fractures, because 3.6% of all pelvic fractures has concomitant bladder injury.[2] Conversely, approximately 70% of traumatic bladder injury is seen with associated pelvic fractures. Bladder rupture is classified according to the location of injury and where leakage of urine occurs. Bladder rupture is considered extraperitoneal if urinary extravasation is confined to the prevesical space. Bladder rupture is classified as intraperitoneal if the peritoneal surface has been breached and there is leakage of urine into the peritoneal cavity.[24] Extraperitoneal bladder rupture occurs most often (60%) as opposed to intraperitoneal rupture (30%). Combined extraperitoneal and intraperitoneal rupture is rare, occurring 5% to 8% of the time.

As is the case with all GU injury, bladder injury is seldom seen in isolation and is associated with multiorgan trauma. Isolated bladder rupture is most often seen in iatrogenic cases and when there is a direct blow to the abdomen in a person with a distended bladder. Iatrogenic injury to the bladder is most often seen in complex obstetric and gynecologic procedures.[25]

Anatomic Considerations

The deep position within the bony pelvis of the bladder shields it from the forces of blunt trauma. When the bladder is distended, however, the bladder is exposed from the bony pelvis and more vulnerable to injury. The bladder dome is the most susceptible to rupture given its weakened area around the urachal attachment.[23] Underdeveloped pelvic bones in children make the bladder more susceptible to rupture from blunt trauma when compared with the adult population.

History and Physical Examination

In assessing for the potential for bladder injury, key historical elements to assess for include difficulty or inability to void, gross hematuria, and suprapubic pain. The mechanism of injury also can point strongly toward the possibility of bladder trauma. Straddle injuries, direct perineal trauma, and known pelvic fractures should raise suspicion for potential underlying bladder injury.[26]

Examination findings suggestive of bladder injury include suprapubic bruising and tenderness, abdominal distention, or perineal wounds in the case of penetrating trauma. It is important to examine for blood at the urethral meatus to assess for the possibility of concurrent urethral injury. In cases of urethral injury, a retrograde urethrogram (RUG) should be performed before assessing for bladder injury with a cystogram.

Diagnostic Studies

A UA with gross hematuria is highly suggestive of bladder rupture and is present 95% of the time. Significant microscopic hematuria (at least >30 red blood cells per high power field [RBC/HPF]) with high-risk pelvic ring fracture patterns warrants targeted investigation for bladder rupture. A completely normal UA does not entirely exclude the possibility of bladder injury, and thus, if a high index of suspicion remains, further investigation must be pursued. Pelvic fracture patterns predictive of potential bladder rupture include pubic symphysis diastasis of greater than 1 cm or obturator ring fracture with greater than 1 cm of displacement.[27] **Box 3** summarizes pelvic fracture patterns that are considered high risk for potential associated bladder or urethral injury. In the presence these particular pelvic fracture patterns, strong consideration should be given to investigating for possible bladder or urethral injury.

A markedly elevated serum creatinine and BUN may be seen in cases of bladder rupture because these substances are reabsorbed into the blood from urine that is spilled into the peritoneum. This "pseudo-renal failure" phenomenon mimics acute kidney injury (AKI) and should be suspected in cases of unexplained AKI and potential bladder injury.[28]

Box 3
Pelvic fracture patterns predicting bladder or urethral injury

- Urethral injury:
  ○ Pubic symphysis diastasis
  ○ Medially displaced inferior pubic rami fractures
  ○ Fractures of all 4 pubic rami ("straddle fracture")
  ○ Vertical shear fracture with SI joint dislocation and pubic rami fractures ("Malgaigne fracture")

- Bladder injury:
  ○ Pubic symphysis diastasis greater than 1 cm
  ○ Obturator ring fracture with displacement >1 cm
  ○ SI joint widening

If bladder injury is suspected, cystography is considered the gold standard for diagnosis. Plain film cystography or CT cystography has similar sensitivity and specificity for bladder injury.[29] Traditional IV contrast-enhanced trauma protocol CT imaging is not sufficient for detecting bladder injury. Nonetheless, before CT or plain film cystography, trauma protocol IV contrast-enhanced CT should be performed first to rule out other solid organ trauma.[30] Combining CT cystography and initial IV-enhanced CT at the same time can lead to diagnostic uncertainty for bladder injury and other solid organ injury. Contrast infused into the bladder during cystography can interfere with IV contrast evaluation of other abdominopelvic organs. A RUG should be performed before CT or plain film cystography to rule out urethral injury before the placement of a Foley catheter for the procedure. Urethral injury can be seen concomitantly 5% to 29% of the time in bladder rupture; thus, a low threshold to perform RUQ before CT cystography should be maintained.[31]

Cystography involves the placement of a Foley catheter to drain the bladder, followed by the instillation of at least 250 mL (350 mL is the ideal volume if the patient can tolerate) of diluted iodinated CT contrast material into the bladder.[30] The Foley catheter is clamped once the bladder is distended sufficiently, and images are subsequently acquired. **Figs.** 4 and **5** are examples of abnormal CT cystograms

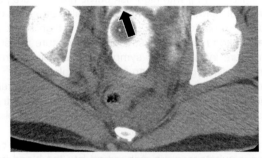

Fig. 4. CT cystogram revealing extraperitoneal bladder rupture. CT cystogram revealing extraperitoneal bladder rupture. Note gross extravasation of contrast into prevesicle space (*black arrow*). (*From* Dane B, Baxter AB, Bernstein MP. Imaging Genitourinary Trauma. *Radiol Clin North Am.* 2017;55(2):321-335; with permission.)

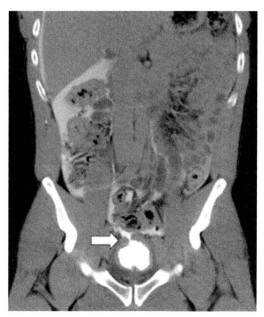

Fig. 5. Intraperitoneal bladder rupture. CT cystogram revealing intraperitoneal bladder rupture. Note gross extravasation of contrast into the peritoneal space (*arrow*). (*From* Dane B, Baxter AB, Bernstein MP. Imaging Genitourinary Trauma. *Radiol Clin North Am.* 2017;55(2):321-335; with permission.)

demonstrating cases of extraperitoneal and intraperitoneal bladder rupture, respectively.

Management

Bladder injury is radiographically classified as contusion or laceration (rupture) and is graded according to the AAST-Organ Injury Scale. Lacerations of the bladder are categorized as either extraperitoneal or intraperitoneal. Extraperitoneal bladder rupture is almost exclusively managed nonoperatively with urinary catheter drainage.[23,32] Operative repair of extraperitoneal bladder rupture may be indicated in a few scenarios. Bone fragments in the bladder tend to delay bladder healing with catheter drainage alone and warrant surgical repair. Concurrent vaginal or rectal laceration predisposes to fistula formation and generally indicates need for primary bladder repair to prevent this complication. Bladder neck injuries also tend to heal poorly with catheter drainage alone, and operative repair should be considered.

Repeat cystography is generally performed in 10 to 14 days to demonstrate resolution of urine leak, at which point the urinary catheter may be removed. Operative repair is indicated if urinary extravasation persists beyond 4 weeks.

Intraperitoneal bladder rupture and penetrating bladder trauma are managed operatively; however, surgical repair is often delayed in the setting of major trauma so as to avoid major pelvic bleeding from concomitant pelvic or other abdominal injuries. In these settings, urinary catheter drainage with eventual surgical repair is indicated[31] (**Box 4**).

Box 4
Key points in bladder trauma

History

- Known pelvic fractures (especially pubic symphysis diastasis >1 cm, SI joint widening, obturator ring fracture with displacement >1 cm), straddle injuries

- Difficulty or inability to void

- Suprapubic pain

- Gross hematuria

Examination

- Suprapubic bruising or tenderness

- Abdominal distention

- Blood at urethral meatus

Diagnostics

- UA: gross hematuria seen often (~95% of the time)

- *CT cystography* preferred imaging modality for diagnosis and should be considered when
  ○ Nonacetabular pelvic fractures (pubic rami, sacrum, ilium) + gross hematuria
  ○ Nonacetabular pelvic fractures + significant microscopic hematuria (>30 RBCs/HPF)
  ○ Unexplained free fluid in pelvis in setting of trauma
  ○ IV contrast-enhanced CT should be performed first to rule out solid organ injury before CT cystogram
  ○ Sufficient volume of contrast (at least 250 mL) needs to be instilled in bladder to detect bladder rupture with adequate sensitivity

- *RUG* should be performed before cystography if associated urethral injury suspected

Management

- Extraperitoneal bladder rupture: largely nonoperative management with urinary catheter drainage

- Intraperitoneal bladder rupture: operative management with urinary catheter drainage

---

URETHRAL TRAUMA
Epidemiology

Trauma to the urethra is most commonly iatrogenic with most occurring owing to urinary catheterization or during surgery involving the urethra. Noniatrogenic trauma to the urethra is rare and only accounts for only ~4% of all GU traumatic injury.

Posterior urethral injury owing to pelvic fractures is the most common noniatrogenic injury to the urethra. Men are 5 times more likely to sustain injury to the urethra because of its longer length and reduced mobility when compared with the female urethra.[1] Anterior urethral injury occurs most commonly during "straddle-type" injuries to the bulbar urethra.

Anatomic Considerations

The urethra is divided anatomically by the perineal membrane into anterior and posterior portions. The posterior portion is proximal to the perineal membrane and the anterior portion distally. The posterior urethra is subdivided into the prostatic and membranous portions. The prostatic urethra extends from the bladder neck to the apex of prostate and is anchored to the anterior pubic arch. This attachment leads to this portion of the posterior urethra being particularly vulnerable to direct injury

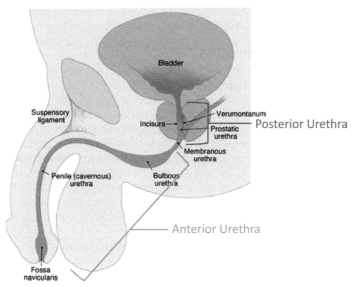

Fig. 6. Normal male urethral anatomy. (*Adapted from* Levin TL, Han B, Little BP. Congenital anomalies of the male urethra. *Pediatric Radiology.* 2007;37(9):851-862; with permission.)

from displaced pubic rami.[33] The membranous urethra extends from beyond the prostatic apex and up to the corpus spongiosum. This portion of the urethra is least protected and most likely to be disrupted within the case of pelvic fractures. **Fig. 6** provides a schematic of the normal male urethral anatomy.

The anterior urethra is subdivided into the bulbous and pendulous parts. The bulbous urethra is more commonly injured by "straddle-type" injuries and penile fractures when compared with the pendulous portion, given its fixation beneath the pubic bone.[33]

History and Physical Examination

Similarly to suspected bladder injury, a history of difficulty voiding is suggestive of possible urethral injury. A straddle-type mechanism of injury to the perineum or known pelvic fractures should alert the clinician to possible underlying urethral trauma.

Classic examination findings indicative of urethral injury include blood at the urethral meatus, gross hematuria, perineal hematoma, and the nonpalpable or "high-riding" prostate.[34] Unfortunately, none of these individual clinical features is particularly sensitive for urethral injury, and most injuries are diagnosed after urinary catheterization. Difficulty with catheter placement or return of gross hematuria upon catheterization often is what prompts investigation for urethral trauma.[35] One study observed no clinical indicators of urethral injury before urinary catheter placement in 60% of patients.[36] These clinical indicators should still be sought out; however, their absence does not exclude the possibility of urethral injury.

Diagnostic Studies

As is the case with other GU injuries, gross hematuria observed on UA of the first spontaneously voided specimen should prompt targeted investigation for urethral as well as other lower GU tract injury. Unfortunately, gross hematuria is not often seen in urethral injury and should not be considered a sufficiently sensitive screening tool for urethral injury. One study reported only 17% of patients with urethral injury had gross hematuria before urinary catheter placement.[36]

The pattern of pelvic fracture seen during the evaluation of a trauma patient should help guide consideration for possible associated urethral injury. Straddle fractures (fractures of all 4 pubic rami), fractures of the inferior pubic ramus with a widened pubic symphysis, and Malgaigne fractures (vertical shear fracture with sacroliaic (SI) joint dislocation and pubic rami fractures leading to upward shifting of hemipelvis) are the most common fracture patterns associated with urethral injury.[37]

The imaging modality of choice for the diagnosis of urethral injury is the RUG. An RUG should be performed before insertion of a Foley catheter in cases of suspect urethral trauma; however, an RUG can still be performed in patients in whom a catheter has already been placed. For male patients, the penis is positioned laterally over the thigh, and a 6- to 8-F Foley catheter with a 5-mL inflatable balloon is placed into the fossa navicularis of the penis. The Foley balloon is then inflated with 1 to 2 mL of saline, and 20 to 30 mL of iodinated contrast is injected slowly into the catheter. Contrast should be injected until visualized fluoroscopically within the bladder at which point images can be acquired.[38] Performing an RUG in female patients is more challenging given the short urethral length; however, the process is the same as with male patients. **Fig. 7** depicts an example of an abnormal RUG.

Management

Given that most urethral injury is seen in the context of other abdominopelvic injuries, definitive management of urethral injury is deferred until patient stability is established. Nonetheless, early diagnosis and prompt urinary diversion are essential in urethral

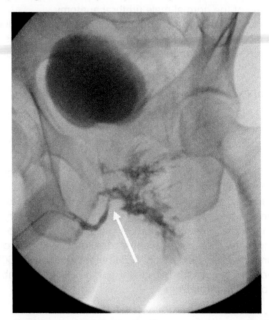

Fig. 7. Posterior urethral injury. RUG demonstrating a posterior urethral injury. Note gross extravasation of contrast at the level of the posterior urethra (*arrow*). (*From* Dane B, Baxter AB, Bernstein MP. Imaging Genitourinary Trauma. *Radiol Clin North Am.* 2017;55(2):321-335; with permission.)

injury so as to prevent infection of extravasated urine and blood, which could spread quickly across fascial planes into the abdomen, chest, perineum, and medial thighs.[39] Long-term consequences of misdiagnosed urethral injury include urethral stricture, sexual dysfunction, urethra-cutaneous fistula formation, or periurethral diverticula.

Urinary diversion in urethral trauma can be accomplished with urethral catheterization or suprapubic catheter placement. Classic teaching advised against attempts at blind urethral catheter placement out of concern for converting a partial urethral tear into a complete tear. Evidence supporting this fear is lacking; moreover, there is some evidence that blind urethral catheterization does not seem to lead to complete urethral disruption.[40]

Nonetheless, blind urethral catheterization in suspected cases of urethral injury remains controversial and is still best avoided, if possible. In cases whereby urgent catheterization is required to help guide resuscitation of a trauma patient, 1 gentle attempt at blind catheterization is reasonable. If the catheter does not pass easily, the procedure should be aborted in favor of suprapubic tube placement or catheter placement of a guidewire.[39] After urinary diversion has been achieved with either careful urethral catheterization or suprapubic tube placement, delayed definitive repair of the urethral injury can be pursued once concomitant abdominopelvic injuries have been stabilized (**Box 5**).

Box 5
Key points in urethral trauma

History

- Straddle-type mechanism of injury to perineum
- Known pelvic fractures
- Difficulty voiding
- Gross hematuria

Examination

- Blood at urethral meatus
- Perineal hematoma
- High-riding prostate

Diagnostics

- UA: gross hematuria not often present ($\sim$17% of the time according to 1 study[36])
- RUG: preferred imaging modality for diagnosis
  - 6- to 8-F Foley catheter placed in fossa navicularis, balloon inflated with 1 to 2 mL of saline
  - 20 to 30 mL of iodinated contrast injected into catheter then fluoroscopic images obtained

Management

- Urinary diversion
  - Suprapubic cystostomy tube
  - Flexible cystoscopy-guided or blind urinary catheter placement (should be performed only with urologic consultation)

EXTERNAL GENITALIA TRAUMA
Penile Fracture

Epidemiology

The vast majority of penile fractures occur during sexual intercourse when the erect penis forcefully hits the female pelvis, accounting for more than 80% of cases of penile fractures. In Africa, Asia, and the Middle East, the "Taghaandan maneuver," which involves forcefully bending the erect penile shaft to achieve rapid detumescence when in unsuitable situations, accounts for a significant portion of penile fractures.[41,42]

Anatomic considerations

A penile fracture is defined as a rupture of the tunica albuginea, corpus cavernosum, or both. A penile fracture may occur in isolation or with an associated urethral injury.[41] The tunica albuginea is thinnest at the ventrolateral aspect of the penile shaft, which explains why most ruptures occur at this site.[43]

History and physical examination

Classic historical signs of a penile fracture include a report of sudden severe penile pain, a simultaneous cracking or popping sound, and immediate rapid detumescence. The examination may reveal gross swelling and hematoma of the penile shaft known as the "eggplant deformity" (**Fig. 8**).[43] Bruising either may be limited to penile shaft or extend to the scrotum and perineum if Buck fascia is breached. A tender, palpable defect may be felt over the area of tunica rupture. Blood at the urethral meatus, gross hematuria, or difficulty voiding may occur and should prompt investigation for possible associated urethral injury.

Diagnostic studies

Penile fracture remains largely a clinical diagnosis highly suggested by classic history and examination findings; however, atypical presentations can occur that may warrant imaging studies. If an associated urethral injury is suspected, RUG should be performed.

Penile US may be highly operator dependent in diagnosing tunica or cavernosum tears, thus limiting its sensitivity in diagnosis when performed by inexperienced sonographers.[44] US can be useful in surgical planning if it successfully locates the defect; however, a negative study does not rule out penile fracture.

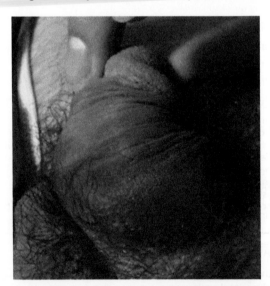

Fig. 8. Penile fracture. Hematoma of the penile shaft, otherwise known as the "eggplant deformity," in a patient with a penile fracture. (*From* Manjunath AS, Hofer MD. Urologic Emergencies. Medical clinics of North America. 2018;102(2):373-385; with permission.)

MRI is considered the most sensitive and specific diagnostic modality for penile fracture, however, because of its cost and limited availability, should be limited to cases whereby the diagnosis is uncertain by history and examination.[44]

Management

Prompt surgical exploration and repair of tunica albuginea defects are recommended in cases of penile fracture. Typically, repair is performed within 24 to 48 hours, but should be performed urgently if associated urethral injury is present[43] (**Box 6**).

Box 6
Key points in penile fracture

History

- Sudden severe penile pain
- Rapid detumescence

Examination

- Gross swelling and hematoma or penile shaft ("eggplant deformity")
- Blood at urethral meatus

Diagnostics

- Largely clinical diagnosis
- Ultrasonography: highly operator dependent and may not be sensitive enough with inexperienced sonographers
- MRI: most accurate for definitive diagnosis
- RUG: should be performed if associated urethral injury suspected

Management

- Urgent surgical repair of tunica albuginea defect and associated urethral injury if present

---

Testicular Trauma

Epidemiology

Blunt trauma to the scrotum accounts for 85% of testicular injury. MVC, physical assaults, and straddle or sporting injuries represent most of the blunt injury to the scrotum. Penetrating trauma to the scrotum is much less common, however is seen most commonly in cases of blast injuries or gunshot wounds.[45]

Anatomic considerations

Testicular injury is overall quite rare given the mobility and elasticity of the testis. The larger volume and more cranial position of the right testicle predisposes it to being trapped against the thigh and pubic bone more often, leading to injury more often than the left testicle.

A variety of injury patterns can be seen in scrotal trauma, depending on which structure is injured. Testicular rupture is the most serious scrotal injury in which the tunica albuginea is torn and testicular parenchyma is extruded. Testicular hematomas may occur with or without associated tunica violation. A hematocele is blood that accumulates between the parietal and visceral layers of the tunica vaginalis. Testicular torsion can also occur in scrotal trauma when sudden cremasteric contraction elevates and rotates the testis.[45]

History and physical examination

Pain and swelling of the scrotum with associated nausea and vomiting may be seen in testicular injury. Examination findings suggestive of testicular injury include scrotal swelling or hematoma, palpable testicular deformity, abnormal testicular lie, or absent cremasteric reflex. Unfortunately, the absence of clinical indicators other than pain after blunt scrotal trauma does not rule out testicular injury, and diagnostic scrotal imaging is required.[46]

Diagnostic studies

Scrotal US is the first-line imaging modality in the diagnosis of testicular injury. US findings suggestive of testicular rupture include loss of testicular contour, heterogenous parenchyma, and visualized tunica albuginea disruption (**Fig. 9**).[45] Testicular hematoma, hematocele, and testicular torsion are all other testicular injuries assessed well by scrotal US.

In cases whereby the US is inconclusive for testicular rupture, MRI is considered highly accurate in identifying disruption of the tunica albuginea.[45] CT is useful in identifying concurrent pelvic trauma; however, its accuracy in the diagnosis of isolated testicular trauma is unclear and generally not considered useful as the first-line imaging modality in scrotal trauma.

Management

In cases of blunt scrotal trauma with confirmed testicular rupture, early surgical exploration and repair are indicated. Small testicular hematomas or hematoceles without disruption of the tunica albuginea may be observed with repeat US to ensure no expansion within 48 hours. If rapid expansion of the hematoma or hematocele is seen, surgical exploration is generally indicated at that time.[43]

In cases of penetrating scrotal trauma, surgical exploration is usually necessary to define extent of injury and control ongoing hemorrhage. US may be performed first in the stable patient to assess injury before surgical exploration. Broad-spectrum antibiotic therapy should be administered as well[43] (**Box 7**).

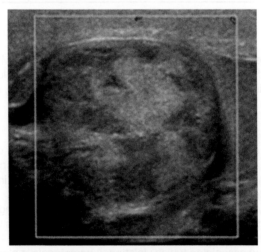

Fig. 9. Testicular rupture. Testicular US demonstrating a heterogenous testicle, loss of vascular flow, and indistinct testicular margins suggestive of testicular rupture. (*From* Dane B, Baxter AB, Bernstein MP. Imaging Genitourinary Trauma. *Radiol Clin North Am.* 2017;55(2):321-335; with permission.)

Box 7
Key points in testicular trauma

History

- Pain and swelling of the scrotum

- Nausea and vomiting

Examination

- Scrotal swelling or hematoma

- Abnormal testicular lie

- Absent cremasteric reflex

Diagnostics

- Scrotal US: imaging modality of choice for diagnosing testicular injury. US findings suggestive of testicular rupture include
  - Loss of testicular contour and vascularity
  - Heterogenous testicular parenchyma
  - Visualized tunica albuginea defect

Management

- Testicular rupture: urgent exploration and surgical repair

- Testicular hematoma or hematocele: serial scrotal US, surgical exploration if rapid expansion within 48 hours

- Testicular torsion: urgent surgical exploration and detorsion

---

Vulvar Trauma

Epidemiology

Injury to the vulva is overall quite rare and can be divided into accidental and nonaccidental traumatic events. Accidental trauma most commonly involves straddle injuries, which is seen often in children and adolescents. Straddle injuries often occur while riding a bicycle but also can occur during other sporting activities. Childbirth, sexual intercourse, and animal bites represent other mechanisms of accidental vulvar trauma.[47]

Nonaccidental trauma to the vulva occurs most commonly in cases of female genital mutilation (FGM) and sexual assault. FGM refers to partial or total removal of the female external genitalia and is a cultural practice seen predominantly in Africa and Asia. The most common form of FGM practiced involves removal of the clitoris and labia minora.[47]

Anatomic considerations

The vulva is a term referring to all of structures of the female external genitalia, including the mons pubis, labia majora and minora, clitoris, and the vaginal vestibule.[48] Because of the relatively concealed location of the vulva, nonaccidental injury to these structures is quite rare.

The structure most commonly injured largely depends on the mechanism of injury. Lacerations to the posterior fourchette and labia minora are most commonly seen during consensual and nonconsensual sexual intercourse. Straddle injuries most commonly will result in vulvar hematomas.[47]

History and physical examination

Careful external examination and subsequent speculum examination will identify most injury to the vulva. Occasionally, examination under anesthesia is required to adequately perform speculum examination and rule out extension of injury to the rectum.

Diagnostic studies

A pelvic radiograph should be performed to rule out associated pelvic fractures in the setting of straddle injuries or MVC that lead to vulvar trauma. RUG should be performed if there is suspicion of concomitant urethral injury.

Management

The management of vulvar hematomas is largely conservative with nonsteroidal anti-inflammatory drugs (NSAIDs), analgesia, and cold compresses. Urinary retention may occur secondary to pain or the degree of swelling, which should be managed with urinary catheterization. Urinary retention in the setting of vulvar trauma should prompt consideration of potential urethral injury however, and retrograde urethrography should be considered. Large or rapidly expanding hematomas rarely may require evacuation by incision and drainage with drainage placement, especially if there is concern for necrosis of overlying skin under high pressure.[47] Lacerations to the labia minora, majora, or vaginal canal itself will require primary closure in a fashion similar to lacerations encountered during childbirth (**Box 8**).

Box 8
Key points in vulvar trauma

History
- Straddle injuries
- Consensual and nonconsensual sexual intercourse
- Female genital mutilation

Examination
- Swelling and tenderness of labia majora or minora
- Laceration of posterior fourchette or vaginal vault
- Need to exclude extension of vaginal laceration to rectum

Diagnostics
- External examination and careful speculum examination
- Examination under anesthesia may be necessary to exclude extension of vaginal laceration to rectum
- Retrograde urethrography should be considered in straddle injuries to rule out associated urethral injury

Management
- Vulvar hematoma: cold compresses and NSAIDs. May require incision and drainage if rapidly expanding or concern for necrosis of overlying skin
- Vaginal laceration: exclude extension to rectum, primary closure similar to repair of childbirth-related laceration

---

SUMMARY

Although rarely posing an immediate threat to the trauma patient, GU injury should be considered in all cases of blunt or penetrating abdominopelvic trauma to avoid misdiagnosis or a delay in diagnosis. A high index of suspicion must be maintained because clinical indicators of GU injury can be subtle, delayed, or completely absent on initial evaluation. IV contrast-enhanced CT should be performed first to screen for life-threatening abdominal and pelvic organ injury. A UA assessing for gross hematuria is helpful in screening for GU injury; however, the absence of hematuria may not be sufficient in ruling out potential GU tract trauma. A careful history and examination should dictate if additional diagnostic studies, such as an RUG, cystography, US, or MRI, are required for targeted investigation of potential GU injury.

REFERENCES

1. McGeady JB, Breyer BN. Current epidemiology of genitourinary trauma. Urol Clin North Am 2013;40(3):323–34.
2. Bjurlin MA, Fantus RJ, Mellett MM, et al. Genitourinary injuries in pelvic fracture morbidity and mortality using the National Trauma Data Bank. J Trauma 2009; 67(5):1033–9.
3. Ter-Grigorian AA, Kasyan GR, Pushkar DY. Urogenital disorders after pelvic ring injuries. Cent European J Urol 2013;66(3):352–6.
4. Erlich T, Kitrey ND. Renal trauma: the current best practice. Ther Adv Urol 2018; 10(10):295–303.
5. Voelzke BB, Leddy L. The epidemiology of renal trauma. Transl Androl Urol 2014; 3(2):143–9.
6. Kansas BT, Eddy MJ, Mydlo JH, et al. Incidence and management of penetrating renal trauma in patients with multiorgan injury: extended experience at an inner city trauma center. J Urol 2004;172(4 Pt 1):1355–60.
7. Chong ST, Cherry-Bukowiec JR, Willatt JMG, et al. Renal trauma: imaging evaluation and implications for clinical management. Abdom Radiol 2016;41(8): 1565–79.
8. Pandyan GVS, Omo-Adua I, Al Rashid, et al. Blunt renal trauma in a pre-existing renal lesion. ScientificWorldJournal 2006;6:2334–8.
9. Shariat SF, Roehrborn CG, Karakiewicz PI, et al. Evidence-based validation of the predictive value of the American Association for the Surgery of Trauma kidney injury scale. J Trauma 2007;62(4):933–9.
10. Dane B, Baxter AB, Bernstein MP. Imaging genitourinary trauma. Radiol Clin North Am 2017;55(2):321–35.
11. Kuan JK, Wright JL, Nathens AB, et al. American Association for the Surgery of Trauma Organ Injury Scale for kidney injuries predicts nephrectomy, dialysis, and death in patients with blunt injury and nephrectomy for penetrating injuries. J Trauma 2006;60(2):351–6.
12. Kozar RA, Crandall M, Shanmuganathan K, et al. Organ injury scaling 2018 update: spleen, liver, and kidney. J Trauma Acute Care Surg 2018;85(6):1119–22.
13. Bjurlin MA, Fantus RJ, Fantus RJ, et al. Comparison of nonoperative and surgical management of renal trauma: can we predict when nonoperative management fails? J Trauma Acute Care Surg 2017;82(2):356–61.
14. Lanchon C, Fiard G, Arnoux V, et al. High grade blunt renal trauma: predictors of surgery and long-term outcomes of conservative management. A prospective single center study. J Urol 2016;195(1):106–11.
15. McCombie SP, Thyer I, Corcoran NM, et al. The conservative management of renal trauma: a literature review and practical clinical guideline from Australia and New Zealand. BJU Int 2014;114(Suppl 1):13–21.
16. Husmann DA, Gilling PJ, Perry MO, et al. Major renal lacerations with a devitalized fragment following blunt abdominal trauma: a comparison between nonoperative (expectant) versus surgical management. J Urol 1993;150(6):1774–7.

17. Siram SM, Gerald SZ, Greene WR, et al. Ureteral trauma: patterns and mechanisms of injury of an uncommon condition. Am J Surg 2010;199(4):566–70.
18. Engelsgjerd JS, LaGrange CA. Ureteral injury. In: StatPearls. Treasure Island (FL): StatPearls Publishing; 2019. Available at: https://www-ncbi-nlm-nih-gov.medproxy.hofstra.edu/books/NBK507817/.
19. Bašić D, Ignjatović I, Potić M. Iatrogenic ureteral trauma: a 16-year single tertiary centre experience. Srp Arh Celok Lek 2015;143(3–4):162–8.
20. Marcelissen TAT, Den Hollander PP, Tuytten TRAH, et al. Incidence of iatrogenic ureteral injury during open and laparoscopic colorectal surgery: a single center experience and review of the literature. Surg Laparosc Endosc Percutan Tech 2016;26(6):513–5.
21. Pereira BMT, Ogilvie MP, Gomez-Rodriguez JC, et al. A review of ureteral injuries after external trauma. Scand J Trauma Resusc Emerg Med 2010;18:6.
22. Taqi KM, Nassr MM, Al Jufaili JS, et al. Delayed diagnosis of ureteral injury following penetrating abdominal trauma: a case report and review of the literature. Am J Case Rep 2017;18:1377–81.
23. Phillips B, Holzmer S, Turco L, et al. Trauma to the bladder and ureter: a review of diagnosis, management, and prognosis. Eur J Trauma Emerg Surg 2017;43(6): 763–73.
24. Guttmann I, Kerr HA. Blunt bladder injury. Clin Sports Med 2013;32(2):239–46.
25. Mendez LE. Iatrogenic injuries in gynecologic cancer surgery. Surg Clin North Am 2001;81(4):897–923.
26. Hsieh C-H, Chen R-J, Fang J-F, et al. Diagnosis and management of bladder injury by trauma surgeons. Am J Surg 2002;184(2):143–7.
27. Avey G, Blackmore CC, Wessells H, et al. Radiographic and clinical predictors of bladder rupture in blunt trauma patients with pelvic fracture. Acad Radiol 2006; 13(5):573–9.
28. Matsumura M, Ando N, Kumabe A, et al. Pseudo-renal failure: bladder rupture with urinary ascites. BMJ Case Rep 2015;2015 [pii:bcr2015212671].
29. Ramchandani P, Buckler PM. Imaging of genitourinary trauma. AJR Am J Roentgenol 2009;192(6):1514–23.
30. Joshi G, Kim EY, Hanna TN, et al. CT cystography for suspicion of traumatic urinary bladder injury: indications, technique, findings, and pitfalls in diagnosis: RadioGraphics fundamentals | online presentation. Radiographics 2018;38(1):92–3.
31. Zinman LN, Vanni AJ. Surgical management of urologic trauma and iatrogenic injuries. Surg Clin North Am 2016;96(3):425–39.
32. Johnsen NV, Young JB, Reynolds WS, et al. Evaluating the role of operative repair of extraperitoneal bladder rupture following blunt pelvic trauma. J Urol 2016; 195(3):661–5.
33. Kommu SS, Illahi I, Mumtaz F. Patterns of urethral injury and immediate management. Curr Opin Urol 2007;17(6):383–9.
34. Mundy AR, Andrich DE. Urethral trauma. Part I: introduction, history, anatomy, pathology, assessment and emergency management. BJU Int 2011;108(3):310–27.
35. Ziran BH, Chamberlin E, Shuler FD, et al. Delays and difficulties in the diagnosis of lower urologic injuries in the context of pelvic fractures. J Trauma 2005;58(3): 533–7.
36. Ball CG, Jafri SM, Kirkpatrick AW, et al. Traumatic urethral injuries: does the digital rectal examination really help us? Injury 2009;40(9):984–6.
37. Basta AM, Blackmore CC, Wessells H. Predicting urethral injury from pelvic fracture patterns in male patients with blunt trauma. J Urol 2007;177(2):571–5.

38. Ingram MD, Watson SG, Skippage PL, et al. Urethral injuries after pelvic trauma: evaluation with urethrography. Radiographics 2008;28(6):1631–43.

39. Barratt RC, Bernard J, Mundy AR, et al. Pelvic fracture urethral injury in males-mechanisms of injury, management options and outcomes. Transl Androl Urol 2018;7(Suppl 1):S29–62.

40. Shlamovitz GZ, McCullough L. Blind urethral catheterization in trauma patients suffering from lower urinary tract injuries. J Trauma 2007;62(2):330–5 [discussion: 334–5].

41. Falcone M, Garaffa G, Castiglione F, et al. Current management of penile fracture: an up-to-date systematic review. Sex Med Rev 2018;6(2):253–60.

42. Mirzazadeh M, Fallahkarkan M, Hosseini J. Penile fracture epidemiology, diagnosis and management in Iran: a narrative review. Transl Androl Urol 2017;6(2):158–66.

43. Rees RW, Brown G, Dorkin T, et al. British Association of Urological Surgeons (BAUS) consensus document for the management of male genital emergencies - penile fracture. BJU Int 2018;122(1):26–8.

44. Agarwal MM, Singh SK, Sharma DK, et al. Fracture of the penis: a radiological or clinical diagnosis? A case series and literature review. Can J Urol 2009;16(2):4568–75.

45. Wang A, Stormont I, Siddiqui MM. A review of imaging modalities used in the diagnosis and management of scrotal trauma. Curr Urol Rep 2017;18(12):98.

46. Wang Z, Yang J-R, Huang Y-M, et al. Diagnosis and management of testicular rupture after blunt scrotal trauma: a literature review. Int Urol Nephrol 2016;48(12):1967–76.

47. Lopez HN, Focseneanu MA, Merritt DF. Genital injuries acute evaluation and management. Best Pract Res Clin Obstet Gynaecol 2018;48:28–39.

48. White C. Genital injuries in adults. Best Pract Res Clin Obstet Gynaecol 2013;27(1):113–30.

Kidney and Ureteral Stones

Jill Corbo, MD, RDMS*, Jessica Wang, MD, RDMS

KEYWORDS

- Renal colic • Kidney stone • Urolithiasis • Nephrolithiasis

KEY POINTS

- There are other conditions that present similar to renal colic with hematuria, that is, abdominal aortic aneurysms.
- Check the urine for infection as well as hematuria. An infection with complete obstruction is a urologic emergency.
- Patients being discharged with an obstructing stone should have close urology follow-up. An obstruction delayed past 2 weeks will progressively worsen the renal outcome.

BACKGROUND

Urinary stone disease (USD) is a generic term that refers to the presence of stones within the urinary tract, commonly known as kidney stones, urolithiasis, or nephrolithiasis. USD is a common disease with annual incidence of approximately 7 to 12 cases/10,000 per year in the United States.[1] Its prevalence has steadily increased in the recent decades with greater than 8% of US population presently being affected.[2] Based on the acute nature of presentation, kidney stones generate a large volume of emergency department (ED) visits and hospital admission. The Healthcare Cost and Utilization Project reported that in 2009 there were 1.3 million ED visits for kidney stones with greater than 3600 ED visits for stones every day.[1] Given the frequent presentation of USD in the ED, it is essential for the emergency practitioner to have the expertise in diagnosis and the management of this disease.

EPIDEMIOLOGY

The prevalence of USD is estimated to be 10% to 15% of the US population, with lifetime risk of stone formation exceeding 12% to 14% in men and 6% in women.[2] There is a high probability of recurrence with up to 50% experiencing a recurrence within 5 years.[3] Its prevalence has doubled over the past 15 years, although it is growing even more rapidly in historically lower-risk groups such as women, children, and Black

The authors do not have any commercial or financial conflicts of interest and funding sources.
Department of Emergency Medicine, Jacobi Medical Center, Building 6, Room 1B25, 1400 Pelham Parkway South, Bronx, NY 10461, USA
* Corresponding author.
E-mail address: Jill.Corbo@nbhn.net

patients.[2] In women it has increased by 75% since 1994, and in Black patients it has increased by greater than 120%.[2] The frequency of USD in children, who are historically low risk, has increased by approximately 4% to 6% yearly, particularly among adolescents,[4] due to multifactorial reasons, which include increase in obesity and changes in diet such as decrease in calcium and increase in fructose intake among adolescents.

This upward trend is significant, resulting in ED visits of greater than 1.3 million annually, repeat ED visits of 11% after initial evaluation, and 20% of the ED visits that result in hospitalization.[5] This increase is associated with significant economic burden. According to the Urologic Disease in America Project funded by the National Institute of Diabetes and Digestive and Kidney Diseases, the annual direct medical cost of USD in the United States is $10 billion, making USD the most expensive urologic condition.[6] The peak incidence occurs between age 20 and 50 years, with male to female ratio of 3:1 and a recurrence rate of approximately 30% in the first 5 years and approximately 50% recurrence rate in 10 years.[2]

Geographic variation has been found to be a risk factor for USD, which is thought to be related to higher ambient temperature.[7] A landmark study characterizing stone formation in the United States using data from the Cancer Prevention Study II[7] identified an increasing prevalence of USD in the United States moving from north to south and west to east[8] establishing the concept of a "stone belt." This is thought to be related to the higher temperature. In fact, studies have demonstrated a correlation of higher ambient month temperatures and the incidence of renal colic and USD worldwide.[9] Many have interpreted the stone belt maps to support the conclusion that higher temperature is associated with an increase risk of stone disease likely from insensible water loss (ie, from perspiration leading to dehydration, urine concentration, and urine supersaturation).[10] Others have postulated that in addition to higher mean temperature, higher precipitation also contributes to the increased risk of USD.[11]

RISK FACTORS

The risk factors for USD are influenced by urine composition, which can be affected by many factors including dietary, systemic illness, and environment. Some are modifiable whereas others are not. Risk factors can be categorized into nondietary, dietary, and urinary. See **Box 1** for summary of risk factors.

Nondietary

Incidence of USD is 3 times more likely in men than in women and predominantly in whites than in Black patients. The risk of USD is 2.5 times more likely if there is a family history likely due to a genetic predisposition and similar environmental and dietary exposures. Prior history of USD and systemic medical conditions such as diabetes, obesity, gout, hypertension, chronic kidney disease, Crohn disease, hyperthyroidism, primary hyperparathyroidism, sarcoidosis, and renal tubular acidosis have all been implicated in increasing the risk of USD. Environmental exposures such as living in warmer climates and certain occupations in which the individual works in higher temperature have been proposed as risk factors for development of USD. This is thought to be related to a combination of factors including insensible water loss from heat and increased vitamin D exposure from living in warmer climates and low fluid intake due to certain occupation's lack of access to bathroom leading to lower urine volume and a higher risk of stone formation.

Box 1
Risk factors of urinary stone disease

Nondietary

- Male sex (3:1 to women)
- White > Asian > Blacks
- Prior history of USD
- Family history
- Systemic conditions: diabetes, obesity, gout, hypertension, chronic kidney disease, Crohn disease, hyperthyroidism, primary hyperparathyroidism, sarcoidosis, renal tubular acidosis, multiple myeloma
- Environmental condition: warmer climate

Dietary

- Low calcium diet
- Low fluid intake
- High sodium diet
- High animal protein diet
- High oxalate diet
- Stone forming medications:
  - Medication stones: indinavir, triamterene, acyclovir
  - Promotes formation of calcium stones: loop diuretic, acetazolamide, theophylline, glucocorticoids
  - Promotes uric acid stones: thiazide, salicylates, probenecid, allopurinol
- Conditions that enhance enteric oxalate absorption often in the setting of malabsorption such as patients with history of gastric bypass, bariatric surgery, and short bowel syndrome.

Urinary

- Low urine volume
- Urine concentration
- Urine composition
- Low urine pH
- Hypercalciuria
- Hyperoxaluria
- Hypocitraturia

Dietary

The composition of urine is influenced by dietary intake and environment, and several dietary factors have been implicated in the development of USD. Nutrients that have been implicated include calcium, animal protein, oxalate, sodium, sucrose, magnesium, and potassium. Certain factors such as low fluid intake, low calcium diet, high animal protein diet, and high sodium diet are known to contribute to the risk of USD. In addition, the use of certain stone-forming medications also increases the risk of stone formation.

Conditions that enhance enteric oxalate absorption often in the setting of malabsorption such as patients with history of gastric bypass, bariatric surgery, and short bowel syndrome are discussed in the next section.

Urinary

Urinary stone formation is intricately related to urine composition, low urine volume, urine concentration, and urine pH. Conditions such as hypercalciuria, hyperoxaluria, and hypocitraturia all increase urinary concentration of these ions and can cause stone formation when the urine becomes supersaturated. The persistent low pH promotes the precipitation of uric acid and is associated with the formation of uric acid stones.

CAUSE

There are 4 main types of urinary stones, with the majority (75%–90%) composed of calcium oxalate, followed by uric acid (5%–20%), calcium phosphate (6%–13%), struvite (2%–15%), and cystine (0.5–1).[12] See **Table 1** for stone types and composition.

The exact pathogenesis of stone formation is complex and involves both metabolic and environmental factors. This pathogenesis is not entirely understood, but it is clear that it is affected by urine composition.[12] Stone formation usually starts in the kidney and is due to urinary supersaturation with free ions (eg, calcium and oxalate in calcium oxalate stones), and this leads to the formation of crystals.[13] It is thought that the process starts with the formation of a nucleus, which is a heterogeneous mixture of substances such as uric acid, and this forms a nidus for nucleation, around which the stone grows. Increased urinary ion excretion and decreased urine volume will favor stone formation.[13] High urine flow rate will reduce supersaturation. However, despite similar degree of urine saturation, stones form in some people whereas not in others, and this may be due to the presence of promoters and inhibitors of crystallization in the urine.[14]

CLINICAL PRESENTATION

The classic presentation of kidney stone is an acute onset, severe unilateral flank pain radiating to the ipsilateral groin; classically it starts at night. The pain is usually

Table 1
Stone composition and causes

Stone Composition	Frequency (%)	Causes
Calcium oxalate and calcium phosphate	90	Hypercalciuria (high dietary sodium and protein, hypercalcemia) Hyperuricosuria (high purine, high protein diet) Hyperoxaluria (low dietary calcium, high oxalate diet or oxalate absorption, genetic hyperoxaluria) Hypocitraturia (chronic metabolic acidosis, inflammatory bowel disease)
Struvite (magnesium-ammonium-phosphate)	2–15	Urine infection from urea-splitting bacteria (ie, *Proteus, Klebsiella, Corynebacterium*) Staghorn formation High urine pH
Uric acid	5–20	Hyperuricosuria (gout) Low urine pH Radiolucent
Cystine	~1	Cystinuria—autosomal recessive disorder of cystine, ornithine, arginine, and lysine Staghorn formation
Others	<1%	Medications (raltegravir, indinavir, triamterene)

Brener ZZ, Winchester JF, Salman H, et al. Nephrolithiasis: evaluation and management. Southern Medical Journal. 2011;104(2):133-9.

episodic, lasting 20 to 60 minutes, and does not completely resolve before the next wave of pain. The typical patient is usually writhing in distress and unable to find a comfortable position. In contrast to the patient with acute abdomen, they do not lie still. As the stone descend into the ureter, the pain may descend to the abdomen corresponding to the location of the stone with associated dysuria, urgency, and frequency. Approximately 30% of patients will report hematuria.[3] Patients will experience nausea and vomiting due to the shared splanchnic innervations of the renal capsule and intestine. Fever is not typically present, unless associated with infection. There are several conditions that may mimic renal colic. **Box 2** lists the most common.

EMERGENCY DEPARTMENT EVALUATION

The diagnosis of the USD includes a history and physical examination, evaluation of patient's risk factors and comorbid conditions, and the likelihood of an important alternate diagnosis. Typically, laboratory evaluations are done, which include a complete blood count, a metabolic panel to assess renal function, and urinalysis to assess for the presence of hematuria and infection. Confirmatory imaging is not always necessary. For example, in a patient with known history of kidney stones, with a typical presentation and low likelihood of an important alternate diagnosis or complications, conservative management may be appropriate.

However, in patients with no prior history of USD and with high risk for complication and alternate diagnosis, diagnostic imaging should be considered.

The development of a clinical prediction rule, the STONE score, aims to evaluate the likelihood of uncomplicated ureteral stones and clinically important alternative diagnosis.[15] This rule uses 5 objective criteria (gender, duration of pain, race, nausea/vomiting, and erythrocytes on urine dipstick) to categorize patients into low, moderate, and high probability of having a ureteral stone. The total score is 0-13 and is divided into 3 groups: low-risk: 0-5, moderate-risk: 6-9, and high-risk: 10-13. This scoring system attempts to predict the likelihood of uncomplicated ureteral stones and is inversely associated with likelihood of an acutely important alternate diagnosis. This clinical prediction rule has the potential to guide decision-making regarding diagnostic

---

Box 2
Differential diagnosis of renal colic

Abdominal aortic aneurysm

Acute myocardial Infarction

Pyelonephritis

Renal artery thrombosis and other renal diseases

Appendicitis

Diverticulitis

Intestinal obstruction

Pelvic and ovarian pathology such as cyst, torsion, ectopic pregnancy

Biliary colic

Herpes zoster

Testicular torsion

Incarcerated hernia

imaging and treatment options. When this prediction rule[15] was attempted to be externally validated, research found that the STONE score can aggregate patients into low-, medium-, and high-risk groups but lacks the sensitivity (53%) to allow clinicians to avoid obtaining a computed tomographic (CT) scan.[16] Further investigation is warranted regarding the utility of this prediction rule.

IMAGING MODALITIES

When a patient presents to the ED with suspected renal colic, there is no consensus on which imaging modality should be obtained or even if imaging is necessary in the ED. The pros to imaging a patient with suspected renal colic include the following: confirm the diagnosis, obtain information about the stone size and location, diagnose complications related to USD, and rule out any potential disorders that mimic renal colic (see **Box 2**). Some physicians image every patient who presents with suspected renal colic, others image only patients with first-time stones. There is a consensus that imaging should be performed in any patient whose abdominal aortic aneurysm is high in the differential. Some clinicians will reserve CT for patients who do not improve with conservative therapy or if another diagnosis is suspected.

CT of the abdomen and pelvis without contrast can be performed using low-radiating dose scanning protocols or standard dose scanning protocols. CT of the abdomen and pelvis without contrast using low-dose radiation scanning is the preferred examination for most adults. It has the highest diagnostic accuracy for renal and ureteral stones. It provides information on the stone size, location, and site of obstruction. CT scan is also useful in determining alternate diagnosis. CT of the abdomen and pelvis without contrast cannot evaluate kidney function. If low-dose radiation CT scan is not available or if the patient has a weight of greater than 130 kg in men and greater than 115 kg in women, then standard dose CT should be performed. Low and standard CT scans have similar diagnostic accuracy with a sensitivity and specificity of greater than 94% and greater than 97%, respectively.[17] The role of intravenous contrast CT of the abdomen and pelvis does decrease the sensitivity of detecting stones less than 3 mm. Of note, stones less than 3 mm have a greater than 85% spontaneous passage rate making the absolute diagnosis of these stones debatable.[18] The elderly population is the subgroup in whom the addition of intravenous contrast may aid in the diagnosis when searching for alternative diagnosis.

Ultrasound of the kidney and bladder can help diagnose renal colic indirectly by detecting hydronephrosis and the symmetry of the ureteral jets. Ultrasound can determine if a patient has unilateral or bilateral hydronephrosis and rarely can visualize presence of ureteral stones. This imaging modality is quick, noninvasive, and does not expose the patient to radiation; therefore, it is the preferred imaging modality in the pregnant patient. In addition, given the recurrent nature of USD, ultrasound should be considered when considering cumulative lifetime exposure of radiation in these patients. The ultrasound has a low sensitivity (54%) and inability to size a stone accurately.[19] Thus, some clinicians will obtain a CT scan after performing an ultrasound, either when an ultrasound is positive to confirm stone size and location in order to formulate a treatment plan or when an ultrasound is negative to confirm the negative test and to determine an alternate diagnosis. A recent multicenter trial with 2759 ED patients presenting with suspected renal colic was randomized to CT scan of abdomen and pelvis without contrast, ultrasound performed by the radiologist, or ultrasound performed in the ED by ED physician at the bedside.[20] After the initial imaging examination, the clinicians can order subsequent examinations at their own discretion. The sensitivity of CT scan was 86%, ultrasound preformed by the radiologist was 57%, and ultrasound preformed by the ED physician was 54%. Physicians ordered a CT scan 41% of the time after the initial test if the initial test was an ultrasound, whereas an ultrasound was ordered only 5% of the time after the initial test being a CT scan. There were no significant differences in high-risk diagnoses with complications, adverse events, and hospitalizations between the 3 arms of the study.[20] Performing an ultrasound as the initial imaging test might decrease the need to order an abdominal and pelvic CT scan and thus decrease the radiation exposure to the patient.

The abdominal radiography at times has been used as an adjunct in the diagnosis of managing patients with nephrolithiasis. The abdominal radiography cannot detect hydronephrosis and has a sensitivity of 57% for stone detection and localization.[21] The abdominal radiography is best when used in conjunction with ultrasound to evaluate progression of conservative therapy and interval stone growth.

An intravenous pyelography (IVP) involves radiographic imaging of the kidney, ureters, and the bladder before and after intravenous contrast dye is administered. It can diagnose hydronephrosis, evaluate renal function, and potentially show the position of the stone. IVP has similar sensitivity to that of ultrasound. This examination generally is not used as a first-line diagnostic imaging examination.

MRI of the abdomen and pelvis is seldom used for nephrolithiasis. MRI poorly detects stones. Currently, MRI is used in nephrolithiasis in pregnant patients with hydronephrosis on ultrasound. In these patients it can help determine the location of the obstruction, while not subjecting these patients to radiation.

MANAGEMENT AND TREATMENT
Analgesia

Management of stone disease should be individualized as well as the decision to consult a urologic specialist. When a patient presents with an acute stone episode, one of the main goal is relief from pain. The pain that renal colic patients experience is from an increase in collecting system pressure and urethral spasm, which is modulated via prostaglandins. Because of this theory, nonsteroidal antiinflammatory drugs (NSAIDs) have been the preferred drug for treatment of renal colic. NSAIDs can decrease smooth muscle tone as well as inhibit prostaglandins. NSAIDs should be avoided in patients with a history of a gastrointestinal bleed or impaired renal function.[22] Narcotics have also been found to be helpful in the treatment of renal colic pain. Narcotics do not help with inhibiting prostaglandins, and in fact some studies found that they increase ureteric muscle tone.[23] Although the European Association of Urology guidelines on urolithiasis recommend NSAIDs as the first choice, many physicians use intravenous opioids as the first-line agents.[24] There have been prospective trials that have shown that the combination of morphine and ketorolac offer pain relief superior to either drug alone and decrease the use of rescue analgesia.[25] Cochrane reviewed the literature of these 2 treatments for renal colic and found that there was equivalent level of analgesia with a slightly higher side effect of vomiting and the need for rescue medication in the opioid group.[24] Lidocaine is an amide local anesthetic that blocks fast-voltage gated sodium channels and thus prevents transmission of afferent pain signals.[26] There was one clinical trial from Iran[26] that found that lidocaine reduced pain intensity better and more quickly when compared with morphine in renal colic patients. Further studies need to be performed with the use of lidocaine for treatment of renal colic.

Hydration and Diuretics

Patients who are dehydrated from either vomiting or decrease in oral intake should receive intravenous hydration. In theory, increase in fluid flow through the affected kidney might expedite stone passage and thus improve the patient's symptoms. Studies have been preformed to prove this hypothesis by high-volume fluid hydration with or without the addition of diuretics to increase urine output. The literature in fact does not support the use of diuretics and high-volume fluid therapy in acute renal colic.[27,28]

Medical Expulsion Therapy

There have been several medical expulsion therapies (METs) that have increased the passage rate of ureteral stones, which include alpha blockers, calcium channel blockers, and antispasmodic agents.[29] Treatments that increase stone passage would benefit the patient by decreasing the need for interventional procedures. The top 2 METs that have been studied for the treatment of renal colic are tamsulosin (an alpha-adrenoceptor antagonist, a smooth muscle relaxant drug) and nifedipine (a calcium channel blocker).[30] A recent multicentre randomized placebo-controlled study compared tamsulosin, nifedipine, or placebo and its effect on intervention for stone clearance.[27] Pickard's study[29] found similar rates of spontaneous stone passage at 4 weeks and even 12 weeks with all 3 arms of the study. In 2018, a meta-analysis of 67 trials showed a small benefit of alpha-blocker therapy with stone passage than with a placebo control (relative risk 1.16, 95% confidence interval 1.07–1.25).[31] A few studies showed a subgroup analysis in patients with larger stones (5–10 mm); there was a higher rate of stone passage with tamsulosin compared with placebo.[32,33] Even though nifedipine has similar rate of passage to tamsulosin, the rate of passage is slower in the nifedipine (28 days vs 14 days) and has more side effects (15% vs 4%).[34] Thus, the use of MET in improving the passage of ureteral stones needs further research. At this time, there is little downside in using tamsulosin in MET, the cost of treatment is low, and there are few side effects.

Prognosis

Most patients who have a ureteral stone can be managed conservatively and discharged home safely with pain management and observation because most of the patients will pass the ureteral stone spontaneously. Factors that affect the spontaneous passage include stone size, stone location, and the degree of obstruction. There is a progressive decrease in stone passage rate because the size of the stone increases. Most stones less than 6 mm in diameter will pass spontaneously, whereas stones greater than 9 mm are unlikely to pass spontaneously.[23] Location of the stone is also a factor in passage rate; approximately 50% of stones pass spontaneously from the proximal ureter compared with 80% of stones at the ureterovesical junction.[23]

Conservative management is appropriate if (1) there is no evidence of sepsis, (2) there is normal renal function, (3) the ureteric stone is unilateral, (4) the contralateral renal unit is normal, (5) it is able to tolerate PO, and (6) there is adequate pain control with oral analgesia.[24] If any of these criteria is not met, a urologic consultation should be requested in the ED.

Patients should be discharged home with pain management and possibility of MET. They should be instructed to strain his/her urine for a several days after discharge from the ED so that the stone can be collected for analysis. This would help the physician determine the stone composition and direct further preventive measures. Even though stone composition is unknown when the patient is discharged from the ED, they should be instructed to increase oral hydration, decrease animal protein consumption, and decrease salt intake.

Patients should be instructed to return to the ED if he/she develops fever, intractable pain, or vomiting or if the pain lasts longer than 2 weeks. Patients should be educated that there is a high (50%) recurrent rate for renal stones.

Outpatient referral to an urologist should be individualized on a case by case basis. In general, patients who have an increase in creatinine level or have a nonobstructing stone with a concurrent urinary tract infection require close follow-up within the next 2 days. Those who have stones greater than 10 mm in size, recurrent renal stones, or failed conservative outpatient management for passage of stones should be referred to a urologist within 1 week.

Urology Consultation

Patients who are not able to be treated conservatively, due to having any one or several criteria in **Box 3**, should consult an urologist in the ED for admission and possible urgent intervention. Patients with an obstructing stone and urinary infection should be admitted for intravenous antibiotics and decompression of the obstruction. Patients with intractable vomiting should be admitted for intravenous hydration and supportive care. As alike, patients with intractable pain who cannot be controlled on oral agents should be admitted for supportive care. Patients with one functioning kidney should also be admitted to the hospital.

COMPLICATIONS
Obstruction

Patients who have a ureteral stone obstruction should have relief of obstruction within 2 weeks. Studies have shown that time to relief of obstruction and the presence of infection were the only significant predictors of outcome of long-term renal damage.[35] If the obstruction was delayed past 2 weeks, renal outcome worsens progressively. Thus, urologists can closely monitor patients with an obstruction that does not have a concurrent infection, if they have a functioning contralateral kidney.

Infection

An infection in the presence of an obstructive stone is a urologic emergency. Antibiotics cannot be excreted unless there is relief of the obstruction. When there is a urinary tract infection with a nonobstructing stone, patients can be treated with oral antibiotics with close follow-up within 24 hours.

Box 3
Admission criteria

1. Urosepsis

2. Intractable vomiting

3. Infection with stone obstruction

4. Stone size greater than 15 mm

5. Bilateral obstruction.

6. Single kidney or transplanted kidney with an obstruction

7. Intractable pain

8. Significantly elevated creatinine level

Stents

Patients with ureteral stents should be evaluated for obstruction, infection, and migration of the stents. This can be done by using abdominal and pelvic CT scan or a KUB ultrasound. Such patients should consult a urologist for their management and disposition.

SPECIAL CONCERNS

Pediatric

Stone disease in the pediatric population is uncommon, although its incidence is increasing especially in teens. The presentation of children with stone disease differs from that of an adult. Children usually present with a vague abdominal pain, not a unilateral colicky flank pain. Gross hematuria is present in 14% to 33% of patients and urinary tract infection affects 8% to 46% of stone pediatric patients.[36] Ultrasound is the study of choice in the pediatric population due to concern over radiation exposure. Indications for admission are the same as for the adults. All children should be referred to a urologist and a work-up for metabolic stone disease should be performed.

Pregnancy

There are anatomic and pathophysiologic changes in pregnancy that increase the risk of renal colic. There is urinary stasis secondary to compression and increase in progesterone levels. There is also hypercalciuria secondary to calcium supplementation and increase in glomerular rate. The renal ultrasound is the study of choice in pregnant patients secondary to the radiation exposure of CT scan. Narcotics are generally required for pain management because NSAIDs are contraindicated in pregnancy. METs can be safely used in pregnancy. Indications for admission are the same as for nonpregnant adults. Close follow-up with obstetrics as well as urologist is needed.

Geriatrics

The first important thing is to make the correct diagnosis. The differential diagnosis for this patient population includes acute myocardial infarction and abdominal aortic aneurysm. The average age of the first presentation for renal colic is 42 years, and it is uncommon for this first presentation to occur in patients older than 60 years.[37] Thus, if a patient older than 60 years presents with no history of USD with symptoms that suggest renal colic, one must have high index of suspicion for an alternate diagnosis.[37] The CT scan is the preferred imaging modality because it can evaluate both the renal collecting system and the aorta as well as other possible alternate diagnoses. The elderly population tend to have comorbid conditions and are on medications that may preclude them from the standard pain management of USD. For example, in patients who have renal failure or peptic ulcer disease, the use of NSAIDs is contraindicated.

REFERENCES

1. Foster G, Stocks C, Borofsky MS. Emergency Department Visits and Hospital Admissions for Kidney Stone Disease, 2009: Statistical Brief #139. Healthcare Cost and Utilization Project (HCUP) Statistical Briefs [Internet]. Rockville (MD): Agency for Healthcare Research and Quality (US); 2006–2012.
2. Scales CD, Smith AC, Hanley JM, et al. Urologic Diseases in America Project: Prevalence of kidney stones in the United States. Eur Urol 2012;62:160–5.

3. Moe OW. Kidney stones: pathophysiology and medical management. Review. Lancet 2006;367:333–44.

4. Tasian GE, Ross ME, Song L, et al. Annual incidence of nephrolithiasis among children and adults in South Carolina from 1997 to 2012. Clin J Am Soc Nephrol 2017;11(3):488–96.

5. Pearle MS, Calhoun EA, Curhan GC. Urologic disease in American project: urolithiasis. J Urol 2005;173:848–57.

6. Litwin MS, Saigal CS. Table 14-47: economic impact of urologic disease. NIH Publication 12-7865. In: Litwin MS, Saigal CS, editors. Urologic diseases in America. Washington, DC: National Institute of Diabetes and Digestive and Kidney Disease, National Institute of Health, Public Health Service, US Department of Health and Human Services; 2012. p. 486.

7. Soucie JM, Thun MJ, CoatesRJ, et al. Demographic and geographic variability of kidney stones in the United States. Kidney Int 1994;46:893–9.

8. Mandel NS, Mandel GS. Urinary tract stone disease in the United States veteran population. I. Geographical frequency of occurrences. J Urol 1989;142:1513–5.

9. Geraghty RM, Proietti S, Traxer O, et al. Worldwide Impact of warmer seasons on the incidence of renal colic and kidney stone disease: evidence from a systematic review of literature. J Endourol 2017;31:729–35.

10. Brinkowski TH, Lotan Y, Pearle MS. Limate-related increase in prevalence of urolithiasis in the United States. Proc Natl Acad Sci U S A 2008;105:9841–6.

11. Dallas KB, Conti S, Liao JC, et al. Redefining the stone belt: Precipitation is associated with increased risk of urinary stone disease. J Endourol 2017;31:1203–10.

12. Yu L, Yuntian C, Banghua L, et al. Epidemiology of urolithiasis in Asia. Asian J Urol 2018;5(4):205–14.

13. Evan AP, Worcester EM, Coe FL, et al. Mechanisms of human kidney stone formation. Urolithiasis 2015;43(Suppl 1):19.

14. Fleisch H. Inhibitors and promoters of stone formation. Kidney Int 1978;13:361–71.

15. Moore CL, Bomann S, Daniels B, et al. Derivation and validation of a clinical prediction rule for uncomplicated ureteral stone- the STONE score: retrospective and prospective observational cohort studies. BMJ 2014;348:g2191.

16. Wang R, Rodriguez R, Moghadassi M, et al. External validation of the STONE score, a clinical prediction rule for ureteral stone: an observational multi-institutional study. Ann Emerg Med 2016;67(4):423–32.

17. Poletti PA, Platon A, Rutschmann OT, et al. Low-dose versus standard-dose CT protocol in patients with clinically suspected renal colic. AJR Am J Roentgenol 2007;188(4):927–33.

18. Coll DM, Varanelli MJ, Smith RC. Relationship of spontaneous passage of ureteral calculi to stone size and location as revealed by unenhanced helical CT. AJR Am J Roentgenol 2002;178:101.

19. Ganesan V, De S, Greene D, et al. Accuracy of ultrasonography for renal stone detection and size determination: is it good enough for management decisions? BJU Int 2017;119:464–9.

20. Smith-Bindman R, Aubin C, Bailitz J, et al. Ultrasonography versus computed tomography for suspected nephrolithiasis. N Engl J Med 2014;371:1100.

21. Fulgham PF, Assimos DG, Pearle MS, et al. Clinical effectiveness protocols for imaging in the management of ureteral calculous disease: AUA technology assessment. J Urol 2003;189(4):1203–13.

22. Safdar B, Degutis LC, Landry K, et al. Intravenous morphine plus ketorolac is superior to either drug alone from treatment of acute renal colic. Ann Emerg Med 2006;48(2):173–81.
23. Cole RS, Fry CH, Shuttleworth KU. The action of the prostaglandins on isolated human ureteric smooth muscle. Br J Urol 1988;61(1):19.
24. Turk C, Petrik A, Sarica K, et al. EAU guidelines on diagnosis and conservative management of urolithiasis. Eur Urol 2016;69:468–74.
25. Holdgate A, Pollock T. Systematic review of the relative efficacy of nonsteroidal anti-inflammatory drugs (NSAIDS) and opioids in the treatment of acute renal colic. BMJ 2004;329(7473):1019.
26. Soleimanpour H, Hassanzadeh K, Vaezi H, et al. Effectiveness of intravenous lidocaine versus intravenous morphine fro patients with renal colic in the emergency department. BMC Urol 2012;12:13.
27. Worster AS, Bhanich Supapol W. Fluids and diuretics for acute ureteric colic. Cochrane Database Syst Rev 2012;(2):CD004926.
28. Kirschner J, Wilbur L. Do fluids facilitate stone passage in acute ureteral colic? Ann Emerg Med 2013;62:36.
29. Pickard R, Starr K, MacLennan G, et al. Medical expulsive therapy in adults with ureteric colic: a multicentre, randomized, placebo-controlled trial. Lancet 2015; 386:341.
30. Hollingsworth JM, Rogers MA, Kaufman SR, et al. Medical therapy to facilitate urinary stone passage: a meta-analysis. Lancet 2006;368:1171–9.
31. Campschroer T, Zhu X, Vernooij RW, et al. Alpha-blockers as medical expulsive therapy for ureteral stones. Cochrane Database Syst Rev 2018;(4):CD008509.
32. Ye Z, Zeng G, Yang H, et al. Efficacy and safety of Tamsulosin in medical expulsive therapy for distal ureteral stones with renal colic: a multicenter, randomized, double-blind, placebo-controlled trial. Eur Urol 2017;73:385–91.
33. Wang RC, Smith-Bindman R, Whitaker E, et al. Effect of tamsulosin on stone passage for ureteral stones: a systematic review and meta-analysis. Ann Emerg Med 2017;69:353.
34. Cao D, Yang L, Liu L, et al. A comparison of nifedipine and tamsulosin as medical expulsive therapy for the management of lower ureteral stones without. Sci Rep 2014;4:5254.
35. Lucarelli G, Ditonno P, Bettocchi C, et al. Delayed relief off ureteral obstruction is implicated in the long-term development of renal damage and arterial hypertension in patients with unilateral ureteral injury. J Urol 2013;189:960–5.
36. Kokorowski PJ, Hubert K, Nelson CP. Evaluation of pediatric nephrolithiasis. Indian J Urol 2010;26(4):531–5.
37. Chauhan V, Eskin B, Allegra JR, et al. Effect of season, age, and gender on renal colic incidence. Am J Emerg Med 2004;22:560–3.

Urinary Retention

Michael Billet, MD[a],*, Thomas Andrew Windsor, MD[b]

KEYWORDS

- Retention • Urinary retention • Catheter • Catheterization • Foley
- Benign prostatic hyperplasia

KEY POINTS

- Urinary retention is caused by obstructive, infectious, pharmacologic/iatrogenic, and neurogenic processes. Obstructive retention due to benign prostatic hyperplasia (BPH) is the most common single cause.
- Bladder decompression is the mainstay of treatment of acute retention; with few exceptions, laboratory workup and imaging should not delay decompression.
- Laboratory workup for acute retention should include urinalysis to exclude infection. Renal function and electrolytes should be obtained in severe or prolonged retention, or with postobstructive diuresis.
- Patients who are hemodynamically stable, have normal postdecompression urine output and renal function, and are capable of maintaining their catheters can be discharged with outpatient follow-up.

INTRODUCTION

Urinary retention is a common problem encountered in the emergency department. Acute urinary retention (AUR) presents as a sudden inability to voluntarily void, and is typically associated with lower abdominal pain. Although the most common cause is prostatic enlargement, particularly benign prostatic hyperplasia (BPH), its etiology can be varied and multifactorial.[1] Treatment of all types of retention aims to decompress the bladder and mitigate the underlying cause of retention. This can generally be accomplished in the emergency department without immediate urologic consultation; however, certain clinical features may require specialist involvement in the emergency department or outpatient setting. This article provides an overview of the common causes of AUR, as well as emergency department evaluation, treatment, and disposition of AUR in men and women.

Disclosure Statement: The authors have nothing to disclose.
[a] Department of Emergency Medicine, University of Maryland School of Medicine, Baltimore, MD, USA; [b] Department of Emergency Medicine, University of Maryland School of Medicine, 110 South Paca Street - Suite 200, Baltimore, MD 21201, USA
* Corresponding author. 110 South Paca Street, Suite 200, Baltimore, MD 21201, USA.
E-mail address: mbillet@som.umaryland.edu

DEFINITION AND PRESENTATION

The International Continence Society defines AUR as, "a painful, palpable or percussable bladder, when the patient is unable to pass any urine."[2] It would therefore be expected that most patients with AUR will describe suprapubic or low abdominal pain and associated difficulty spontaneously voiding. While true in most patients, this presentation is not guaranteed; those with acute on chronic retention, acute spinal cord compression, or those with underlying neuropathy may be less sensitive or insensitive to the pain associated with bladder overdistension.[3] These patients will also be more likely to have overflow incontinence, which can rarely be mistaken for continued spontaneous voiding, and sometimes even frequent urination. A history of prior retention or other lower urinary tract symptoms such as straining, terminal dribbling, or nocturia can be helpful in identifying patient at risk for painless retention.

The physical examination may reveal suprapubic distension and dullness to percussion. In urology literature, bladder volumes greater than 300 mL are often cited as the minimum value necessary to identify a distended bladder on examination in the non-obese patient.[4] Examiner proficiency and issues blinding have made validation of this claim difficult, and patient habitus can completely preclude palpation or percussion of a distended bladder.[5] In the American Urologic Association's consensus statement on chronic urinary retention (CUR), 300 mL is the minimum postvoid residual volume necessary to diagnose CUR.[6] The statement also emphasizes the largely historical underpinnings of this threshold, and recommends a symptom-based approach to acute and chronic retention. Bedside ultrasound and automated bladder volume devices can quickly differentiate retention from other causes of urinary incontinence, discussed more in the workup section.

BACKGROUND AND PREVALENCE

The incidence of AUR has been estimated as 3.0 to 6.8 cases per 1000 person-years in the general male population.[7] Most cases of AUR occur in men because of the longer urethra and presence of the prostate. Furthermore, there is a clear increase in the prevalence of AUR with aging, secondary to prostatic hypertrophy that occurs in essentially all men as part of the aging process. By the eighth decade of life, the incidence of AUR in men increases fivefold to tenfold from rates in middle age, with an estimated 1 case per 10 men in their 70s, and 1 case per 3 men in their 80s experiencing AUR at some point.[8] The increased incidence with age is not limited to men with prostatic hypertrophy; diabetes-related nerve damage and retention secondary to medication effects similarly increase with age. Cases of AUR that occur in women or younger men are often infection related, iatrogenic, or a consequence of medication effects.[9]

ETIOLOGY
Obstructive

Obstructive urinary retention is caused by any process leading to narrowing or compression of the urinary tract at or distal to the neck of the bladder. This obstruction can be divided into intrinsic causes, with the obstruction coming from within the urinary tract, and extrinsic causes, with the obstruction arising from compression by an external structure or mass. Among intrinsic causes, BPH is overwhelmingly the most common cause of urinary retention in men.[1] Other intrinsic processes leading to AUR include lower urinary tract malignancy, blood clots, urethral stricture, and bladder stones. The presence of blood clots leading to obstruction should prompt consideration of urinary tract malignancy.

A detailed history and physical examination should be performed in any patient with suspected or confirmed urinary retention. This should include thorough examination of the external genitalia in men, and pelvic examination in women. Extrinsic causes of AUR include abdominal and pelvic tumors, phimosis, and paraphimosis in men, and pelvic organ prolapse in women. Paraphimosis is a true urologic emergency because of the high risk of vascular compromise; immediate manual reduction should be attempted after adequate analgesia. Compression of the glans can aid in manual reduction. If initial attempts are unsuccessful, further attempts should be limited because of the risk of worsening inflammation, and a urologist should be emergently consulted to perform a dorsal slit procedure.[10] Although rare, pelvic organ prolapse can cause vascular compromise or ureteral kinking and upper urinary tract obstruction.[11] Pelvic organ prolapse can be manually reduced by the emergency physician with essentially no contraindications. A more extensive list of obstructive causes of AUR can be found in **Table 1**.

Infectious

Genitourinary infection can lead to urinary retention through various mechanisms. Inflammation of the urinary tract at any level can cause narrowing and obstructive urinary retention. Patients with underlying urinary tract pathology, particularly BPH, are more susceptible to have infection lead to obstruction compared with the general population.[12] Recurrent urinary tract infections are therefore a risk factor for future retention and a consequence of inadequately treated retention. The most common causative organism leading to UTI is *Escherichia coli,* cultured in 75% to 95% of uncomplicated UTIs in adults.[13] Among patients with underlying urinary tract pathology, *E coli* remains the most common causative organism; other less common organisms include *Enterococcus* spp., *Klebsiella pneumoniae*, *Candida* spp., *Staphylococcus aureus*, *Proteus mirabilis*, *Pseudomonas aeruginosa*, and group B streptococcus.[14] Because of high regional variability in antibiotic resistance, local antibiograms should be consulted when possible to determine the optimal antibiotic regimen.[15] Sexually transmitted infections can also cause retention, through direct inflammation of the urinary tract, pain leading to sympathetic overactivity, or stricture development caused by chronic or frequent infection.

Neurogenic

The innervation of the bladder and lower urinary tract is complex, with voluntary voiding (micturition) requiring sympathetic, parasympathetic, and somatic pathways.[16] Sensation of bladder fullness is mediated through pelvic sensory nerves, and

Table 1	
Causes of obstructive urinary retention	
Level of Obstruction	**Example**
Bladder	Calculi, malignancy, hemorrhage
Prostate	BPH, prostatic calculi, abscess, malignancy
Urethra	Stricture, calculi, diverticulum, urethral valve, periurethral abscess
External male genitalia	Phimosis, paraphimosis, meatal stenosis
Female genitalia	Atrophic vaginitis, vulvovaginitis, pelvic organ prolapse
Any level	Abdominal or pelvic tumor, abdominal aortic aneurysm, pelvis fracture

Data from Klahr S. Obstructive nephropathy. Intern Med. 2000;39(5):355-61.

processed centrally through the pontine storage and micturition centers. Once the sensation to void is processed, the action of micturition requires a closely coordinated interaction between bladder contraction (detrusor muscle stimulation) and relaxation of the bladder outlet (**Fig. 1**). As such, these pathways are highly susceptible to neurologic insult, which can be acute or chronic. Alteration of activity at the neuromuscular junction in any of these sites can also lead to AUR; further discussion of pharmacologic causes of AUR is provided.

Acute causes of neurogenic bladder include compression of the spinal cord or nerve roots in the cauda equina. In fact, AUR is considered to be the earliest and most sensitive examination finding in patients with acute cauda equina syndrome (CES), with AUR identified on presentation in 50% to 70% of patients with CES.[17] Other studies have shown a postvoid residual volume greater than 200 mL to have a sensitivity of 90% and specificity of 95% when combined with a history consistent for acute CES.[18] Patients with acute central nervous system emergencies, particularly stroke, are also susceptible to developing urinary retention; the incidence of AUR after ischemic stroke has been reported to be 21% to 29% at 3 weeks after infarction.[19] Chronic insult can also lead to dysfunction of the pathways regulating voiding, particularly diabetic neuropathy. Nearly half of diabetics will experience some form of lower urinary tract symptoms.[20] Although detrusor overactivity is the most common form of urinary dysfunction among diabetics, 23% will experience detrusor areflexia and are subsequently prone to retention, which can present acutely or chronically.[21]

Iatrogenic/Pharmacologic

Iatrogenic causes of AUR can be grouped into pharmacologically and nonpharmacologically mediated processes. All patients presenting with AUR should undergo a thorough medication history, as the complex innervation of the urinary tract makes

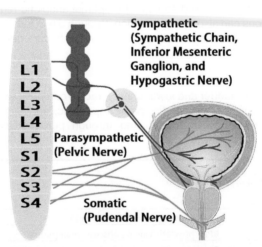

Fig. 1. Innervation of the lower urinary tract. Sympathetic innervation arises from the lower thoracic and upper lumbar spinal nerve roots, passing through the sympathetic chain, and innervates the bladder and internal sphincter via the hypogastric nerves. Parasympathetic fibers arise from the sacral nerve roots and provide innervation to the bladder via the pelvic nerve. Somatic innervation is provided to the external sphincter via the pudendal nerve. *Adapted from* Wikimedia Commons. Available at: https://commons.wikimedia.org/wiki/File:Diagram_showing_the_layers_of_the_bladder_CRUK_304.svg.

retention a common adverse effect of many frequently prescribed medications. Particular attention should be given to medications with anticholinergic properties, both those that are used specifically for those properties and the wide variety of medications with anticholinergic effects. A list of common medications that have been implicated in AUR can be seen in **Table 2**; those with anticholinergic properties are specifically noted.

Recent surgeries should also be noted, particularly those involving general anesthesia, large volumes of fluid administration, or intraoperative urinary catheterization, as these are all independent risk factors for developing postoperative urinary retention.[22] Postoperative AUR is not limited to surgeries involving the urinary tract or even the abdomen; AUR is a frequently encountered complication of nearly all types of surgery. This specific subtype of iatrogenic retention may be less frequently encountered in the emergency department, as postoperative retention typically presents in the immediate postoperative period. One study demonstrated that nearly half of all patients who will go on to develop postoperative retention are able to be identified by ultrasound in the postanesthesia care unit.[23]

A history of lower urinary tract surgery or prior urinary catheterization should also be noted, as this history increases the likelihood of urethral stricture development. Iatrogenic causes are the leading etiology of urethral strictures, accounting for 32% to 45% of all cases.[24] The most common surgeries and procedures leading to stricture development are hypospadias correction, transurethral surgery, and repeated passage of large catheters. Open or laparoscopic prostatectomy and simple cystoscopy have a relatively lower rate of this complication.[25]

Table 2
Medications with urinary retention as a known adverse effect

Class	Implicated Medications
Anticholinergic	Atropine, cyclopentolate, homatropine, tropicamide, scopolamine, ipratropium, tiotropium
Antihistamines (anticholinergic mediated, class-wide effect)	Diphenhydramine, hydroxyzine, doxepin, promethazine, cetirizine, fexofenadine, loratadine
Analgesics	Opioids (class-wide effect), nonsteroidal anti-inflammatory drugs (class-wide effect)
Benzodiazepines	Class-wide effect
Calcium channel antagonists	Class-wide effect
Antidepressants	Tricyclic antidepressants (A), fluoxetine, reboxetine
Antipsychotics, antiparkinsonians	Chlorpromazine (A), thioridazine (A), clozapine (A), risperidone (A), ziprasidone (A), amantadine (A), haloperidol (A)
Antiarrhythmics	Disopyramide (A), flecainide
Sympathomimetic (alpha-adrenergic)	Phenylephrine, pseudoephedrine
Sympathomimetic (beta-adrenergic)	Isoproterenol, terbutaline, epinephrine, norepinephrine
Muscle relaxants	Baclofen, cyclobenzaprine

Medications with anticholinergic properties are noted with (A).
Data from Verhamme KM, Sturkenboom MC, Stricker BH, Bosch R. Drug-induced urinary retention: incidence, management and prevention. Drug Saf. 2008;31(5):373-88.

EVALUATION
Laboratory Workup

Laboratory studies are not required to diagnose AUR, but may be useful in identifying associated complications. Concern for significant or prolonged obstruction that may cause hydroureteronephrosis warrants a chemistry panel to evaluate for a postrenal acute kidney injury (AKI). Urinalysis and urine culture should be obtained in patients with AUR, for the main purpose of evaluating for urinary tract infection. Microscopic and gross hematuria following decompression are typically benign and self-limited.[26]

Imaging

Imaging studies can be helpful to identify the presence, cause, or degree of AUR. Several commercial products exist to quickly estimate bladder volume (eg, Bladder-Scan, Verathon Incorporated [Bothell, Washington]). These automated point-of-care devices utilize 3-dimensional ultrasound to estimate bladder volume, and can be useful both on presentation and after attempted decompression. These devices may be limited by patient habitus or the presence of hemoperitoneum, ascites, or other extra-vesicular fluid that can artificially increase the calculated bladder volume.[27] Bedside point-of-care ultrasound (POCUS) is commonly available in the emergency department and can rapidly identify and quantify bladder volume. Furthermore, POCUS can identify bladder clots, prostatic hypertrophy, bladder or urethral stones, and hydronephrosis in a way that automated devices cannot.[28]

Computed tomography (CT) may be particularly helpful to evaluate for abdominal or pelvic masses, yet it is less sensitive than MRI if there is suspicion for a spinal cord compression or cauda equina syndrome.[29] Although recent literature suggests that venous-phase iodinated contrast may not pose a significant risk for contrast-induced nephropathy, institutional policy may limit the use of intravenous contrast to patients with normal renal function, precluding use of contrast-enhanced CT in patients with acute or chronic kidney disease.[30] Conversely, noncontrast-enhanced ultrasound can be performed in patients with acutely or chronically impaired renal function, with essentially no contraindications. For nontraumatic cases of AUR, laboratory testing and imaging need not delay prompt relief of the obstruction.[31]

TREATMENT

Prompt bladder decompression is the mainstay of treatment for nearly all etiologies of AUR. This can be accomplished by urethral or suprapubic catheterization. Both routes have advantages, disadvantages, and contraindications. If imaging studies are unavailable or inconclusive regarding the degree of retention, catheterization can be diagnostic and therapeutic.

Urethral Catheterization

Urethral catheterization is the most common type of catheterization in the emergency department. For adult patients, initial attempts should be made with a standard tip 16-French Foley catheter, but the clinical scenario may necessitate other sizes or types of catheter (**Fig. 2**). Sterile procedure should be observed to limit the exposure to catheter-related urinary tract infections (CAUTIs).[32] Although catheter advancement should occur with minimal force, conditions that decrease urethral diameter, such as prior stricture or BPH, can make placement more difficult. If the initial attempt is unsuccessful in a patient who is unlikely to have BPH, or in a patient with history of urethral stricture, it is reasonable to attempt to pass a smaller catheter. In the setting of prostate enlargement, the increased rigidity of a larger catheter (18- or 20-French)

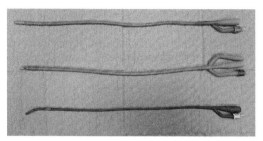

Fig. 2. Indwelling urethral catheters. Top: 16-French, standard tip; middle: 18-French 3-way, short tip; bottom: 14-French, Coudé tip (Tiemann type). (© 2019 C. R. Bard, Inc. Used with permission.)

may aid successful placement.[33] A semirigid angulated Coudé catheter may aid in advancing past the prostatic lobes, because it is designed to match the curvature of the bulbar urethra.[34] For the patient with gross hematuria or passage of clots contributing to AUR, a 3-way catheter allows for continuous bladder irrigation if output remains bloody after the initial flushing.[35]

Blind urethral catheterization is contraindicated in patients with recent urologic surgery, or confirmed or suspected urethral trauma.[31] Urologic consultation may be necessary if passage of a catheter consistently fails despite a reasonable number of attempts. Excessive attempts in the face of resistance or patient-reported discomfort are inappropriate as this can worsen underlying urinary tract pathology or inflammation. For this reason, clean intermittent self-catheterization (CISC) is not recommended for AUR, particularly obstructive AUR. This is in contrast to chronic retention, where CISC is the preferred method of bladder decompression.[36,37]

Suprapubic Catheterization

Suprapubic catheterization, although less common than urethral catheterization, can be performed by adequately trained emergency physicians.[35] The suprapubic approach is typically reserved for situations in which placement of a urethral catheter is either contraindicated or unsuccessful despite appropriate attempts. The decision to perform this procedure should be made in conjunction with a consulting urologist. To place a suprapubic catheter, the bladder must be identified through palpation, and ideally visualized in real-time with ultrasound. Several techniques exist to place the catheter; the 2 main approaches are a percutaneous Seldinger technique with passage of a guidewire into the bladder, dilation of the tract, and over-wire catheter insertion; and insertion of a trocar, through which a catheter is subsequently placed.[38] A risk unique to the suprapubic approach is bowel injury, occurring with a reported incidence of 2.4% to 2.7%.[39]

Pharmacotherapy

Medications do not typically resolve AUR by themselves, but they are commonly initiated in the immediate treatment phase and continued for ongoing prevention, particularly when prostatic obstruction is the suspected etiology. The two main classes of medications used for AUR due to an enlarged prostate are alpha blockers and 5-alpha reductase inhibitors.[40] Contraction of the bladder neck, urethra, and prostate are mediated through alpha-1 adrenergic activity.[41] As such, blockade of alpha-1 receptors is a mainstay of pharmacotherapy in both acute and chronic urinary retention. Alpha blockers have been demonstrated to reduce rates of catheter reinsertion after a trial without catheter.[42,43] Caution should be taken when using alpha blockers in patients at risk for orthostatic hypotension, as alpha-1 blockade reduces vascular responsiveness to postural changes.[41] 5-alpha reductase inhibitors act by decreasing the conversion of testosterone to dihydrotestosterone, which has a higher affinity for the androgen receptor present in the prostatic urethral epithelium; this blockade has the long term effect of slowing prostate growth.[44] Due to their hormone-mediated mechanism of action, 5-alpha reductase inhibitors are unlikely to improve AUR in the short-term, but are beneficial in preventing ongoing prostate hypertrophy and future episodes of retention.[45]

Surgical Treatment

Several surgical options exist for the management of patients with recurrent symptoms, failed trial without catheter, or underlying urinary tract pathology that is unlikely to improve with conservative management. Surgical or procedural intervention is most commonly used for obstructive AUR. Transurethral prostate ablation is a commonly performed procedure for mild or intermittent retention or other lower urinary tract symptoms related to BPH. For more severe cases of AUR caused by underlying prostatic enlargement, transurethral radical prostatectomy (TURP) is a traditionally successful surgery.[46] In recent decades, several minimally invasive and robotic assisted procedures have been developed.[47] Urethral dilation or stenting can be of benefit if urethral stricture or external compression is the suspected etiology. Women with retention secondary to atrophic vaginitis or pelvic organ prolapse should be referred to a urogynecologist after treatment of the acute retention.

POSTDECOMPRESSION MANAGEMENT
Complications

The most common acute complications of bladder decompression include hematuria, infection, and postobstructive diuresis. Urinalysis obtained after catheterization will commonly demonstrate at least some degree of microscopic hematuria, with the incidence depending on factors such as time since catheterization, underlying pathology, technical difficulty, or number of attempts.[48] Gross hematuria is a less common finding, but may also be suggestive of underlying urinary tract pathology. If caused by the catheterization procedure, hematuria is usually self-limited. Hemodynamically significant hematuria is a rare occurrence.[49,50]

Although conventional wisdom has taught that urethral catheterization is associated with an increased rate of CAUTIs compared with the suprapubic route, no statistical difference in rates of CAUTI has been found in short-term catheterization.[51] Furthermore, likelihood of CAUTI may be of less importance for AUR, which is expected to be brief or self-limited. However, compared with subrapubic catheterization, urethral catheterization catheterization is associated with increased noninfectious complications, particularly patient-reported discomfort.[52]

Postobstructive diuresis is a condition in which elevated renal tract pressure impairs the kidneys' ability to concentrate urine, leading to diuresis when pressure is normalized. It is defined as a urinary output greater than 200 mL for at least 2 hours after decompression, or greater than 3 L in 24 hours.[53] Hemodynamic instability has been reported secondary to volume losses, particularly in patients with decreased intravascular reserve. Patients should be rehydrated orally or intravenously, with some sources advocating replacement of 75% of urinary losses, although high-quality evidence on this topic is lacking.[54] Despite advocacy by some practitioners, there is no evidence that gradual or intermittent decompression decreases the risk of hematuria, hemodynamic instability, hydronephrosis, or postobstructive diuresis compared with immediate decompression.[55]

Indications for Hospitalization

Most patients who experience successful decompression with a catheter can be discharged home with plans for appropriate urology follow up. Patients that present with urosepsis, retention secondary to trauma, AKI, or have other associated inpatient needs should be hospitalized. Hematuria that is, self-limited or resolves after continuous bladder irrigation does not necessitate admission.[26]

Discharge and Follow-up

Patients with normal postobstructive urine output, reassuring vital signs, and no indications for further emergent workup after placement of a catheter can typically be discharged. Patients should be counseled on catheter care, how to change the drainage bag, and when to follow-up. Most patients who are discharged should follow-up with a urologist for a spontaneous voiding trial without a catheter. As previously mentioned, alpha-1 blockers decrease rates of catheter reinsertion, and should be started if no contraindications exist.[42] The optimal time for catheter removal remains a subject of debate. An observational study of over 2600 men with BPH showed that patients whose catheters were removed in fewer than 3 days were more likely to spontaneously void than those with longer periods of catheterization.[56] Previous randomized trials indicated that patients were more likely to void during a trial without a catheter if left in place for 1 week.[57]

SUMMARY

Acute urinary retention is a common condition encountered in the emergency department. Prompt bladder catheterization is indicated for the vast majority of cases, and most patients can be safely discharged after bladder decompression. A focused laboratory evaluation should be performed to identify the underlying cause of obstruction. At the very least, this should include urinalysis to exclude urinary tract infection. Laboratory studies to evaluate renal function and electrolyte status may be indicated based on clinical features and patient risk factors. Those with serious infections, ongoing postobstructive diuresis, hemodynamic instability, significant electrolyte abnormalities, or AKI should be hospitalized for fluid and electrolyte replacement and specialist evaluation, if indicated.

REFERENCES

1. Emberton M, Anson K. Acute urinary retention in men: an age old problem. BMJ 1999;318(7188):921–5.
2. Abrams P, Cardozo L, Fall M, et al. The standardisation of terminology of lower urinary tract function: report from the Standardisation Sub-committee of the International Continence Society. Neurourol Urodyn 2002;21(2):167–78.
3. Sylvester PA, Mcloughlin J, Sibley GN, et al. Neuropathic urinary retention in the absence of neurological signs. Postgrad Med J 1995;71(842):747–8.
4. Abrams PH, Dunn M, George N. Urodynamic findings in chronic retention of urine and their relevance to results of surgery. Br Med J 1978;2(6147):1258–60.
5. Negro CL, Muir GH. Chronic urinary retention in men: how we define it, and how does it affect treatment outcome. BJU Int 2012;110(11):1590–4.

6. Stoffel JT, Peterson AC, Sandhu JS, et al. AUA white paper on nonneurogenic chronic urinary retention: consensus definition, treatment algorithm, and outcome end points. J Urol 2017;198(1):153–60.

7. Fong YK, Milani S, Djavan B. Natural history and clinical predictors of clinical progression in benign prostatic hyperplasia. Curr Opin Urol 2005;15(1):35–8.

8. Jacobsen SJ, Jacobson DJ, Girman CJ, et al. Natural history of prostatism: risk factors for acute urinary retention. J Urol 1997;158(2):481–7.

9. Mevcha A, Drake MJ. Etiology and management of urinary retention in women. Indian J Urol 2010;26(2):230–5.

10. Kessler CS, Bauml J. Non-traumatic urologic emergencies in men: a clinical review. West J Emerg Med 2009;10(4):281–7.

11. Miyagi A, Inaguma Y, Tokoyoda T, et al. A case of renal dysfunction caused by pelvic organ prolapse. CEN Case Rep 2017;6(2):125–8.

12. Speakman MJ, Cheng X. Management of the complications of BPH/BOO. Indian J Urol 2014;30(2):208–13.

13. Gupta K, Hooton TM, Naber KG, et al. International clinical practice guidelines for the treatment of acute uncomplicated cystitis and pyelonephritis in women: a 2010 update by the Infectious Diseases Society of America and the European Society for Microbiology and Infectious Diseases. Clin Infect Dis 2011;52(5): e103–20.

14. Flores-mireles AL, Walker JN, Caparon M, et al. Urinary tract infections: epidemiology, mechanisms of infection and treatment options. Nat Rev Microbiol 2015; 13(5):269–84.

15. Zhanel GG, Hisanaga TL, Laing NM, et al. Antibiotic resistance in Escherichia coli outpatient urinary isolates: final results from the North American Urinary Tract Infection Collaborative Alliance (NAUTICA). Int J Antimicrob Agents 2006;27(6): 468–75.

16. Fowler CJ, Griffiths D, De groat WC. The neural control of micturition. Nat Rev Neurosci 2008;9(6):453–66.

17. Gardner A, Gardner E, Morley T. Cauda equina syndrome: a review of the current clinical and medico-legal position. Eur Spine J 2011;20(5):690–7.

18. Small SA, Perron AD, Brady WJ. Orthopedic pitfalls: cauda equina syndrome. Am J Emerg Med 2005;23(2):159–63.

19. Kong KH, Young S. Incidence and outcome of post-stroke urinary retention: a prospective study. Arch Phys Med Rehabil 2000;81:1464–7.

20. Liu G, Daneshgari F. Diabetic bladder dysfunction. Chin Med J 2014;127(7): 1357–64.

21. Golbidi S, Laher I. Bladder dysfunction in diabetes mellitus. Front Pharmacol 2010;1:136.

22. Koch CA, Grinberg GG, Farley DR. Incidence and risk factors for urinary retention after endoscopic hernia repair. Am J Surg 2006;191(3):381–5.

23. Keita H, Diouf E, Tubach F, et al. Predictive factors of early postoperative urinary retention in the postanesthesia care unit. Anesth Analg 2005;101(2):592–6.

24. Lumen N, Hoebeke P, Willemsen P, et al. Etiology of urethral stricture disease in the 21st century. J Urol 2009;182(3):983–7.

25. Fenton AS, Morey AF, Aviles R, et al. Anterior urethral strictures: etiology and characteristics. Urology 2005;65(6):1055–8.

26. Etafy MH, Saleh FH, Ortiz-vanderdys C, et al. Rapid versus gradual bladder decompression in acute urinary retention. Urol Ann 2017;9(4):339–42.

27. Cooperberg MR, Chambers SK, Rutherford TJ, et al. Cystic pelvic pathology presenting as falsely elevated post-void residual urine measured by portable

ultrasound bladder scanning: report of 3 cases and review of the literature. Urology 2000;55(4):590.

28. Tsze DS, Kessler DO. Rapid evaluation of urinary retention and penile pain using point-of-care ultrasound. Pediatr Emerg Care 2014;30(8):580–2.

29. Mcnamee J, Flynn P, O'Leary S, et al. Imaging in cauda equina syndrome–a pictorial review. Ulster Med J 2013;82(2):100–8.

30. Hinson JS, Ehmann MR, Fine DM, et al. Risk of acute kidney injury after intravenous contrast media administration. Ann Emerg Med 2017;69(5):577–86.e4.

31. Chapple C, Barbagli G, Jordan G, et al. Consensus statement on urethral trauma. BJU Int 2004;93(9):1195–202.

32. Assadi F. Strategies for preventing catheter-associated urinary tract infections. Int J Prev Med 2018;9:50.

33. Willette PA, Coffield S. Current trends in the management of difficult urinary catheterizations. West J Emerg Med 2012;13(6):472–8.

34. Shah J. Catheterisation. Ann R Coll Surg Engl 2012;94(1):5–7.

35. Jahn P, Beutner K, Langer G. Types of indwelling urinary catheters for long-term bladder drainage in adults. Cochrane Database Syst Rev 2012;(10):CD004997.

36. Weynants L, Hervé F, Decalf V, et al. Clean intermittent self-catheterization as a treatment modality for urinary retention: perceptions of urologists. Int Neurourol J 2017;21(3):189–96.

37. Aguilera PA, Choi T, Durham BA. Ultrasound-guided suprapubic cystostomy catheter placement in the emergency department. J Emerg Med 2004;26(3): 319–21.

38. Goyal NK, Goel A, Sankhwar SN. Safe percutaneous suprapubic catheterisation. Ann R Coll Surg Engl 2012;94(8):597–600.

39. Ahluwalia RS, Johal N, Kouriefs C, et al. The surgical risk of suprapubic catheter insertion and long-term sequelae. Ann R Coll Surg Engl 2006;88(2):210–3.

40. Chapple CR. A comparison of varying alpha-blockers and other pharmacotherapy options for lower urinary tract symptoms. Rev Urol 2005;7:S22–30.

41. Michel MC, Vrydag W. Alpha1-, alpha2- and beta-adrenoceptors in the urinary bladder, urethra and prostate. Br J Pharmacol 2006;147(Suppl 2):S88–119.

42. Fisher E, Subramonian K, Omar M. The role of alpha blockers prior to removal of urethral catheter for acute urinary retention in men. Cochrane Database Syst Rev 2014;(6):CD006744.

43. Poon IO, Braun U. High prevalence of orthostatic hypotension and its correlation with potentially causative medications among elderly veterans. J Clin Pharm Ther 2005;30(2):173–8.

44. Kim EH, Brockman JA, Andriole GL. The use of 5-alpha reductase inhibitors in the treatment of benign prostatic hyperplasia. Asian J Urol 2018;5(1):28–32.

45. Roehrborn CG. Alfuzosin 10 mg once daily prevents overall clinical progression of benign prostatic hyperplasia but not acute urinary retention: results of a 2-year placebo-controlled study. BJU Int 2006;97(4):734–41.

46. Wasson JH, Reda DJ, Bruskewitz RC, et al. A comparison of transurethral surgery with watchful waiting for moderate symptoms of benign prostatic hyperplasia. The Veterans Affairs Cooperative Study Group on Transurethral Resection of the Prostate. N Engl J Med 1995;332(2):75–9.

47. Christidis D, Mcgrath S, Perera M, et al. Minimally invasive surgical therapies for benign prostatic hypertrophy: The rise in minimally invasive surgical therapies. Prostate Int 2017;5(2):41–6.

48. Petursson SR, Weintraub M. Incidence and range of microscopic hematuria in patients with indwelling urinary catheters. Res Commun Chem Pathol Pharmacol 1975;12(3):513–20.
49. Nyman MA, Schwenk NM, Silverstein MD. Management of urinary retention: rapid versus gradual decompression and risk of complications. Mayo Clin Proc 1997; 72(10):951–6.
50. Naranji I, Bolgeri M. Significant upper urinary tract hematuria as a rare complication of high-pressure chronic retention of urine following decompression: a case report. J Med Case Rep 2012;6:254.
51. Kidd EA, Stewart F, Kassis NC, et al. Urethral (indwelling or intermittent) or suprapubic routes for short-term catheterisation in hospitalised adults. Cochrane Database Syst Rev 2015;(12):CD004203.
52. Saint S, Trautner BW, Fowler KE, et al. A multicenter study of patient-reported infectious and noninfectious complications associated with indwelling urethral catheters. JAMA Intern Med 2018;178(8):1078 85.
53. Vaughan ED, Gillenwater JY. Diagnosis, characterization and management of post-obstructive diuresis. J Urol 1973;109(2):286–92.
54. Halbgewachs C, Domes T. Postobstructive diuresis: pay close attention to urinary retention. Can Fam Physician 2015;61(2):137–42.
55. Boettcher S, Brandt AS, Roth S, et al. Urinary retention: benefit of gradual bladder decompression - myth or truth? A randomized controlled trial. Urol Int 2013;91(2): 140–4.
56. Desgrandchamps F, De La Taille A, Doublet JD, RetenFrance Study Group. The management of acute urinary retention in France: a cross-sectional survey in 2618 men with benign prostatic hyperplasia. BJU Int 2006;97:727.
57. Djavan B, Shariat S, Omar M, et al. Does prolonged catheter drainage improve the chance of recovering voluntary voiding after acute urinary retention (AUR)? Eur Urol 1998;33(Suppl. 1):110.

Approach to Acute Kidney Injuries in the Emergency Department

Tanveer Gaibi, MD, FACEP[a],*, Aditi Ghatak-Roy, MD[b]

KEYWORDS

- Acute kidney injury • Emergency department • Renal emergency
- Clinical management

KEY POINTS

- Comprehensive overview and evidence-based acute management of kidney injuries in the emergency department setting.
- Summary of causes of acute kidney injuries, and clinical evaluations that should prompt urgent interventions.
- Management of specific acute conditions, such as rhabdomyolysis and contrast-induced acute kidney injuries, and higher risk populations, such as the elderly.

INTRODUCTION

Acute kidney injury (AKI) is a common health issue worldwide that presents as a spectrum of diseases. It has been associated with increased risk of mortality and often progression to chronic kidney disease, particularly in the elderly population. There are several other derangements associated with AKI, including metabolic acidosis, and body fluid volume disturbances. The epidemiology of AKI in hospitalized or critically ill populations is well known and studied, but the prevalence in the general emergency department (ED) population is not well characterized. As such, management of AKI in the acute setting and appropriate outpatient follow-up has not been optimized. This article provides a review of key principles regarding renal disease and an evidence-based approach to the management of AKI in the emergency setting.

Disclosure Statement: The authors have no disclosures of any relationship with a commercial company that has a direct financial interest in subject matter or materials discussed in the article or with a company making a competing product.

[a] Department of Emergency Medicine, Inova Fairfax Medical Center, 3300 Gallows Road, Falls Church, VA 22042, USA; [b] Department of Emergency Medicine, George Washington University, 900 23rd Street Northwest, Washington, DC 20037, USA
* Corresponding author.
E-mail address: tgaibi@yahoo.com

Emerg Med Clin N Am 37 (2019) 661–677
https://doi.org/10.1016/j.emc.2019.07.006
0733-8627/19/© 2019 Elsevier Inc. All rights reserved.

emed.theclinics.com

The population seen in the emergency or acute setting is often diverse with complex medical histories and without effective primary care follow-up. One-third of community-acquired AKIs may be first identified in the ED. Thus, ED providers see a substantial amount of AKI that can be intervened on if identified, managed, and discussed appropriately with these patients.

DEFINITION

A variety of definitions for AKI have been proposed. To reach a universal consensus, in 2012, the Kidney Disease: Improving Global Outcomes (KDIGO) group defined AKI based on the urine output and the serum creatinine (SCr) concentration. This definition is an increase in SCr of greater than or equal to 0.3 mg/dL within 48 hours or an increase in SCr greater than 1.5 times baseline within 7 days or decreased urine output for 6 hours (**Table 1**).[1] Other classification systems of AKI, such as RIFLE (risk, injury, failure, loss, end-stage) and Acute Kidney Injury Network (AKIN), can also be used. The advantage of KDIGO is that it covers parameters in AKIN and RIFLE, taking into account changes in creatinine levels within 48 hours or decline in glomerular filtration rate (GFR) over 7 days. Realistically, prospective cohort studies support that all three criteria are effective tools for predicting mortality without significant differences among them.[1]

AKI is defined as a sudden reduction in kidney function that is characterized by a diminished GFR as manifested by an increased SCr or reduced urine output. AKI is further divided into three categories: (1) prerenal, or a decrease in kidney blood flow; (2) intrarenal, or injury to the kidney parenchyma itself; and (3) postrenal, or obstructed urine flow. Intrarenal AKI is subdivided based on which part of the kidney is involved: glomeruli, vasculature, or interstitium. Determining the source of AKI is important because the cause and treatment vary based on the type of insult.

However, SCr concentration may not provide an accurate, real-time assessment of patients with AKI. Creatinine clearance measures how well the glomeruli filter creatinine from the plasma and is a close approximation of the GFR. These concentrations

Table 1
KDIGO guidelines for acute kidney injuries

Kidney Disease: Improving Global Outcomes (KDIGO) Guidelines

AKI Stage	Serum Creatinine	Urine Output
1	1.5–1.9 × baseline OR ≥0.3 mg/dL increase	<0.5 mL/kg/h for 6–12 h
2	2.0–2.9 × baseline	<0.5 mL/kg/h for ≥12 h
3	3.0 × baseline OR serum creatinine increase ≥ mg/dL OR initiation of renal-replacement therapy	<0.3 mL/kg/h for ≥24 h OR anuria for ≥12 h

Risk, Injury, Failure, Loss, End-Stage (RIFLE) Criteria

AKI Stage	Serum Creatinine	Urine Output
1	Increase in Cr ≥150% mg/dL	<0.5 mL/kg/h for 6–12 h
2	Increase in Cr ≥200–300%	<0.5 mL/kg/h for ≥12 h
3	Increase in Cr ≥300% OR creatinine >4 mg/mL with acute increase ≥0.5 mg/dL or initiation of renal-replacement therapy	<0.3 mL/kg/h for ≥24 h OR anuria for ≥12 h

Data from Moore PK, Hsu RK, Liu KD. Management of acute kidney injury: core curriculum 2018. Am J Kidney Dis 2018;72(1):136–48.

may lag behind the acute changes from baseline. Furthermore, SCr values are confounded by dilution, volume overload states, and reductions of creatinine production during the acute phases of an illness. Finally, muscle mass can alter relative SCr levels, which fluctuate in critical and acute care settings.

For these reasons, and to more accurately apply steady-state kinetics, other biomarkers, such as serum cystatin C, neutrophil gelatinase-associated lipocalin, kidney injury molecule-1, are being studied as potential surrogates for acute kidney function. However, in the acute setting, SCr remains the most validated estimation of GFR to determine kidney function.

CLINICAL EVALUATION

AKI may lead to life-threatening complications. These complications include severe metabolic acidosis; hyperkalemia; and volume overload states, such as pulmonary edema or pericardial tamponade. Essential elements from the history and physical examination can help identify these complications. It is important to determine if kidney function abnormalities are at baseline or truly represent an acute injury. This is difficult to accomplish in the acute setting; occasionally the patient knows his or her baseline kidney function, or a baseline is ascertained via record review.

Once AKI is identified, ascertain the source of the injury. It is important to first rule out prerenal and postrenal sources before considering intrarenal sources. Prerenal causes occur in the setting of recent volume losses, such as hemorrhage, gastrointestinal or urinary fluid losses, and recent postoperative courses during which the patient was either hypotensive or exposed to iodinated contrast for imaging (although this is controversial). Postrenal sources may be considered in patients with signs of nocturia, or urinary frequency, which may be suggestive of prostatic or other obstruction and retention. Also, consider obstructive sources in cancer or trauma patients, or those known to have a solitary kidney. It is rare to have bilateral, obstructive ureteral calculi and so, in general, any injury caused by obstructive kidney stones will be offset by the secondary kidney.

Next, search for exposure to nephrotoxic agents, especially, in patients with reduced GFR. Common offending pharmacologic agents include antibiotics, such as vancomycin; aminoglycosides; nonsteroidal anti-inflammatory drugs; and angiotensin-converting enzyme (ACE) inhibitors/angiotensin receptor blockers. Iodinated radiocontrast was once thought to be nephrotoxic; however, recent studies have shown that this association is not as strong as previously believed.[2]

On physical examination, evaluate patients in terms of hemodynamic and volume status. Check for dry mouth, reduced skin turgor, cool peripheral extremities, and delayed capillary refill times. Examine vital signs for evidence of shock, which may warrant invasive hemodynamic monitoring with arterial lines, central venous pressure monitoring, and so forth. Ultrasonography of the inferior vena cava at end expiration and the internal diameter of the right ventricle at end diastole may indicate hypovolemia and underfilling, respectively.[3] These patients may require a wide range of therapies from intravenous (IV) fluids to diuretics or, in most critical situations, renal-replacement therapy (RRT).

RISK FACTORS FOR ACUTE KIDNEY INJURY

There are multiple, well-studied, and well-defined risk factors for developing AKI, which an emergency physician should assess in all patients, but particularly those in critical condition.[4] Elderly patients (65 years or older) are more prone to AKI than younger patients and have a poorer prognosis, despite advances in treatments, such as dialysis. Older patients, have chronic diseases that lead to structural changes to kidneys over the years (discussed later). This vulnerable population has less kidney reserve as a consequence and is more susceptible to developing AKI after insult.

Other risk factors for developing AKI include ischemia caused by volume depletion, surgical procedures, sepsis or acute infections, and nephrotoxic agents. Chronic underlying diseases, such as hypertension, diabetes, congestive heart failure, atherosclerosis, chronic kidney disease, and obstructive (postrenal) uropathy are notable medical conditions that place patients at higher risk for developing AKI. In patients with these risk factors who go on to develop AKI, there have been significant differences in further complications, such as delay to discharge from hospital, ventilator use, and concomitant diseases.

CAUSES OF ACUTE KIDNEY INJURY

More than 75% of patients with AKI have either prerenal azotemia or acute tubular necrosis (ATN). Prerenal failure may be caused by fluid losses, fluid sequestration, decreased cardiac output, or renal artery narrowing. Intrarenal causes include ATN, interstitial, glomerular, and small vessel disease. Postrenal causes are those secondary to obstruction. Ultrasound can assess for masses, hydronephrosis, ureteral dilatation, and the absence of ureteral jets entering the bladder (90% positive predictive value for complete obstruction) (**Table 2**).[5]

Acute Glomerulonephritis

Glomerulonephritis, one of the intrinsic causes of AKI, is caused by autoimmune damage to the kidneys themselves, that progress to inflammatory changes leading to renal failure. Following diabetes and hypertension, it accounts for 10% to 15% of end-stage renal diseases in the United States.[4,6] These disease processes are defined by nephrotic and nephritic syndromes. Nephritic syndrome is a constellation of symptoms including hematuria, proteinuria, decreased renal function, and high blood pressure. Emergency physicians should consider intrinsic renal disease in patients who present with these symptoms, because hematuria/proteinuria are often overlooked, but may be a critical consideration in managing patients appropriately. Even mild elevations in kidney function, high blood pressure, or urinary issues can signal rapid loss of renal function, if not identified or managed quickly. With prompt and early

---

Table 2
Etiologies of acute kidney injuries

Prerenal	Intrarenal	Postrenal
Low systemic volume	Glomerular	Bladder obstruction
Congestive heart failure	Tubular	Prostate enlargement
Liver failure	Ischemia	Urinary retention
Hypovolemia	Infection	Malignancy
Low cardiac output	Nephrotoxins	Bilateral obstructive
Dysfunctional kidney	Vascular	nephrolithiasis
autoregulation		Obstruction of single functioning
Angiotensin-converting enzyme		kidney
inhibitors/angiotensin		
receptor blockers		
Nonsteroidal anti-inflammatory		
drugs		

Data from Waikar SS, Bonventre JV. Acute Kidney Injury. In: Jameson JL, Fauci AS, Kasper DL, et al, editors. Harrison's Principles of Internal Medicine, 20e Edition. New York, NY: McGraw-Hill.

management, one can hope to prevent chronic renal failure from acute glomerulone-phritis syndromes.

Briefly, the pathophysiology of acute glomerulonephritis involves autoimmune-mediated inflammation that leads to subsequent fibrosis of the glomerular apparatus. For example, in post-streptococcal glomerulonephritis, antibodies formed against streptococcal antigen adhere to glomeruli at the time of infection. Inflammatory path-ways initiate complement and coagulation cascades, which leads to cell lysis, fibrin deposition, and ultimately damage to the native structure of the glomeruli. In the long term, intraglomerular hypertension and destruction of the normal anatomy can lead to permanent scarring.

The various types of acute glomerulonephritis are outside of the scope of this re-view. Examples include postinfectious glomerulonephritis, IgA nephropathy, micro-scopic polyangiitis, and lupus nephritis. There are several specialized laboratory studies, such as complement levels, that assist nephrologists in final diagnoses. The laboratory studies can be deferred to a specialist and are not critical in the emer-gency setting. However, it is prudent for an emergency physician to consider clinical presentations in patients who present with the constellation of nephrotic syndrome: hypertension, periorbital swelling or lower leg edema, and AKI. Also consider appro-priate age groups, because several types of acute glomerulonephritis or nephrotic syndrome manifest more in pediatric patients. For example, postinfection glomerulo-nephritis is considered in a patient who reported a sore throat or skin infection, typi-cally 1 to 12 weeks before presentation. Most commonly, postinfectious glomerulonephritis presents in young children between 2 and 12 years old and more often in boys than girls. Patients with respiratory infections, purpura, and arthritis with signs of nephritic syndrome may be suffering from Wegener granulomatosis or microscopic polyangiitis.

The treatment of acute glomerulonephritis includes supportive care and immunosuppressive therapies to counteract the autoimmune cascade causing intrinsic renal damage. Supportive treatment initiated early in the ED, with blood pressure control and, at times, dialysis, can be lifesaving. Blood pressure control is important in the acute setting because it can help slow the decline in GFR or proteinuria. ACE inhibitors have antiproteinuric and antifibrotic effects, but, acutely, can cause further renal dysfunction. ACE inhibitors are typically used in the chronic phase (ie, chronic kidney disease). Other supportive measures include use of diuretics and management of hyperkalemia, acidosis, uremia, and fluid overload.

These supportive measures do not reverse the underlying pathophysiology. Immu-nosuppressive treatments, such as steroids, aim to prevent glomerular inflammation, but come at the risk of infection. Other medications include mycophenolate mofetil, cyclophosphamide, pulse steroids, or IV immunoglobulins. These therapies are often complex and require management with specialists.

Sepsis

The leading cause of death among patients with AKI is sepsis and accounts for more than 40% of mortality.[7] A study done by Levy and colleagues[8] demonstrated an odds ratio for mortality of 6.5 for patients who had AKI in the setting of sepsis. In this study, 45% of patients with AKI who died had developed sepsis.[8] Mehta and colleagues[9] also demonstrated similar findings through the Program to Improve Care in Acute Renal Disease database which showed 40% of patients with AKI went on to develop sepsis. These studies and analyses suggest that patients with AKI should be closely monitored for the development of infection.

Currently there are many theories on how hemodynamics are altered during sepsis. It is unclear whether it is an ischemic phenomenon or systemic vasodilation. Studies have shown in cardiac arrest patients that AKI is uncommon. In animal studies where the subjects were exposed to massive hemorrhage there was no evidence of increased AKI.[10] It is now thought that inflammatory responses represent the dominant abnormality in sepsis-associated AKI.[11,12]

Currently, treatment of the patient with sepsis remains supportive with fluid resuscitation remaining as the hallmark of care. Recently, studies comparing early goal-directed therapy have not been able to demonstrate a benefit to protocolized resuscitation with Early goal directed therapy in septic shock compared with usual care. The PROMISE trial did not show significant differences in outcomes.[13]

In randomized controlled studies of nonsurgical patients with sepsis, colloids have not improved patient outcomes and may actually worsen them. There is no evidence to support the use of colloids, and therefore isotonic solutions should be used.[14] Waechter and colleagues[15] demonstrated that the focus of resuscitation in the first 1 hour with aggressive fluid administration and initiation of vasoactive agents within the first 6 hours have produced the best patient outcomes. Finally, the VANISH trial showed no difference in AKI or mortality when comparing vasopressin with norepinephrine as the initial vasopressor for septic shock.[16] Evidence continues to show no benefit of dopamine and its agonist for the prevention of AKI. Patients with AKI should be monitored closely for infection and prompt treatment is indicated to reduce mortality.

Drug-Induced Acute Kidney Injury

Drug-induced kidney disease is a frequent cause of renal dysfunction. Drugs account for nearly 20% of acute episodes of acute renal failure.[17] Among older adults, the incidence of drug-induced nephrotoxicity may be as high as 66%.[18] There are four major phenotypes of therapeutic drug-induced AKI including tubular injury, glomerular injury, interstitial injury, and crystal induced injury (**Table 3**). It is important that the emergency physician understand these mechanisms and which patient-related risk factors whether it be age, diabetes, or underlying renal insufficiency coupled with drug interactions can help prevent AKI secondary to medications. There are too many drugs to list and many cause AKI through multiple injury pathways. Many drugs work together to cause AKI. For example, many patients are on calcium channel blockers for their hypertension, but for an acute respiratory process may be started on a macrolide.[19] There is a clear correlation that concurrent administration of these drugs is associated with a higher risk for hospitalization with AKI. Surveillance in the ED with pharmacists who can check for nephrotoxic medication and real-time AKI analysis may lead to reductions in harm.[20,21]

Healthy young adults typically have a GFR 120 mL/min, and the kidney autoregulates GFR to preserve GFR and urine output. Certain drugs can interfere with the kidneys' ability to autoregulate glomerular pressure and decrease GFR.[20]

Renal tubular cells are susceptible to the toxins because their role in reabsorbing glomerular filtrate exposes them to high levels of circulating toxins.[22] Drugs associated with this pathogenic mechanism of injury include aminoglycosides, contrast, and vancomycin. These agents cause injury by impairing mitochondrial function.[23] The presence of "muddy brown casts" of epithelial cells found in the urine is pathognomonic for ATN. The overall prognosis for ATN is good if the cause is identified and corrected early.

Acute interstitial nephritis, which can result from a hypersensitivity reaction, is caused by an inflammatory injury that is often non-dose-related. Many drugs have

Table 3
Drug-induced AKI phenotypes

			Type of Injury			
Tubular	Contrast	Aminoglycosides	Vancomycin			
Interstitial	Penicillin	Proton pump inhibitor	Vancomycin	Loop and thiazide diuretic	Nonsteroidal anti-inflammatory drugs	Ranitidine Quinolones Acyclovir
Glomerular	Hydralazine	Bisphosphonates	Lithium			
Crystal-induced	Sulfa	Indinavir				

been thought to cause acute interstitial nephritis, including allopurinol; β-lactams, quinolones, sulfonamides, and acyclovir; diuretics (loops, thiazides); nonsteroidal anti-inflammatory drugs; proton pump inhibitors (PPIs); and ranitidine (Zantac).[24] Of note PPIs have been associated with an increased risk for AKI.[25] After excluding other causes of kidney dysfunction, PPI exposure should be considered in patients with worsening SCr. The two main electrolyte abnormalities that are associated with PPI include hyponatremia and hypomagnesemia.[26]

Certain medications that are insoluble in human urine are known to precipitate in the renal tubules. Clinical settings that enhance the risk of precipitation include volume depletion, underlying kidney disease, and metabolic disturbances that promote changes in urinary pH favoring precipitation. Commonly prescribed drugs associated with production of crystals include ampicillin, ciprofloxacin, sulfa drugs, indinavir, and methotrexate.[27]

There are many drugs that can cause glomerular injury and inflammatory disease and present as nephritic syndrome. Some of the more important drugs include bisphosphonates and hydralazine.[28] These drugs can also typically cause ATN. Thus we recommend monitoring SCr before treatment and holding therapy in the setting of renal insufficiency.

It is worth noting that illicit drugs, specifically synthetic cannabinoids, may lead to AKI in addition to myocardial infarction, psychosis, seizures, and hyperemesis.[29] Interestingly, creatinine kinase (CK) does not go up as high as in methamphetamine- or cocaine-induced rhabdomyolysis. The most common injury was acute tubular injury in these patients. Treatment is supportive and rarely requires steroids.

DIAGNOSTIC TESTING

AKI is diagnosed using laboratory values. Evaluate urinalysis, urine sediment, and urine chemistries. A high ratio of blood urea nitrogen to creatinine is considered a sign of prerenal azotemia. In this setting, sodium is inappropriately retained so a urine sodium concentration of less than 20 mEq/L is also indicative of prerenal cause. If obstruction is suspected, ultrasound of the kidneys and postvoid bladder volumes are warranted. Further investigation of intrarenal causes include urine electrolytes and urine osmoles. Kidney biopsy is at the discretion of the nephrologist and typically reserved for patients suspected for intrarenal cause. Examples of these etiologies include systemic lupus erythematosus, glomerulonephritis, and ATN.

ACUTE MANAGEMENT IN THE EMERGENCY DEPARTMENT
Volume Status

During normal physiologic stress response, the body is able to autoregulate blood flow to the kidneys despite acute changes in blood pressure; this mechanism is disrupted in AKI. Patients may present with hypervolemia, such as peripheral edema, pulmonary edema, respiratory distress, heart failure, pericardial effusion, or cardiac tamponade. These states should be managed with diuretics, fluid restriction, RRT, or appropriate procedures to alleviate the volume. Conversely patients with hypovolemia should be fluid resuscitated because it is essential to maintain organ perfusion.

The use of IV fluids in hypovolemic patients is a delicate balance. Patients who receive fluids may become acutely volume overloaded. The use of vasopressors can further reduce blood flow to the kidneys. In several large trials, it was shown that early goal-directed therapy in patients with sepsis who received crystalloid fluids had no effect on mortality or the need for RRT.[5] Several retrospective studies have demonstrated associations between volume overload states and mortality in critically ill patients.[30] For this reason, frequent monitoring for volume changes is important. If clinical history supports large volume losses, such as vomiting and severe diarrhea, and physical examination supported hypovolemia, administer IV fluid therapy. Consider using vasopressors for patients who do not respond to fluid resuscitation.

The constitution of IV fluids should also be considered. Crystalloids, such as lactated Ringer or normal saline, equilibrate solutes across cell membranes. Colloid fluids often contain albumin, gelatins, or starches, which depend on oncotic gradients to increase volume in an intravascular space. Several studies have examined crystalloids versus colloids in AKI. Notably, in the Crystalloid versus Hydroxyethyl Starch (CHEST) trial, where intensive care unit patients were randomly assigned saline solution versus colloids, there was an increased risk of RRT in the colloid group. Although the crystalloid group overall had more incidences of AKI by RIFLE criteria driven by urine output, the colloid arm of the study had more severe AKI and therefore a trend toward RRT.

Recent literature regarding balanced fluid resuscitation versus normal saline demonstrates mixed reviews depending on acuity of the patient. The SMART trial examined outcomes including adverse kidney events, time to discharge, and mortality in critically ill adult patients who received saline (0.9% normal saline) versus balanced crystalloids (lactated Ringer solution or Plasma-Lyte A). This study demonstrated a marginal superiority in secondary outcomes of balanced crystalloids, particularly patients who received large volumes of resuscitation.[31] However, another recent study, dubbed the SALT-ED trial, examined adult ED patients who received a minimal of 500 mL of IV isotonic crystalloids and were hospitalized outside of the intensive care unit, which was essentially a negative trial.[32] The primary outcome showed no difference in the number of hospital-free days in both treatment groups, although the secondary outcome (incidence of major adverse kidney events at 0 days) was in favor of balanced crystalloids. From a practical standpoint and in the context of weaknesses of both studies, it is prudent to consider balanced crystalloids in critically ill, high-volume resuscitated patients; otherwise there is no outstanding practical difference in balanced crystalloids versus normal saline.

Colloids are beneficial for some AKI subgroups. For instance, in situations of large volume depletion, such as paracentesis or end-stage liver disease, albumin administration has been shown to lower risk for AKI.[9,33]

In assessing volume status, the overall goal in the emergent setting is to improve cardiac output and therefore improve tissue oxygenation. Physiologic end points, such as urine output or mean arterial pressure, should be monitored closely in the inpatient setting. In the ED, consider starting with 75 to 100 mL per hour (1–3 L total) with frequent clinical evaluations for pulmonary congestion.

Metabolic Derangements

Kidneys maintain the body's electrolyte balance. In AKI, patients often develop hyperkalemia, hyperphosphatemia, hypocalcemia, metabolic acidosis, or symptoms of uremia because of reduced filtration. This may lead to bleeding, pericarditis, or altered mental status.

Clinical manifestations of hyperkalemia include, most critically, muscle weakness/paralysis and cardiac arrhythmias secondary to conduction abnormalities. These occurs at potassium levels greater than 7.0 mEq/L. Hyperkalemia causing conduction abnormalities is detected on electrocardiograms (ECG). There is a wide variety of ECG changes; however, the most common findings are tall peaked T waves with shortened QT interval, lengthening of PR interval and QRS duration, absence of P waves, and ultimately sine wave pattern as the QRS progresses in duration.

In patients with hyperkalemia and ECG changes administer calcium gluconate or calcium carbonate (1 g IV over minutes, repeat as needed) to stabilize the cardiac membrane. Then use regular insulin (10 U IV or weight-based and administered with glucose), β_2-adrenergic agonists (nebulized albuterol), or sodium bicarbonate (50 mEq/50 mL IV). These drugs promote potassium ions to shift intracellularly. One can then use loop diuretics (furosemide, 40–60 mg IV) only if the patient's volume status has been assessed and determined to be hypervolemic or euvolemic with appropriate supportive fluids provided; or cation resins (sodium polystyrene sulfonate, 15 g orally) to eliminate potassium in the urine and stool (**Table 4**).

The use of cation resins, such as sodium polystyrene sulfonate (Kayexalate), is controversial because there is limited evidence regarding its efficacy and there are some potential untoward effects that may outweigh benefits.[34] This substance works by exchanging sodium for ammonium, calcium, potassium, and magnesium with the main goal to encourage excretion of potassium via the feces. It is suspended with sorbitol, which is an osmotic cathartic, to increase gastrointestinal transit time because the resin swells with hydration and can cause severe constipation or bowel obstruction. However, despite this combination, this medication may result in colonic necrosis. In fact, the US Food and Drug Administration has issued a "black box" warning because of the potential for colonic necrosis and other proven acute treatments for hyperkalemia should be prioritized. Other disadvantages of sodium polystyrene sulfonate include a long onset of action (minimum 2 hours) and sodium load in the medication, which is a trigger for acute exacerbation of congestive heart failure.

Recent studies have examined newer binding agents, such as patiromer and sodium zirconium cyclosilicate (ZS-9). Patiromer is a synthetic polymer of nonabsorbable beads that exchanges calcium for potassium excretion in the stool in the distal colon.[35] However, this polymer does not swell with hydration and therefore does not necessitate an ancillary fecal cathartic. Recent literature has examined the efficacy of eliminating potassium in cardiac and chronic kidney disease patients with promising results. Theoretically this polymer can cause hypercalcemia and thus has a "black box" warning against administering calcium-containing agents within 6 hours of administration.

ZS-9 is a nonabsorbable cation exchanger; however, it is not a polymer and able to selectively bind to nine times the amount of potassium as Kayexalate.[36] Side effects include urinary tract infection and edema from sodium retention from the exchange

Table 4
Dose, onset, and duration for hyperkalemia drug treatments

Effect	Treatment	Dose	Onset	Duration
Stabilize membrane	Calcium gluconate/ carbonate	10 mL IV over 10 min	Immediate	30–60 min
Shifters	Albuterol	10–20 mg nebulized	30 min	2 h
	Insulin	10 units IV with dextrose 25–50 g	20 min	4–6 h
	Sodium bicarbonate	150 mmol IV	Hours	Hours
Excretors	Furosemide	40–80 mg IV	15 min	2–3 h
	Sodium polystyrene sulfonate	15–30 g in 15–30 mL	Hours	4–6 h
Definitive	Hemodialysis		Immediate	3 h

effects. A recent meta-analysis investigating patiromer and ZS-9 found that these agents were more efficacious compared with Kayexalate, although further studies are warranted to test side effects, use in specific patient populations, and medication interactions.[37]

Metabolic acidosis can occur with the inability to excrete acids (eg, renal ammonium) via the renal system or from hypoperfusion leading to lactic acidosis, which then is unable to be metabolized by the injured kidneys. Consider bicarbonate or base equivalents depending on the severity of acidosis (pH <7.1). Uremia may present with encephalopathy, vomiting, or even platelet dysfunction.

Blood Pressure Management

Patients with kidney disease typically present with hypertension. The pathophysiology of hypertension depends on the duration of disease, acute versus chronic, and type of kidney disease (ie, vasculitides vs intrinsic kidney disease). In a true hypertensive emergency causing organ ischemia, for example, with evidence of AKI, patients are likely habituated to higher blood pressures. Thus, mean arterial pressures should be reduced slowly, by no more than 20% in the first hour and gradually by no more than 15% over the subsequent 24 hours. Consider adrenergic-blocking agents, such as labetalol given in 20-mg IV bolus initially, followed by 20 to 80 mg every 10 minutes to a total dose of 300 mg. Hydralazine, a direct arteriolar vasodilator, given in doses of 10-mg IV boluses is an alternative, although patients have more unpredictable fluctuations and responses to this medication.

In acute glomerulonephritis, patients manifest with volume overload caused by sodium retention from increased reabsorption in the collecting tubules. The exact mechanism of how nephrotic syndrome or acute glomerulonephritis induces the changes in volume status remains unclear. However, this expanded volume affects two systems: suppresses the renin-angiotensin-aldosterone system, and enhances release of atrial natriuretic peptide.[38] Because volume overload is the primary driving mechanism for hypertension in acute glomerulonephritis, the preferred initial therapy are diuretics. Loop diuretics, such as furosemide, are particularly effective in patients with reduced GFR. Second-line therapy are ACE inhibitors because these drugs activate the otherwise pathologically suppressed renin-angiotensin-aldosterone system mechanism (**Box 1**).

Organ Damage

AKI is increasingly recognized for affecting other vital organs systems, particularly the heart, liver, and lungs. Myocardial contractility is reduced in metabolic acidosis. Hypoperfusion of the heart leads to myocardial stunning and has been shown to promote apoptosis of myocardial tissue within 72 hours.

Complex interactions also exist between the kidneys and liver, leading to development of hepatorenal syndrome. This is a form of kidney injury, unresponsive to fluids, in chronic liver disease that causes systemic and splanchnic vasodilation and kidney

---

Box 1
Antihypertensive medications

Furosemide

Lisinopril

Labetalol

Hydralazine

---

vasoconstriction. Diagnosis of this syndrome typically occurs in the inpatient setting as the patient is tested for response to diuretic withdrawal, absence of macroscopic kidney injury (measured by proteinuria and renal ultrasound), and other criteria. However, in recognizing the potential for hepatorenal syndrome in patients with cirrhosis in the emergency setting, providers should focus on volume resuscitation, avoidance of diuretics and early treatment of bacterial infections. The International Club of Ascites also provides careful guidance regarding vasoconstrictors use (eg, terlipressin, norepinephrine, or midodrine plus octreotide).[30]

Renal failure can cause noncardiogenic pulmonary edema (acute respiratory distress syndrome), which in contrast to cardiogenic pulmonary edema resulting from volume overload is direct lung injury mediated by proinflammatory cytokines. As such, these conditions do not respond to fluid diuresis. These patients often require mechanical ventilation. Fluid diuresis in these patients can potentially delay recovery from the original AKI.

Diuretics

Loop diuretics are considered in hypervolemic states because these medications not only prevent volume overload, but also minimize ischemic tubular injury by decreasing metabolic demand from the activation of the sodium-potassium-chloride cotransporter in the renal medulla. However, multiple studies have failed to demonstrate benefits of diuretics in AKI. The current KDIGO recommendation is to avoid these medications except in frank hypervolemia or in early AKI to promote urine output, demonstrating functional renal tubular system.[1]

Glycemic Control

The KDIGO group recommends maintaining blood sugar concentrations between 110 and 149 mg/dL. These guidelines are based off multiple large multicenter trials examining AKI, mortality, and various other outcomes. The largest of these is the Normoglycemia in Intensive Care Evaluation - Survival Using Glucose Algorithm Regulation (NICE-SUGAR) study. This study examined glycemic control in critically ill patients and found that between intensive glycemic control (81–108 mg/dL) and conventional glycemic control (<180 mg/dL), there was no difference in RRT rates. However, the intensive glycemic control group was associated with higher mortality.[39] The kidneys serve an important role in glucose excretion and insulin metabolism. Thus, patients with AKI are higher risk for severe hypoglycemia.

Renal-Replacement Therapy

The ultimate treatment of severe AKI leading to critical life-threatening derangements, such as volume overload, acidosis, hyperkalemia, and toxin accumulation, is RRT or dialysis. In dialysis, solutes and fluids are removed from the body by either diffusion (ie, hemodialysis) or convection (hemofiltration), or a combination of the two. The decision to start RRT should be done in conjunction with nephrology consultation because volume and electrolyte management exceeds the scope of core emergency medicine. However, initiation of consultation is important to consider for emergent dialysis. Indications for emergent dialysis are shown in **Box 2**.

Contrast-Induced Acute Kidney Injury

Contrast-induced nephropathy refers to a type of AKI that results within a few days of exposure to iodinated contrast for imaging studies. This is the third most common cause of new AKI in hospitalized patients after hypoperfusion and nephrotoxic drugs.[2]

Box 2
Indications for emergent dialysis
Acidosis (pH <7 1)
Electrolytes (potassium >6.5 refractory to treatment)
Ingestions of dialyzable drugs (salicylates, lithium, toxic alcohols)
Overload (especially with hypertension, increasing oxygen requirements)
Uremia (bleeding, pericarditis, encephalopathy)

The AKI insult is self-limited but has been associated with increased mortality and even progression to chronic kidney disease. Patients with an estimated GFR less than 60 mL/min/1.73 m^2 are higher risk for contrast-induced AKIs.

Multiple recent publications demonstrated that the degree over injury is perhaps not as critical as once believed.[2] Aycock and colleagues[40] published a robust systematic review and meta-analysis in 2017 looking at rates of AKI, need for RRT, or mortality in patients receiving IV contrast versus patients who received no contrast. The study found no significant differences in outcomes in the two groups and thus use of IV contrast does not seem to be associated with increased AKI. In clinical practice, radiologists are cautious in administering potentially harmful contrast and take into consideration comorbidities, other nephrotoxic medications the patient is currently taking, and other reasons the patient's kidney perfusion may be inhibited during their clinical course. In such cases, minimize nephrotoxic agents, use the lowest possible radiocontrast concentrations, administer IV hydration pre-exposure and postexposure, and consider RRT in critical cases.

A study published in 2014 examined discharged patients in the ED who received computed tomography of the abdomen and pelvis with IV contrast and where the authorities measured rates of contrast nephropathy.[41] This single-center study included patients with comorbidities, such as hypertension; diabetes; or nephrotoxic medications, such as ACE inhibitors. The study demonstrated 28% of patients followed up within 1 week, and only 7.5% had a laboratory work-up. The overall incidence of contrast-induced nephropathy was 15.3%. This condition seemed to be associated with risk factors, such as advanced age, diabetes, and hypertension, rather than an acutely new SCr derangement. As discussed in the disposition section, it is important to screen patients for reliable follow-up.

RHABDOMYOLYSIS

Rhabdomyolysis is a syndrome characterized by skeletal muscle injury. Muscle damage is measured with myoglobin, CK, and lactate dehydrogenase. Muscle injury may be secondary to trauma, myositis, medications, and muscle dystrophies and can cause significant life-threatening electrolyte disorders and acute renal injury. Renal injury is particularly common in patients suffering from hypovolemia. This leads to renal vasoconstriction to maintain perfusion, and concomitant accumulation of muscle breakdown products filtering through renal tubules.

Clinically, patients present with a history of myalgias, muscle weakness, and dark colored urine in the setting of muscle overuse; occasionally nausea, vomiting or fever may manifest. However, the history may be misleading in the acute care setting. For example, patients may present after a seizure, undisclosed medication use, or a spectrum of activity level from prolonged immobilization to running a marathon. Diagnostically, CK levels are elevated with a five-fold or greater increase from upper limit of normal (1000 IU/L), and myoglobin is detected in the urine. Myoglobin is a heme-containing protein released from damaged muscle. Urine dipstick detects blood but generally an absence of red blood cells on microscopy, which distinguishes myoglobin from hemoglobin. However, the half-life of myoglobin is 2 to 3 hours. Because of the rapid metabolism of myoglobin to bilirubin, serum levels may return to baseline within 6 to 8 hours.[42] By contrast, CK levels increase 2 to 12 hours after muscle injury and peak at 24 to 72 hours. Studies have shown a correlation of CK levels greater than 5000 IU/L and 50% chance of progression to AKI.[42]

The management of rhabdomyolysis includes aggressive fluid resuscitation and electrolyte correction in the early phase to improve renal perfusion and promote adequate urine output. This is primarily how azotemia is prevented. Although controversial, consider sodium bicarbonate, 50 mmol for each 2 to 3 L of IV fluid therapy. There is no clear benefit regarding balanced crystalloids versus normal saline, so either IV fluids may be used. The role of sodium bicarbonate or sodium acetate is to alkalinize the urine, although this practice is not currently evidence based.[43] Damaged muscle cells release potassium and phosphorus, which should be monitored. RRT may be considered based on electrolyte derangements, such as hyperkalemia, hypercalcemia, anuria, hyperazotemia, or kidney injury not responding to volume resuscitation. Treatment goals include urinary output goal of 200 mL/h, urine pH greater than 6.5, and plasma pH 7.5.[44]

Elevated CK
↓
IV hydration with normal saline or 5% dextrose in normal saline
↓
Goal urine output 200 mL/h, plasma pH <7.5
↓
Serial evaluations for worsening AKI, electrolyte disturbances, compartment syndrome
↓
Consider admission for CK >5000 IU/L or patients at high risk for AKI (see section Risk Factors for AKI)

SPECIAL POPULATIONS
Elderly

In elderly patients, there is a physiologic change in the kidney and change in muscle mass, which may affect estimated GFR. The metabolism of creatine from muscles to creatinine and the rate of the secretion of creatinine differs in older age. Multiple studies have examined other biomarkers for more accurate reflections of estimated GFR, but in the acute setting SCr continues to be the standard. Be mindful that elderly patients are more susceptible to AKIs and may not always be reflected in immediate laboratory results.[45]

Cardiac Disease

Patients with acute coronary syndrome (ACS) have complex factors that can impact kidney function.[46,47] Not only does ACS impair cardiac output and increase venous congestion, but medical interventions can also lead to impaired GFR. Patients with ACS also activate several neurohormonal systems that serve to vasodilate and vasoconstrict vasculature in the body, which can profoundly affect kidney function and perfusion. Furthermore, the body undergoes rapid fluctuations in fluid status from resuscitation, bleeding, drug therapies, and effects from such procedures as percutaneous coronary intervention or intra-aortic balloon pumps. Thus, these patients are at high risk for developing AKI in acute cardiac disease settings. The development and severity of AKI in patients with ACS has been independently associated with increased morbidity and mortality in short- and long-term follow-up; thus, it is important to note and trend abnormalities in kidney function for this hospitalized patient population.

DISPOSITION

The disposition of patients with AKI who present in the acute setting is varied. In most cases, an AKI is indicative of kidney insult either from prerenal, intrarenal, or postrenal sources. It is typically appropriate to admit these patients to the hospital to ascertain the source of insult and observe for correction of kidney function because patients are at increased risk for subsequent AKI, progression to chronic kidney disease, and increased mortality. In patients who have an isolated AKI and are otherwise appropriate for discharge, arrange solid follow-up. If the patient has reliable follow-up, he or she should have their kidney function checked in 3 months.

An examination of risk factors, prevalence, management, and outcomes in the ED patient population has sparse data. To explore this lack of data, one Canadian study looked at the prevalence of AKI in two urban EDs, and secondarily discharged patients without renal-specific follow-up and rate of death or renal replacement at 30 days.[48] The prevalence of AKI was 5.5% but of the one-third of patients discharged home, only 12.9% were given renal-specific follow-up (ie, repeat bloodwork with primary physician), suggesting that emergency physicians should extend management to informing patients of kidney injury findings.

Consultation to nephrology or urology services may be indicated in the emergent setting. Most commonly, consultation for emergent dialysis is appropriate for life-threatening acidosis, medically unresponsive electrolyte derangements, toxic ingestion, volume overload, or uremia. Nephrologists should be consulted (typically as an inpatient) for AKIs suspected secondary to intrinsic kidney disease, such as acute glomerulonephritis. Consult urology for AKIs suspected secondary to postrenal causes, such as obstructive nephrolithiasis. Specialty services, such as interventional radiology, may be available on an institution-specific basis for procedures, such as nephrostomy tube placement.

REFERENCES

1. Moore PK, Hsu RK, Liu KD. Management of acute kidney injury: core curriculum 2018. Am J Kidney Dis 2018;72(1):136–48.
2. Hassen GW, Hwang A, Liu LL, et al. Follow up for emergency department patients after intravenous contrast and risk of nephropathy. West J Emerg Med 2014; 15(3):276–81.
3. Nee PA, Bailey DJ, Todd V, et al. Critical care in the emergency department: acute kidney injury. Emerg Med J 2016;33(5):361–5.
4. Ostermann M, Joannidis M. Acute kidney injury 2016: diagnosis and diagnostic workup. Crit Care 2016;20(1):299.
5. Gong Y, Zhang F, Ding F, et al. Elderly patients with acute kidney injury (AKI): clinical features and risk factors for mortality. Arch Gerontol Geriatr 2012;54(2): e47–51.
6. Vinen CS. Acute glomerulonephritis. Postgrad Med J 2003;79(930):206–13.
7. Selby NM, Kolhe NV, McIntyre CW, et al. Defining the cause of death in hospitalized patients with acute kidney injury. PLoS One 2012;7:e48580.

8. Levy EM, Viscoli CM, Horwitz RI. The effect of acute renal failure on mortality. A cohort analysis. JAMA 1996;275:1489–91.

9. Mehta RL, Pascual MT, Soroko S, et al. Program to improve care in acute renal disease: spectrum of acute renal failure in the intensive care unit. The PICARD experience. Kidney Int 2004;66:1613–21.

10. Chua HR, Glassford N, Bellomo R. Acute kidney injury after cardiac arrest. Resuscitation 2012;83:721–7.

11. Siegemund M, van Bommel J, Stegenga ME, et al. Aortic cross-clamping and re-perfusion in pigs reduces microvascular oxygenation by altered systemic and regional blood flow distribution. Anesth Analg 2010;111:345–53.

12. Martensson J, Bellomo R. Sepsis-induced acute kidney injury. Crit Care Clin 2015;31:649–60.

13. Nguyen HB, Jaehne AK, Jayaprakash N, et al. Early goal directed therapy in se-vere sepsis and septic shock: insights and comparisons to ProCESS, ProMISe, and ARISE. Crit Care 2016;20:160.

14. Raghunathan K, Bonavia A, Nathanson BH, et al. Association between initial fluid choice and subsequent in-hospital mortality during the resuscitation of adults with septic shock. Anesthesiology 2015;123:1385–93.

15. Waechter J, Kumar A, Lapinsky SE, et al. Cooperative antimicrobial therapy of septic shock database research group: interaction between fluids and vasoactive agents on mortality in septic shock: a multicenter, observational study. Crit Care Med 2014;42:2158–68.

16. Gordon AC, Mason AJ, Thirunavukkarasu N, et al, VANISH Investigators. Effect of early vasopressin vs norepinephrine on kidney failure in patients with septic shock: the VANISH randomized clinical trial. JAMA 2016;316:509–18.

17. Nash K, Hafeez A, Hou S. Hospital-acquired renal insufficiency. Am J Kidney Dis 2002;39(5):930–6.

18. Kohli HS, Bhaskaran MC, Muthukumar T, et al. Treatment-related acute renal fail-ure in the elderly: a hospital-based prospective study. Nephrol Dial Transplant 2000;15(2):212–7.

19. Gandhi S, Fleet JL, Bailey DG, et al. Calcium-channel blocker-clarithromycin drug interactions and acute kidney injury. JAMA 2013;310:2544–53.

20. Goldstein SL, Mottes T, Simpson K, et al. A sustained quality improvement pro-gram reduces nephrotoxic medication-associated acute kidney injury. Kidney Int 2016;90:212–21.

21. Schoolwerth AC, Sica DA, Ballermann BJ, et al. Renal considerations in angio-tensin converting enzyme inhibitor therapy: a statement for healthcare profes-sionals from the Council on the Kidney in Cardiovascular Disease and the Council for High Blood Pressure Research of the American Heart Association. Cir-culation 2001;104(16):1985–91.

22. Markowitz GS, Perazzella MA. Drug-induced renal failure: a focus on tubulointer-stitial disease. Clin Chim Acta 2005;351(1–2):31–47.

23. Mehta RL, Awdishu L, Davenport A, et al. Phenotype standardization for drug-induced kidney disease. Kidney Int 2015;88:226–34.

24. Raghavan R, Eknoyan G. Acute interstitial nephritis: a reappraisal and update. Clin Nephrol 2014;82:149–62.

25. Brewster UC, Perazzella MA. Proton pump inhibitors and the kidney: critical re-view. Clin Nephrol 2007;68:65–72.

26. Perazzella MA. Drug-induced nephropathy: an update. Expert Opin Drug Saf 2005;4(4):689–706.

27. Perazella MA, Markowitz GS. Bisphosphonate nephrotoxicity. Kidney Int 2008;74: 1385–93.

28. Pendergraft WF 3rd, Herlitz LC, Thornley-Brown D, et al. Nephrotoxic effects of common and emerging drugs of abuse. Clin J Am Soc Nephrol 2014;9: 1996–2005.

29. Zhao A, Tan M, Maung A, et al. Rhabdomyolysis and acute kidney injury requiring dialysis as a result of concomitant use of atypical neuroleptics and synthetic cannabinoids. Case Rep Nephrol 2015;2015:235982.

30. Özdemir S. Evaluation of rhabdomyolysis cases that apply emergency service. Istanbul: Northern Clinics of Istanbul; 2017:4(3).p. 257–61

31. Semler MW, Self WH, Wanderer JP, et al, for the SMART Investigators and the Pragmatic Critical Care Research Group. Balanced crystalloids versus saline in critically ill adults. N Engl J Med 2018;378(9):829–39.

32. Self WH, Semler MW, Wanderer JP, et al. Balanced crystalloids versus saline in noncritically ill adults. N Engl J Med 2018;378(9):819–28.

33. Chawla LS, Busse L, Brasha-Mitchell E, et al. Intravenous angiotensin II for the treatment of high-output shock (ATHOS trial): a pilot study. Crit Care 2014;18:534.

34. Sterns RH, Rojas M, Bernstein P, et al. Ion-exchange resins for the treatment of hyperkalemia: are they safe and effective? J Am Soc Nephrol 2010;21:733–5.

35. Weir MR, Bakris GL, Bushinsky DA, et al. Patiromer in patients with kidney disease and hyperkalemia receiving RAAS inhibitors. N Engl J Med 2015;372: 211–21.

36. Packham DK, Rasmussen HS, Lavin PT, et al. Sodium zirconium cyclosilicate in hyperkalemia. N Engl J Med 2015;372:222–31.

37. Meaney CJ, Beccari MV, Yang Y, et al. Systematic review and meta-analysis of patiromer and sodium zirconium cyclosilicate: a new armamentarium for the treatment of hyperkalemia. Pharmacotherapy 2017;37:401–11.

38. Rodríguez-Iturbe B, Colic D, Parra G, et al. Atrial natriuretic factor in the acute nephritic and nephrotic syndromes. Kidney Int 1990;38(3):512–7.

39. Koyner JL, Adhikari R, Edelson DP, et al. Development of a multicenter ward-based AKI prediction model. Clin J Am Soc Nephrol 2016;11(11):1935–43.

40. Aycock RD, Westafer LM, Boxen JL, et al. Acute kidney injury after computed tomography: a meta-analysis. Ann Emerg Med 2018;71(1):44–53.e4.

41. Gabow PA, Kaehny WD, Kelleher SP. The spectrum of rhabdomyolysis. Medicine 1982;61(3):141–52.

42. Khan FY. Rhabdomyolysis: a review of the literature. Neth J Med 2009;67(9): 272–83.

43. Cereda M, Horak J, Neligan PJ. Renal diseases. In: Fleisher LA, editor. Anesthesia and uncommon diseases. 5th edition. Philadelphia: Saunders Elsevier; 2006. p. 229–60.

44. Torres PA, Helmstetter JA, Kaye AM, et al. Rhabdomyolysis: pathogenesis, diagnosis, and treatment. Ochsner J 2015;15(1):58–69.

45. Raman M, Middleton RJ, Kalra PA, et al. Estimating renal function in old people: an in-depth review. Int Urol Nephrol 2017;49(11):1979–88.

46. Marenzi G, Cosentino N, Antonio L, et al. Acute kidney injury in patients with acute coronary syndromes. Heart 2015;101(22):1778–85.

47. Goldberg RJ, Weng FL, Praveen K. Acute and chronic allograft dysfunction in kidney transplant recipients. Med Clin North Am 2016;100(3):487–503.

48. Scheuermeyer FX, Grafstein E, Rowe B, et al. The clinical epidemiology and 30-day outcomes of emergency department patients with acute kidney injury. Can J Kidney Health Dis 2017;4. 205435811770398.

Evaluation of the Renal Transplant Recipient in the Emergency Department

John David Gatz, MD, Ryan Spangler, MD*

KEYWORDS

- Renal transplant • Rejection • Surgical complication • Transplant emergency

KEY POINTS

- Renal transplant patients are a unique population requiring evaluation for complex conditions.
- Timing of transplant, medications, and comorbid conditions can play a role in both medical and surgical complications.
- Appropriate treatment and disposition of these patients are crucial to maintaining a functional transplanted kidney.

INTRODUCTION

Organ transplantation has revolutionized the management of chronic kidney disease. In 2017, kidney transplantation accounted for approximately 20,000 of the 35,000 solid organ transplants (SOTs) performed in the United States.[1] As the survival rates for recipients and grafts continue to improve, a growing and specialized population of patients is emerging. They inevitably come to emergency departments (EDs) with complications specifically related to their transplant.

Prior studies demonstrated that more than half (57%) of renal transplant recipients seek help in EDs within the first 2 years after transplant and that approximately a third of recipients require readmission within 30 days after their initial discharge.[2–4] A review of more than 10,000 patients in 3 states found that renal transplant recipients average 126.9 ED visits per 100 patient-years (95% CI, 125.1–128.8), with approximately half (48%) of ED visits resulting in admission. Importantly, only 57% of ED visits requiring admission occurred at the medical facility where the transplantation had been performed. Visits to nontransplant centers become increasingly common as the time after transplantation increases. The most common ED diagnoses resulting in admission and discharge are summarized in **Table 1**.[2]

Disclosure Statement: The authors have nothing to disclose.
Department of Emergency Medicine, University of Maryland School of Medicine, 110 South Paca Street, Sixth Floor, Suite 200, Baltimore, MD 21201, USA
* Corresponding author.
E-mail address: rspangler@som.umaryland.edu

Emerg Med Clin N Am 37 (2019) 679–705
https://doi.org/10.1016/j.emc.2019.07.008
0733-8627/19/© 2019 Elsevier Inc. All rights reserved.

Table 1	
The most common diagnoses in renal transplant recipients presenting to an emergency department	
Admitted Patients	**Discharged Patients**
1. Complication of device, implant, or graft	1. Abdominal pain
2. Essential hypertension	2. UTIs
3. Diabetes mellitus with complications	3. Fluid and electrolyte disorders
4. Septicemia	4. Nonspecific chest pain
5. Fluid and electrolyte disorders	5. Genitourinary symptoms and ill-defined conditions
6. Acute and unspecified renal failure	6. Nausea and vomiting
7. Congestive heart failure; nonhypertensive	7. Fever of unknown origin
8. Pneumonia	8. Diabetes mellitus with complications
9. UTIs	9. Other gastrointestinal disorders
10. Complications of surgical procedures or medical care	10. Superficial injury; contusion

Adapted from Schold JD, Elfadawy N, Buccini LD, et al. Emergency department visits after kidney transplantation. Clin J Am Soc Nephrol 2016;11:674-83.

This article reviews the critical differential diagnoses and management considerations in this unique and growing population. The emergency care provider must be familiar with the potential surgical and medical pitfalls, because misdiagnosis or mismanagement can have significant implications on graft and recipient survival.

SURGICAL ANATOMY OF KIDNEY TRANSPLANTATION

Understanding postsurgical complications in a renal transplant patient requires knowledge of a patient's new anatomy. Patient-specific factors might have dictated the surgical placement and techniques that were used. Ideally, the transplanted kidney is placed in the iliac fossa extraperitoneally via a Gibson incision in the lower quadrant (left or right).[5] This approach provides adequate access to the necessary vasculature and space for the kidney. If the patient is small or the donor kidney is large, the kidney might need to be placed intraperitoneally. Laparoscopic transplantation was first described in 2009 and, based on a small case series, seems to achieve short-term and long-term outcomes similar to those associated with open transplantation. Larger studies of the less invasive technique are warranted.[6,7]

The graft vasculature could differ depending on the donor type (living or deceased). In most circumstances, the donor's renal vein is anastomosed to the recipient's external iliac vein and the donor's renal artery is anastomosed to the recipient's external iliac artery.[5]

The preferred approach for connecting the kidney to the bladder is ureteroneocystostomy. The end of the donor's ureter is usually sutured into the side of the bladder. Based on the surgeon's preference, a stent is or is not placed to prevent obstruction. If the donor's ureter is not long enough to reach the bladder, ureteroureterostomy can be performed, connecting the donor's ureter to the recipient's ureter. In some cases, the recipient's ureter is sutured directly to the donor's kidney renal pelvis[5] (**Fig. 1**).

IMMUNOSUPPRESSIVE THERAPY

In the early days of transplant medicine, failure of the transplant caused by cellular rejection was commonplace. It was not until the advent of antirejection immunosuppressant drugs that the transplant field could take off. There have been and will continue to be advancements and improvements in these regimens. The goal of

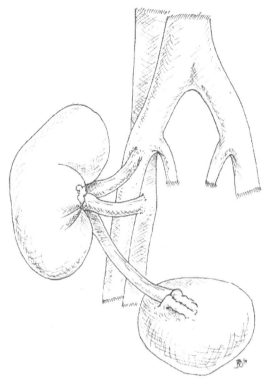

Fig. 1. Common surgical anatomy of the transplanted kidney. (*Courtesy of* Ben Dunning.)

therapy is to prevent acute rejection, but care must also be taken to reduce the risk of medication toxicity and side effects to prolong the life of the transplant. Current standard therapies are summarized:

1. Induction therapy
2. Subsequent therapy
   a. Calcineurin inhibitors (CNIs)
   b. Antimetabolite agents
   c. Corticosteroids

Induction therapy is used at the time of transplant and only for a short time. There are multiple classes of induction medications, most of them geared toward depleting or inactivating T cells. Some patients do not require induction therapy, but this decision is unlikely to be relevant to the emergency physician. In the ED, it is unlikely to encounter these medications. They have side effects that can increase a patient's risk for some infections or cancers, but these same risks exist for patients who do not undergo induction therapy.

The transplant world was revolutionized by CNIs, notably cyclosporine and more recently tacrolimus. These most important antirejection drugs come with significant side effects, notably renal toxicity (**Table 2**). To prevent their undesirable effects, their levels must be monitored closely. Consensus has not developed on the best timing for measurement of cyclosporine levels: some centers use C2 levels (obtained 2 hours after administration) and others use a trough level. Both seem to be effective; however, it is functionally easier to measure trough levels, so that method is often preferred.[8,9]

Table 2
Side effects and drug interactions of common transplant medications

Medications	Common Side Effects	Important Medication Interactions
Cyclosporine	Nephrotoxicity, hypertension, hepatotoxicity, hyperlipidemia, nausea, vomiting, diarrhea, and pain syndromes	Anticonvulsants (eg, phenytoin and carbamazepine) can decrease activity Diltiazem, verapamil, and amiodarone increase activity/toxicity Digoxin levels might increase and lead to digoxin toxicity
Tacrolimus	Headache, nausea, vomiting, diarrhea, hypertension, nephrotoxicity, lymphoproliferative disorders, abdominal pain, and alopecia	See "Cyclosporine"
Mycophenolic acids	Diarrhea, nausea, vomiting, constipation, pain, anemia, and insomnia	Magnesium- and aluminum-containing antacids decrease absorption Decreased clearance of acyclovir and related compounds, especially in renal failure PPI may cause early release in the stomach
Azathioprine	Bone marrow suppression	Allopurinol can increase activity/toxicity Might inhibit warfarin activity
Sirolimus	Hyperlipidemia, arthralgia, hirsutism, diarrhea, hypertension, lymphocele, tachycardia, thrombocytopenia, and anemia	See "Cyclosporine"
Prednisone	Headache, delayed wound healing, hyperglycemia, peptic ulcer	NSAIDs/EtOH increase the risk of peptic ulcer Digoxin increases the risk of arrhythmia due to hypokalemia Decreased effectiveness of insulin and other antidiabetic medications

Abbreviations: EtOH, alcohol; NSAID, nonsteroidal antiinflammatory drug; PPI, proton pump inhibitors.

Adapted from BC Transplant. Clinical Guidelines for Transplant Medications. Revised January 2019. Available at http://www.transplant.bc.ca/Documents/Health%20Professionals/Clinical%20guidelines/Clinical%20Guidelines%20for%20Transplant%20Medications.pdf. Accessed March 4, 2019.

Random measurements of tacrolimus levels are of little utility, so this drug should be monitored as a trough (1–3 hours before the next dose).[10,11]

Mycophenolate mofetil is an antimetabolite prodrug that is synthesized to mycophenolic acid, and mycophenolate sodium is another formulation in the mycophenolic acid family.[11] They are used in conjunction with other immunosuppressant medication classes to prevent rejection by suppressing proliferation of T lymphocytes and B lymphocytes.[11] Side effects include anemia, nausea, and diarrhea, sometimes debilitating enough to require dose reduction or discontinuation of this medication entirely. Levels usually are checked initially to ensure appropriate dosing and should be checked in the event of rejection or severe gastrointestinal or other side effects. Generally, a trough level obtained 12 hours after the last dose is used.[12]

Corticosteroids are a mainstay of transplant antirejection therapy, but their use varies among patients and centers. Prednisone is the corticosteroid that is encountered most often when assessing renal transplant recipients in the ED. Although one of the most commonly encountered medications, it may be tapered and withdrawn or, in rare cases, not used at all.[11] Some patients report that they took it after their surgery and have finished their prescribed course. Prednisone is prescribed for a wide range of conditions, so its side effects are well documented. Some of the more common ones are peptic ulcer, weight gain, myopathy, hyperglycemia, and adrenal suppression. Patients on long-term corticosteroid therapy might need supplemental corticosteroid treatment if they experience trauma, sepsis, or another illness, because their native adrenal response has been diminished.[11]

Sirolimus and everolimus, mammalian target of rapamycin (mTOR) inhibitors that have been developed over the past 20 years, could be encountered as well. Their use is less defined than the other medication classes noted.[13,14] Despite the decreased risk of certain malignancies related to the use of mTOR inhibitors compared with cyclosporine, adoption of this class of medication in standard regimens is variable and inconsistent. Side effects related to these medications are discussed later in this article, related to specific organ systems.

KEY POINTS

1. When assessing a renal transplant recipient in the ED, review the medications being taken by the patient as well as their side effects, which could be the cause of the presenting symptoms.
2. Be cognizant of drug interactions, including effects on transplant medications.

RENAL AND URINARY TRACT PROBLEMS
Acute Allograft Dysfunction

Although a renal transplant recipient may present to an ED for any reason, all chief complaints should be viewed in the context of how a patient's allograft could be affected. In most cases, a basic chemistry panel should be requested. It is imperative for the emergency care provider to compare a patient's current renal function to the patient's historic values. Laboratory measurements of creatinine levels are known to be inconsistent[15] and can result in a 10% to 20% increase in the reported value. Although it may be appropriate for patients with small variations in serum creatinine to be followed as outpatients, an acute increase of 25% or more should prompt further work-up.[16]

The differential diagnosis for acute allograft dysfunction is broad. As for any other patient, prerenal and postrenal causes should first be excluded, including any unique structural surgical complications (discussed later). Additionally, a seemingly simple prerenal etiology, such as diarrhea, does not absolve a clinician from further investigation, because it can represent a significant medical complication in the immunosuppressed patient (discussed later). Patients can experience recurrence of the initial glomerular disease process that led to renal failure. Recurrence rates of conditions, such as focal segmental glomerulosclerosis, are as high as 50% and associated with a 50% rate of graft loss.[16]

The ED assessment of allograft dysfunction often includes the following:

1. History and examination: assessment of vital signs, volume status, and graft tenderness
2. Diagnostics: assessment for urinary infection (urinalysis and culture), proteinuria, CNI levels, and renal ultrasound (for hydronephrosis or fluid collection) with Doppler (to assess vascular compromise)

Rejection

A provider must always consider immunologic rejection with alterations in renal function. Some patients are asymptomatic during this process, whereas others have generalized signs and symptoms, such as hypertension, fever, malaise, decreased urine output, and graft pain or tenderness. The threshold to consider rejection should

Table 3
Types of renal transplant rejection

Type	Etiology	Presentation	Management
Hyperacute	A type II hypersensitivity reaction Mediated by preformed antibodies against the donor tissue, leading to complement activation and rapid thrombosis	Occurs within minutes to hours after vascularizing the transplanted graft (not an ED presentation) Rapid thrombosis causes a dark and cyanotic kidney. Rare but ultimately catastrophic for the renal graft	Compatibility screening largely prevents these reactions. Ultimately, patients require explanation.
Acute	Acute rejection has 2 major types: 1. Humoral (antibody-mediated) 2. Cellular These processes can occur simultaneously.	Acute humoral rejection: increased serum creatinine and symptoms that include oliguria, fever, and tenderness over the graft; most common in the first few weeks or after reduction in immunosuppression Acute T-cell–mediated rejection: much more common than acute humoral rejection; presents as rapid loss of allograft function; can occur any time after transplantation (especially if immunosuppression is reduced)	Mainstay of treatment is pulse corticosteroids (up to 1000 mg methylprednisolone, given gradually over 30–60 min). There is no standardized protocol; and treatment is best done in conjunction with an admitting transplant team.
Chronic	Similar to acute rejection, a combination of humoral and cellular-mediated processes	Often has a more insidious presentation (gradual rise in serum creatinine and accompanying proteinuria) Renal allograft may begin to appear atrophic on ultrasound Remains difficult to distinguish from acute rejection	Biopsy typically is required for diagnosis. No acute management considerations Should exclude concomitant processes contributing to allograft dysfunction

always be low. Concern about rejection should prompt transfer/admission for further evaluation, such as HLA testing, for donor-specific antibodies and/or allograft biopsy. Types of rejection are compared in **Table 3**.

Acute rejection is the most emergent consideration. The mainstay of treatment is pulse corticosteroids. Doses should be given gradually (over 30–60 minutes), because bolus administration has been associated with cardiac arrhythmias, likely due to ventricular repolarization disturbances.[17] Additional therapies generally are beyond the scope of ED practice. Such therapies include antilymphocyte antibody therapy for acute cellular rejection and intravenous immunoglobulin and plasmapheresis for acute antibody-mediated rejection. Consequently, any patient whose presentation sparks concern about acute rejection should be transferred to a facility capable of these therapies and staffed with transplant specialists.

Asymptomatic Bacteriuria

There are no decisive data on the management of asymptomatic bacteriuria in renal transplant recipients. A Cochrane review on the subject, published in 2018, did not identify any benefit in administering antibiotics intended to prevent subsequent symptomatic urinary tract infection (UTI), mortality, graft loss, acute rejection, hospitalization, or graft function.[18] The same investigator group demonstrated considerable variability in antibiotic practice patterns among the European nephrologists, transplant surgeons, and infection disease physicians they surveyed.[19] The Infectious Diseases Society of America does not recommend routine screening for asymptomatic bacteriuria beyond the first posttransplant month.[20]

Urinary Tract Infection

Infections of the renal allograft carry significant risk. Renal transplant recipients may have multiple risk factors that predispose them to UTIs (**Table 4**). Reflux into the renal cavity can profoundly increase the risk that a lower UTI will progress to pyelonephritis (80% vs 10%).[21] There also are important temporal differences in the bacterial pathogens implicated in UTIs. *Enterococcus* spp make up a disproportionate amount of infections in the first month. The ability to form biofilms and the frequent use of cephalosporins during the perioperative period are theorized to cause this increased prevalence. After the first month, gram-negative species (eg, *Escherichia coli*, *Proteus* spp, *Klebsiella* spp, *Enterobacter* spp, and *Pseudomonas* spp) make

Table 4	
Risk factors associated with urinary tract infections	
Transplant-independent factors	Preexisting urinary flow impairment
	Preexisting urinary tract anomaly
	Diabetes
	Female gender
Transplant-dependent factors	Deceased-donor grafts
	Ureteral stents
	Bladder instrumentation
Posttransplant factors	Vesicoureteral reflux
	Strictures
	Immunosuppression

From Gołębiewska J, Dębska-Ślizień A. Chapter 3: Urinary tract infections in renal transplant recipients. In Jarzembowski T, Daca A, Dębska-Ślizień MA (eds). Urinary Tract Infection: The Result of the Strength of the Pathogen, or the Weakness of the Host. London: InTech Open; 2018.

Table 5
Typical antibiotic regimens for urinary tract infection

Infection	Antibiotic
Mild UTI	Ciprofloxacin $\pm$ amoxicillin for 7 d
Moderate UTI	Ciprofloxacin vs ceftriaxone vs augmentin for 14 d after culture sensitivity
Severe UTI	Piperacillin-tazobactam vs cefepime for 14–21 d after culture sensitivity
Candida	Asymptomatic: no treatment Symptomatic: fluconazole for 14 d

From Nigam LK, Vanikar AV, Patel RD, et al. Chapter 4: Urinary tract infection in renal allograft recipients. In Jarzembowski T, Daca A, Dębska-Ślizień MA (eds). Urinary Tract Infection: The Result of the Strength of the Pathogen, or the Weakness of the Host. London: InTech Open; 2018.

up the preponderance of infections.[22] Common antibiotic regimens are shown in **Table 5**. Fungal infections are possible but are often asymptomatic. The most commonly implicated pathogen is *Candida*, which can cause ascending infections and obstructive fungal balls.[23]

Key points regarding the antibiotic treatment of urinary infections are as follows:

1. Review both local and patient-specific susceptibility data.
2. Patients with recurrent UTIs are likely to have multidrug-resistant pathogens. Review any available previous culture data.
3. Treat patients with a known history of pathogens that produce extended-spectrum β-lactamase with a carbapenem.
4. All infections are considered complicated. Treat patients with lower UTIs for at least 7 days.
5. Treat patients with upper UTIs for 2 weeks to 3 weeks.
6. Pay attention to potential drug interactions, especially with CNIs (**Table 6**).

Nephrolithiasis

Although common in the general complication, kidney stones are relatively rare among renal transplant recipients. A recent systematic review and meta-analysis estimated

Table 6
Effects of common renal antibiotics on calcineurin inhibitor levels

Antifungal agents Ciprofloxacin Erythromycin	Can increase CNI levels
Levofloxacin Ofloxacin	Typically do not affect CNI levels
Cephalosporin Imipenem Rifampin	Can reduce CNI levels
Aminoglycosides Amphotericin	Can have synergistic nephrotoxic effects when paired with CNI medications

Significant elevations should prompt concern about viral infections, such as CMV, HBV, and HCV. Viral assessment when severe.

From Nigam LK, Vanikar AV, Patel RD, et al. Chapter 4: Urinary tract infection in renal allograft recipients. In Jarzembowski T, Daca A, Dębska-Ślizień MA (eds). Urinary Tract Infection: The Result of the Strength of the Pathogen, or the Weakness of the Host. London: InTech Open; 2018.

the incidence of kidney stones in renal transplant recipients at 1.0%, often occurring several years after transplantation (compared with a lifetime incidence of 13% among men and 7% among women). Several reasons have been proposed, among them being that the comparatively low glomerular filtration rate of a transplanted kidney essentially protects the kidney from stone formation.[24]

Nephrolithiasis is a rare disorder that can have significant implications. Relevant to emergency medicine, many patients do not experience pain, owing to denervation of the transplanted graft. Therefore, stones tend to be found incidentally or during work-up for other symptoms, such as oliguria, renal failure, gross hematuria, and infection.[25,26] Because of the lack of typical pain and atypical presentation, nephrolithiasis can be mistaken for acute rejection.[25] Importantly, struvite stones, which are associated with infectious urea-splitting bacteria, represent a slightly higher proportion of observed stones in transplant recipients than in the general population.[24] Fortunately, all traditional methods of treating urolithiasis are considered safe for kidney transplant recipients. Patients requiring admission should be transferred to specialty centers with all available resources.[25]

Nephrotoxicity

Although many medications demonstrate nephrotoxicity, those of greatest interest in regard to renal transplant recipients are CNIs. This class of drugs revolutionized immunosuppression in SOT. Unfortunately, they can affect almost every aspect of a transplanted kidney, causing reductions in flow and glomerular filtration rate, triggering thrombotic microangiopathy, and leading to various forms of fibrosis and atrophy. Consequently, it can be helpful to measure cyclosporine or tacrolimus concentrations, because acute toxicity can resolve within days after dose adjustment (discussed previously).

Renal Cell Carcinoma

The risk of renal cell carcinoma is already elevated in patients with end-stage renal disease (ESRD). It is even further heightened by in the transplant patient, with an approximate 15-fold increase in incidence[27] (ultimately, a 100-fold greater incidence than in the general population). Consequently, any unexplained hematuria found during evaluation should prompt work-up for malignancy.

SURGICAL COMPLICATIONS AFFECTING THE ALLOGRAFT
Hematoma

Bleeding of the transplanted kidney and at the surgical site occurs most often in the early postoperative period (**Table 7**). Allograft hemorrhage occurs primarily within the first 1 day or 2 days after transplant, often from small vessels that had previously spasmed.[5,28] It is rare, occurring in less than 2% of cases.[28] Secondary hemorrhage can occur as well, documented as occurring in 0.3% to 3% of transplant patients.[29] Patients can present with a variety of predictable symptoms: pain, a bulging incision, blood oozing from the incision, tachycardia, and hypotension are all possible together or individually.[28] When patients present with these complaints in the early postoperative period or even a few weeks out, the possibility of bleeding/hematoma should be evaluated promptly.

The work-up of these patients should include laboratory analyses and imaging. A complete blood cell count to determine a patient's hemoglobin/hematocrit is decreasing and coagulation studies are recommended in preparation for possible surgery. Both ultrasound and computed tomography (CT) scan have been used

Table 7
Surgical complications affecting the renal allograft

Surgical Emergency	Symptoms	Diagnosis	Treatment
Hematoma	Pain, hypotension, tachycardia	CT scan	Nothing Surgical evacuation
Lymphocele	Swelling of site, leg swelling, DVT, urinary obstruction	Ultrasound Scintigraphy	Aspiration, sclerotherapy, surgical fenestration
TRAS	Hypertension, flash pulmonary edema	Ultrasound Angiography	Hypertension control, angioplasty, or revision
Urine leak	Decrease urine output, swelling, leakage	Ultrasound Scintigraphy	Foley catheter[a] Stenting vs surgery
Torsion	Fatigue, nausea/vomiting, decrease urine output	Ultrasound, CT Laparoscopy	Surgical detorsion
Obstruction	Pain, swelling, decreased urine output	Ultrasound	Foley catheter,[a] stenting, or surgical revision

[a] Should be initiated in the ED.

to assess for the presence and size of a hematoma. Because the sensitivity of ultrasound is only 73%,[30] CT is preferred to identify a hematoma and accurately estimate its size.

Intervention may not be needed for small nonexpanding hematomas that are not causing significant pain or renal dysfunction. They often are found incidentally. A large or actively bleeding hematoma that is compressing the kidney, vessels, or ureters requires surgical evacuation and control of bleeding.

Lymphocele

A lymphocele is a collection of lymph fluid in the transplant bed, generally occurring from either recipient or donor lymphatics that fail to close off during surgery. This complication can occur at almost any time but is most common 2 weeks to 6 months after transplantation.[31] Reports of its incidence range from 0.6% to 26%, making it relatively frequent.[31–33] In some patients, a lymphocele is asymptomatic and noted as an incidental finding. In others, it can lead to outflow obstruction and urinary retention. Significant lymphoceles can lead to leg swelling, deep vein thrombosis (DVT), secondary hypertension (via compression of the transplant's renal artery), and even graft ischemia due to decreased blood supply.[34] The most common findings and complaints are abdominal swelling, wound leakage, obstructive renal injury, edema of leg, and infection.[33]

Ultrasound is the recommended initial imaging to identify a suspected lymphocele. CT, magnetic resonance imaging (MRI), and scintigraphy are additional options, but the latter 2 often are neither readily available nor necessary during ED evaluation. Further imaging, or even aspirating the fluid for measurement of the creatinine level, might be helpful to distinguish lymphocele from urinary leak. A high creatinine level indicates a urine collection. Ideally, aspirations are performed by the transplant team, who should always at least be consulted before undertaking such a procedure. A clinically significant collection should be evaluated at a center with the experience and capability to surgically manage these patients. Because a patient requiring aspiration frequently requires transfer regardless of the result of the aspirate, it seems reasonable for smaller EDs to transfer the patient without performing the procedure.

A variety of treatment options are available for a lymphocele. Depending on its size and level of complexity, they range from observation to drainage, sclerotherapy, aspiration, or even fenestration to allow drainage into the peritoneum.[35] These therapies are typically performed by a transplant surgery team, although some centers use interventional radiology.

Transplant Renal Artery Stenosis

Transplant renal artery stenosis (TRAS) is the most common vascular complication of renal transplantation, with an incidence ranging from less than 1% to 23%.[36,37] Theoretically, it can occur any time after transplantation but is most commonly seen 3 months to 2 years after the procedure.[36] Early on, patients tend to be asymptomatic. Over time, intractable hypertension, graft dysfunction, and elevated hematocrit may be noted.[5] In the emergency setting, patients may present with new or recurrent pulmonary edema, congestive heart failure, or another acute hypertensive crisis.[36] If other causes of the symptoms are ruled out, TRAS must be considered.[5,36,37] Ultrasound is the preferred initial diagnostic approach, because it is commonly available and noninvasive. Its sensitivity is operator dependent and it can be nonspecific. Angiography remains the gold standard to confirm TRAS, as it is diagnostic and could be therapeutic as well.[36,37]

Besides treating the acute hypertensive crisis, there are no specific recommendations for work-up and treatment of TRAS in the ED. If it is mild, medication for hypertension and close monitoring of a patient's renal function and blood pressure are sufficient. If this treatment fails, the patient may need angioplasty/stenting or surgical reconstruction of the vessels.

Urinary Leak

Urinary leak is a rare, early complication caused by anastomotic leak or necrosis of the distal ureter resulting from inadequate blood supply.[5] It occurs in 2% to 6% of cases.[38] Surgical technique can play a role in its causation and certain studies suggest that risk can be decreased by stenting at the time of anastomosis.[39] In some cases, severe obstruction has led to calyceal rupture and urine leakage.[38] Patients with a urinary leak may develop pain, swelling of the transplant site, and decreased urine output. A bulge may be identified on examination and sometimes, if early, urine leaking from the wound may be noted.[5]

Ultrasound is the recommended imaging to identify the extrarenal collection. Often, it may not be clear if the fluid is a urinary collection or lymphocele, and ultimate diagnosis is made by radionucleotide scintigraphy or aspiration of fluid, as previously discussed (a high creatinine level indicating urine collection).[38] Foley catheter placement is required immediately on identification of a urinary leak, and surgical intervention often is necessary. Ultimately, reconstruction may be deemed necessary, but stenting suffices in some situations. If an obstruction is causing or contributing to the leak, treating it with Foley catheter insertion or stenting at the point of obstruction is required.

Torsion

The true incidence of torsion is not known, but it is thought to be very rare. It has been reported primarily in case reports. Theoretically, torsion occurs more frequently with intraperitoneal placement of the kidney.[40] A suspected cause is a decrease in adhesions, often seen in patients taking sirolimus. Torsion can occur at any time after transplant.[40] Risk factors include a long vascular pedicle, excess fluid in the perinephric space, and a long ureter. Some surgeons perform prophylactic nephropexy, particularly for intraperitoneal placement.

The symptoms of torsion are nonspecific. Complaints are rarely related to the torsion itself, because the transplanted kidney is denervated; they are more likely to be secondary effects of renal dysfunction and graft edema. Abdominal pain, oliguria/anuria, nausea/vomiting, diarrhea, weight gain, edema, and fatigue have all been described.[41] Similar to testicular or ovarian torsion, the kidney can torse intermittently,[42] which, coupled with nonspecific symptoms, makes this a challenging diagnosis.

A diagnosis of torsion can be suggested by ultrasound, CT, or even renal scintigraphy. In patients in whom it is strongly suspected, surgical exploration might be necessary. Treatment of torsion is exclusively surgical, with possible nephrectomy if the artery is thrombosed or the kidney is not salvageable. Because torsion is difficult to diagnose, it is often found late, when the transplant is not salvageable. Long-term graft survival Is possible if the torsion is intermittent and surgical intervention is prompt.[43]

Obstruction

Urinary outlet obstruction occurs in 2% to 10% of patients, making it one of the more frequent complications. It is generally caused by ureteric ischemia, kinking, or stenosis.[28] Clots in the bladder can lead to urinary obstruction as well and should be considered in patients with frank hematuria.[5] Prompt diagnosis of the obstruction is important to prevent injury and graft loss. Symptoms include those typical of urinary obstruction in the general population, for example, decreased urinary output as well as swelling of the transplant site. Outlet obstruction in renal transplant patients rarely causes pain; a patient who is experiencing pain probably has an obstruction below the bladder.

Urinary obstruction is diagnosed by the finding of hydronephrosis or bladder distension on ultrasound imaging.[28] It is important to obtain images of both the kidney and the bladder to determine the location of the obstruction. Hydronephrosis and a distended bladder indicate a distal obstruction, as caused by, for example, prostatic hyperplasia, whereas an underdistended bladder indicates ureteral obstruction.

Treatment is based on the cause and location. Foley catheter placement might be indicated for bladder obstruction. Bladder irrigation could be necessary to remove clots. Care must be taken to not disrupt the ureteric anastomosis by overdistending the bladder, especially in patients who recently had surgery. In a case of ureter stricture or kinking, several percutaneous or periurethral surgical options are available, whereas open revision may be required for severe cases.[5]

INFECTION IN RENAL TRANSPLANT RECIPIENTS

Like other SOT recipients, a renal transplant recipient is at risk of a predictable spectrum and timing of infections[44] Most significant infections occur within the first 6 months. Infections can be challenging to diagnose in transplant patients because their inflammatory responses are impaired. Patients with a severe infection might present with only vague complaints and new fever. It is imperative that the emergency physician maintain a low threshold for infectious work-up in this population.[21] One comprehensive analysis of mortality among renal transplant recipients in the United States identified infection as the second most common cause of death.[45] Another study identified it as the leading cause of death 4 years to 10 years after transplantation.[46] Specific risk factors for infection include age greater than 65, deceased-donor graft, and diabetes.[45]

System-specific infections are discussed in further detail in their respective sections. General principles are discussed regarding unique infectious risks at the 3 major time periods (early, intermediate, and late).

Early Infections (0–30 Days Posttransplant)

Nosocomial infections associated with the surgery and concomitant procedures (eg, intubation and catheterization) should be anticipated.[21] During the initial 30 days, technical problems affecting the functional integrity of the renal allograft, such as vesicoureteral reflux, could contribute to the development of infection. Nosocomial infections can also develop from current or recent indwelling cannulas, such as urethral catheters, or from prolonged endotracheal intubation.[44,47] Emergency physicians should consider both superficial and deep surgical site infections (SSIs), recognizing that a patient's decreased inflammatory response might cause such infections to appear mild (discussed later). Donor-derived infections (both bacterial and fungal) also are possible.[44]

Intermediate Infections (30–180 Days Posttransplant)

The 6 months after transplant is a vulnerable time. Within this window, the emergency physician should consider 2 specific categories of infection: immunomodulator-related viral infections and opportunistic infections. Cytomegalovirus (CMV) is the best-known infection; others include BK polyomavirus, Epstein-Barr virus (EBV), hepatitis B virus (HBV), hepatitis C virus (HCV), and human herpesvirus 6.[21]

CMV deserves special attention, because it is one of the most common SOT complications and is capable of triggering or worsening organ rejection.[21,48] CMV infections most commonly occur 1 month to 3 months after transplantation.[49] Fortunately, there have been important advances in managing CMV in the past several years, and many patients are on some form of prophylaxis.[44,48] CMV syndrome is a flulike generalized infection unique to SOT recipients. Probable diagnosis requires detectable viral replication levels in addition to at least 2 constitutional symptoms (fever [temperature $\geq 38^\circ$C for at least 2 days]; new or increased malaise or fatigue; or laboratory findings, such as leukopenia, neutropenia, atypical lymphocytosis [$\geq 5\%$], thrombocytopenia, or new transaminitis). CMV infection also can present as an end-organ disease, such as CMV pneumonia, gastrointestinal disease, hepatitis, retinitis, encephalitis/ventriculitis, nephritis, cystitis, myocarditis, and pancreatitis.[50] The infection can affect multiple organ systems simultaneously, but pneumonitis remains its most common presentation.[21]

EBV infection can present similarly, and even simultaneously, during this timeframe. As in nontransplant patients, EBV can manifest along a spectrum from asymptomatic viremia to a mononucleosis-like syndrome that includes fever, malaise, lymphadenopathy, and even hepatosplenomegaly.[21,44] The most significant EBV-associated complication is posttransplant lymphoproliferative disorder, a potentially life-threatening condition (discussed later).[51] The seriousness of this condition makes suspicion for EBV infection even more important.

The second major category is opportunistic infections. Invasive fungal infections (such as disseminated aspergillus and candidiasis) can present as subacute respiratory symptoms or severe, life-threatening infections. Another opportunistic pulmonary infection is *Pneumocystis jirovecii* pneumonia (PJP), which can be clinically indistinguishable from CMV infection.[21,52] Mycobacterial diseases and other opportunistic organisms, such as *Strongyloides stercoralis*, can have varied pulmonary presentations as well.[53] *S stercoralis* can cause hemorrhagic enterocolitis, as can infections with

Salmonella and *Listeria*, which can more easily invade the mucosa in immunosuppressed transplant patients.[21,54]

Ideally, acute treatment of any infection during this window should be initiated in consultation with the admitting service or a transplant pharmacist. Opportunistic infections might require complex treatment regimens, because many antimicrobials pose the risk of nephrotoxicity. Acute episodes of CMV infection typically are treated with oral valganciclovir for mild/moderate disease (900 mg every 12 hours) and intravenous ganciclovir for severe disease (5 mg/kg every 12 hours if the patient has normal renal function).[48]

Late Infections (>180 Days Posttransplant)

After the initial 6 months, patients' vulnerability will, in part, be determined by their initial infection history and graft success. The ideal healthy transplant recipient has not developed any of the previously discussed immunomodulator-related infections and is not experiencing any significant rejection, allowing a comparably minimal immunosuppressive regimen. As such, these patients have only slightly elevated susceptibility to community-acquired infections. The most common are caused by community-acquired respiratory and gastrointestinal viral pathogens.[52]

In contrast, patients with active immunomodulator-related infection or the need for long-term immunosuppression can display progressive disease processes. Examples include recurrent or acquired viral hepatitis and other viral activations, such as latent varicella zoster virus (VZV) or herpes simplex virus (HSV). Finally, patients with chronic rejection require aggressive immunosuppression and are consequently at high risk of opportunistic infections. These include the pathogens discussed previously regarding intermediate infections.

KEY POINTS

1. Infection risk changes throughout a patient's posttransplant course.
2. Attention should be paid to the timing of the transplant and to any recent treatment of acute rejection.

CARDIOVASCULAR DISORDERS

Although patients receiving renal transplants reap many benefits from the procedure, their risk of death from cardiovascular disease (CVD) is up to 20 times higher than in the general population, at 3.5% to 5%.[55] The reasons for this increased risk for CVD are multifactorial. Renal disease itself increases the risk for CVD, and, although renal transplant decreases this risk, it was still found to be higher than among nondialysis/renal transplant recipients in age-matched controls.[56] Some of the complication comes from antirejection medications, which worsen hyperlipidemia.[57]

Many conditions that lead to renal disease also contribute to CVD: hypertension, diabetes, and hyperlipidemia. One study suggests that the increased risk of ischemic heart disease imposed by these conditions, specifically diabetes, might be greater in transplant recipients than in the general population.[58] The same study noted that the risk for ischemic heart disease for diabetic women was 5-fold higher than in the nontransplant population (3-fold for men). Congestive heart failure is a known complication of chronic kidney disease; approximately 70% of patients starting dialysis have abnormal heart structure or function.[59] Patients who receive a transplant often have improved function and functional status on the New York Heart

Association chart, but the longer the patients are on dialysis, the less likely they are to normalize heart function.[60] Although this improvement with transplant is promising, congestive heart failure is still a highly morbid condition affecting transplant patients.

KEY POINTS

1. Renal disease is a significant cardiac risk factor yet frequently is not present in common risk stratification tools.
2. Diabetes confers a greater cardiovascular risk to renal transplant patients than the general population, but it is unclear how this association should be incorporated into frequently used risk stratification tools (Thombolysis in Myocardial Infarction (TIMI); History, EKG, Age, Risk factors, and Troponin (HEART) score/pathway, and so forth).

PULMONARY PROBLEMS

Pulmonary complications in renal transplant patients tend to be caused directly by the immunosuppression drugs they need to take and their side effects. Renal transplant patients lack the immune support necessary to fight off infections, putting them at risk of pneumonia from bacteria, tuberculosis, and fungi.[61] In addition, complications from medication, specifically sirolimus, have been indicated in pulmonary disease in the transplant patient. Thankfully, in the absence of other confounding factors, renal transplant patients tend to have few other respiratory abnormalities. Some studies suggest that posttransplant patients have improved lung function testing compared with pretransplant dialysis patients.[62]

Pneumonia is the most common life-threatening infection in renal transplant patients, although it tends to occur less frequently than in other transplant groups. The overall risks of pneumonia and its associated mortality are estimated be 8% and 15%, respectively.[63] Identification and treatment of these infections are critical and can be more difficult than in immunocompetent patients. For this reason, high-resolution CT scan is often recommended because of its increased sensitivity over plain radiography and the additional information it provides, especially if the chest radiograph is normal, but clinical suspicion for pneumonia remains.[64] When infection is suspected, empiric antibiotics are recommended due to the high mortality rate of untreated pneumonia.

Caution should be taken in the symptomatic patient with normal CT findings. CMV pneumonia can be present without revealing CT findings.[64] Opportunistic infections, such as Pneumocystis and tuberculosis, also are more likely in this population. PJP tends to be limited relatively well by prophylactic medications. Tuberculosis is also relatively uncommon, to the point that routine prophylaxis in non–high-risk patients is not recommended.[65] Prophylaxis against CMV is often given, but this pathogen should remain a consideration after prophylaxis has been ended, especially in a patient with fever, pancytopenia, or pulmonary disease.

Infection can be difficult to differentiate from drug side effects, which can also present with abnormal findings on radiograph or CT scan. Sirolimus can cause pneumonitis, appearing as bilateral interstitial infiltrates on chest films and CT scans.[66] In patients without infectious symptoms, pneumonitis should remain a consideration, and the ultimate diagnosis may require bronchial alveolar lavage.[61] Fortunately, if the diagnosis is made, most patients make full recovery in 3 months to 6 months after cessation of sirolimus.[67]

KEY POINTS

1. Pneumonia in transplant patients can be deadly and should be treated early and aggressively.

2. Strongly consider CT imaging for suspected pneumonia and other pulmonary pathology given the poor sensitivity of plain chest radiographs.

GASTROINTESTINAL PROBLEMS

Gastrointestinal symptoms, from dyspepsia to diarrhea, are common in this population, owing to both infectious pathogens and medication side effects. The symptoms can have significant consequences: an acute bout of gastroenteritis has the potential to affect medication compliance or lead to dehydration. Chronic diarrhea can be easily dismissed as unimportant but deserves attention, because posttransplant diarrhea has been associated with an increased risk of graft loss and death. An immunosuppressed state, specific immunosuppression medications, and frequent exposure to broad-spectrum antibiotics can all predispose a renal transplant recipient to diarrheal illness. Some of the most common infectious sources include *Clostridium difficile*, CMV, bacterial overgrowth, and norovirus. Posttransplant diarrhea has many noninfectious causes as well, the most common being the immunosuppressive medication mycophenolate mofetil.[68]

With regard to management in the ED, all transplant patients must be able to tolerate medications consistently by mouth prior to discharge. Chronic diarrhea does not automatically necessitate admission, but it is reasonable to coordinate initial studies so that they can be followed-up by the transplant specialist on an outpatient basis. Those studies include standard stool cultures; examination for parasites and fungi; and evaluation for *C difficile*, rotavirus, adenovirus, and norovirus (some tests may be send-outs).

HEPATOBILIARY AND PANCREATIC DISORDERS
Hepatobiliary Disease

Liver disease is common among renal transplant recipients. Hepatotrophic infections with HBV, HCV, and hepatitis E virus are common. The prevalence of HCV is as high as 40% in some studies; its presence has been associated with worse outcomes in renal transplant recipients (graft loss and death from sepsis). Acute hepatitis (donor-derived or otherwise) warrants immediate work-up. The manifestation of infection with a non-hepatotrophic pathogen, such as CMV, EBV, HSV, and VZV, can resemble acute liver disease. In immunosuppressed patients, hepatic abscesses and mycobacterial infections are possible.

Many of the medications that often are prescribed for renal transplant patients induce toxicity. Given the complexity of these patients' medication regimens, new medications should be started with close attention to drug–drug interactions. Commonly implicated medications are listed in **Table 2**.

A patient with severe polycystic kidney disease also can have liver polycystic disease, which can cause abdominal pain depending on the size of the masses and infection, hemorrhage, and rupture in extreme cases.

New-Onset Posttransplant Diabetes

New-onset diabetes after transplantation (NODAT) is an important complication associated with increased cardiovascular complications and infection risk.[69] The available prevalence data vary, but, overall, NODAT is estimated to occur in one-quarter of renal transplant recipients and is associated with medications, such as glucocorticoids and CNIs.[70] From an emergency physician's perspective, it is important to know that no hypoglycemic agent is contraindicated for the renal transplant patient. No significant drug interactions between common diabetes medications and standard immunosuppressive medications have been reported.[69] Despite the relatively high rate of NODAT, comparatively few reports of patients presenting with diabetic ketoacidosis have been published. Several case reports have suggested that tacrolimus contributed to diabetic ketoacidosis presentations.[71]

NEUROLOGIC AND PSYCHOLOGICAL DISORDERS

Neurologic symptoms in the renal transplant recipient may come from infection, metabolic derangements, malignancies, complications of immunosuppressive medications, and stroke. An individual's presentation may be secondary to multiple processes, because these pathologies are not mutually exclusive.

In the setting of immunosuppression, infectious etiologies remain one of the greatest neurologic concerns. The list of possible central nervous system (CNS)-relevant donor-derived transmissions alone is beyond the scope of this review; it includes bacterial, viral, fungal, parasitic, and oncologic processes. Reactivation of viral infections (with, for example, HSV and VZV) within the recipient may result in meningoencephalitis. As discussed previously, immunomodulator-related viruses (CMV, EBV, and so forth) not only can cause neurologic symptoms on their own but also increase the risk of additional opportunistic infections. Asymptomatic respiratory colonization with pathogens, such as *Aspergillus*, *Cryptococcus*, and *Nocardia*, can present as pulmonary-brain syndromes with CNS metastasis in the setting of immunosuppression.[72] The emergency physician should have a low threshold for lumbar puncture (LP) in symptomatic patients. Given the high prevalence of abnormal findings, it has been argued that all immunocompromised patients should undergo noncontrast head CT prior to LP.[73] Large volumes of cerebrospinal fluid may increase the sensitivity of certain laboratory tests.

Clinical symptoms alone are rarely diagnostic. Patients might require extensive laboratory and imaging work-ups that likely will continue outside the ED. Empiric antimicrobial therapy is best initiated in consultation with an admitting transplant team. It should be CNS penetrating and broad spectrum and should include specific coverage for *Pneumococcus*, *Listeria*, *Cryptococcus*, and HSV. Patients boarded in the ED should continue to receive their existing immunosuppressive regimen unless the emergency physician is specifically directed otherwise. An abrupt cessation, especially of corticosteroids, can precipitate immune reconstitution inflammatory syndrome, can worsen CNS symptoms, and might cause hydrocephalus.[72]

A focal neurologic deficit can result from either an infectious or a malignant space-occupying lesion. In addition, many of the same risk factors that contribute to development of ESRD increase the likelihood of stroke in this population. A renal allograft is not a contraindication to administration of tissue plasminogen activator.[74] In contrast, the presentation of a generalized metabolic encephalopathy, especially in the setting of oliguria, should prompt concern for acute graft failure related to any of the previously described surgical, infectious, and immunologic etiologies.

Depression and anxiety can be underappreciated in transplant patients. Observed rates of these conditions are substantially higher than in the general population and even greater than in individuals with other chronic medical conditions. One specific area of interest is the association between depression and morbidity or mortality. Dew and colleagues[75] found an increased relative risk (RR) of death (RR, 1.65; 95% CI, 1.34–2.05) among SOT recipients with depression. Further analysis of renal transplant recipients revealed an increased risk of death-censored graft loss (RR, 1.65; 95% CI, 1.21–2.26), defined as graft failure with either return to dialysis or retransplantation while excluding patient death with a functioning graft. Consequently, it behooves the emergency physician to provide psychosocial resources and inform a patient's primary transplant team if there is any concern for psychological/mood disorder.

KEY POINTS

1. Transplant patients are at elevated risk for a variety of unique neurologic infections not commonly seen in immunocompetent patients.
2. The threshold for LP should be low.

HEMATOLOGIC DISORDERS

Blood disorders are, fortunately, relatively uncommon. They can have devastating effects on renal transplant recipients. Complications may be related to the transplant itself (graft-versus-host disease or passenger lymphocyte syndrome), a patient's antiviral and immunosuppressive medications, or opportunistic infections.[76,77]

Immunosuppressant medications can contribute to lymphoproliferative disorders in kidney transplant patients. A majority of cases of lymphoma have been linked to B cells infected with EBV, which tends to be held in check with normal immune status but has to potential to proliferate with high levels of immunosuppression.[78] Renal transplant patients may be at a 20-fold greater risk for lymphoma than the general population.[77] The most significant manifestation of EBV is posttransplant lymphoproliferative disorder, which can occur along a spectrum ranging from indolent localized growths to fulminant presentations. The most common symptoms are fever and lymphadenopathy, but the presentation can include the full range of constitutional and systemic symptoms, gastrointestinal symptoms (including obstruction), and even focal neurologic findings. The allograft itself can also be affected, resulting in renal dysfunction.[52]

Thrombotic microangiopathy can occur after transplantation in response to rejection, medications, or a variety of other factors. The presentation can be similar to the disorder in patients without transplant, manifesting as a triad of thrombocytopenia, microangiopathic hemolytic anemia, and acute kidney injury. It should be considered in patients with acute kidney injury and biopsy results that are negative for rejection.[79] Unfortunately, the prognosis is poor, with graft loss of approximately 50% at 2 years and 50% mortality at 3 years.[80,81] Treatment is aimed at eliminating the cause, so switching medications away from CNIs may be helpful.[82] Plasmapheresis may be indicated in some cases, and if the diagnosis is known, this may necessitate transfer to a capable facility.[83]

Although the presenting symptoms of lymphoproliferative disorders can be nonspecific, evidence of new anemia or pancytopenia on CBC evaluation in the early posttransplant period should be investigated aggressively. In patients with new anemia, diseases, such as hemophagocytic syndrome or passenger lymphocyte syndrome, may have other signs of hemolysis, such as elevated lactic acid dehydrogenase or unconjugated hyperbilirubinemia.[84] Early identification and treatment of the cause of the abnormality should be explored early, often with bone marrow biopsy, because early treatment can improve outcomes.

KEY POINT

- When a renal transplant patient has abnormal hematology test results during the ED evaluation, further work-up is required. It is unlikely that a definitive diagnosis will be made in the ED.

MUSCULOSKELETAL AND ARTICULAR COMPLICATIONS

Due to comorbid conditions and the medical therapy that transplant patients need, musculoskeletal problems can be a cause of significant morbidity. The most frequently implicated factors are preexisting renal osteodystrophy and corticosteroid use, leading to osteopenia and osteoporosis.[85] In the patients studied by Sessa and associates,[86] the combination of sirolimus and steroids was particularly implicated. This pathology can lead to an increased fracture risk; however, how great an increase is debatable and may be minimal compared with similar groups in the general population.[87]

CNI-induced pain syndrome causes pain in the feet, ankles, and lower legs. It is worse with weight bearing and ambulation but is relieved by rest and feet elevation.[88] Standard radiographs and physical examination results are normal. The diagnosis typically is made with MRI and a decrease in pain when CNI levels are adjusted. CNI trough levels are elevated in most, but not all, of these patients.[89] Adding a calcium channel blocker might help alleviate the discomfort; nonsteroidal anti-inflammatory drugs (NSAIDs) and opioids are likely to have little effect.[88,89] The definitive treatment is CNI management or discontinuation.

KEY POINTS

1. Consider CNI-induced pain and referral for definitive management or medication adjustment in situations with no other explanation.
2. The transplant population may have an increased risk for fracture, so clinical suspicion for it should be high.

CUTANEOUS PROBLEMS IN RENAL TRANSPLANT RECIPIENTS

SSI is a significant concern in the immediate postoperative period after SOT. In general, renal transplantation has a lower incidence of SSI compared with procedures involving other organs but with reasonable variability within reported rates in the literature. Studies vary in their reported incidence of SSIs, ranging from 7.5% to 15%. Most infections occur at the superficial-incisional level. On average, SSIs are diagnosed 11 days after transplantation and are most commonly caused by coagulase-negative staphylococci.[90,91] In the setting of immunosuppression, the emergency care provider must maintain a high level of suspicion, because such infections can appear deceptively mild on clinical examination. Other opportunistic complications, including *Cryptococcus* infection and mucormycosis, can present as cutaneous infections.

From a more chronic perspective, SOT significantly increases the risk of several malignancies. The greatest increase in incidence (approximately 20-fold) is observed in carcinomas of the skin.[27] A vast majority are squamous or basal cell carcinomas, which usually occur on sun-exposed areas and have a mean time to development of 8 years to 10 years after transplantation. When a suspicious lesion is identified during the ED examination, the patient should be referred for prompt dermatology follow-up.

COMMON LABORATORY ABNORMALITIES

Similar to ESRD, several hematologic and electrolyte abnormalities are common among renal transplant recipients. They are listed in **Table 8**.

THE CRASHING RENAL TRANSPLANT PATIENT

Renal transplant recipients are vulnerable to severe illness because of their comorbid conditions and immunosuppressed state. Although rates of hospitalization seem to be

Table 8
Common laboratory abnormalities in renal transplant recipients

Abnormality	Cause	Management Concerns
Anemia	ESRD patients often require erythropoietin before transplant; its discontinuation after transplant might cause mild anemia that gradually resolves. Significant posttransplant anemia could be postoperative bleeding. Immunosuppression allows infections, such as parvovirus B19, to cause severe anemia and even pancytopenia.[92]	Significant changes should prompt evaluation of surgical and/or infectious sources.
Erythrocytosis	Elevated hemoglobin and/or hematocrit is observed in a quarter of patients and can be caused by a variety of issues.	Excessive levels (hemoglobin $\geq$17–18 g/dL or hematocrit $\geq$52%–55%) are associated with an increased risk of thromboembolic complications.
Leukopenia and thrombocytopenia	Observed with viral infections, such as parvovirus B19 and CMV Known side effects of several common medications, including azathioprine, mycophenolate mofetil, sirolimus, trimethoprim-sulfamethoxazole, and alemtuzumab	Review potential causes. Assess for neutropenia.
Potassium	CNIs commonly cause mild, episodic hyperkalemia.[93] Sirolimus has been associated with decreased potassium levels.	Assess for electrocardiographic changes. Mild hyperkalemia rarely requires treatment. Severe hyperkalemia may be treated with insulin, but some advocate a reduced dose (5 units instead of 10 units) in patients with diminished renal function.[94] The potassium exchange resin sodium polystyrene sulfonate (kayexalate) should not be used for hyperkalemia; it is a risk factor for colonic perforation.[95]
Hypophosphatemia	Mild hypophosphatemia is common in renal transplant recipients. The cause often is multifactorial but can be secondary to CNIs.[93]	Severe hypophosphatemia should prompt evaluation because it could represent a correctable injury to the renal graft.

(continued on next page)

Table 8 (continued)		
Abnormality	**Cause**	**Management Concerns**
Hypercalcemia	Common in patients with a prolonged prior history of hemodialysis, due to persistent secondary hyperparathyroidism	Most cases resolve spontaneously within a year after transplantation.
Hypomagnesemia	Common in setting of CNIs	Dietary supplementation is common. Intravenous repletion is reasonable for severe hypomagnesemia (<1.0 mg/dL).[93]
Transaminitis	Often secondary to medications Significant elevations should prompt concern about viral infections, such as CMV, HBV, and HCV.	Viral assessment when severe

decreasing over time, up to 10% of renal transplant recipients require intensive care unit admission, most often for treatment of sepsis.[96] The most severe infections typically are pneumonia (50% to 60% of cases) and acute graft pyelonephritis (17%–25%).[96] One single-center review of sepsis in renal transplant recipients in Brazil found that, in cases of an identifiable source, gram-negative pathogens accounted for 45% of presentations whereas gram-positive and fungal sources were responsible for 20% and 24%, respectively.[97] PJP is the most common opportunistic pneumonia. In contrast to AIDS patients, renal transplant patients derive no clear benefit from adjunctive steroid therapy.[98]

Pulmonary edema is observed frequently in critically ill renal transplant recipients. Its frequency might be due to associated acute graft dysfunction, leading to volume overload. A patient's fluid status should be assessed before large fluid boluses are administered empirically. If central venous access is required, it best to avoid subclavian central venous catheters (to preserve arteriovenous fistulas) and, if possible, to avoid femoral central venous catheters on the side of the renal graft.[99]

A universal strategy for managing immunosuppression during critical illness has not been delineated. There is understandable concern that reduction of immunosuppression could help recovery during sepsis but at the risk of damage to the renal graft. Given this complexity, managing immunosuppressants in this population necessitates immediate coordination between the EM physician, the intensivist, and a transplant specialist.[96]

KEY POINTS

1. Assess fluid status and monitor closely due to the increased risk of pulmonary edema.
2. Avoid subclavian central venous catheters, if possible, and try to avoid placing central access on the side of the transplanted kidney.

FINAL THOUGHTS

Renal transplant recipients are a growing population that can present to any ED. Although a chief concern might not be directly related to a patient's renal allograft, the potential interplay between the patient's presentation and the transplant should always be considered. Four key concepts to keep in mind are as follows:

1. Infection versus rejection: these are recurrent issues in this population, and clinically occult presentations hold the potential to be catastrophic.
2. Transplantation explanation: always ask when and why patients received their renal transplantation, because this information can narrow what pathology to suspect.
3. Medication alteration: changes in the level of immunosuppression are key to understanding potential complications. Emergency care providers should identify any recent increases or decreases in a patient's immunosuppression regimen and should ask about the patient's compliance with instructions.
4. Situation communication: the emergency care provider should be willing to communicate concerns with the transplant team, because these are complicated and vulnerable patients.

ACKNOWLEDGMENTS

The article was copyedited by Linda J. Kesselring, MS, ELS.

REFERENCES

1. Organ donation statistics. US Department of Health & Human Services. Available at: https://www.organdonor.gov/statistics-stories/statistics.html#glance. Accessed January 8, 2019.
2. Schold JD, Elfadawy N, Buccini LD, et al. Emergency department visits after kidney transplantation. Clin J Am Soc Nephrol 2016;11:674–83.
3. McAdams-Demarco MA, Grams ME, Hall EC, et al. Early hospital readmission after kidney transplantation: patient and center-level associations. Am J Transplant 2012;12:3283–8.
4. Unterman S, Zimmerman M, Tyo C, et al. A descriptive analysis of 1251 solid organ transplant visits to the emergency department. West J Emerg Med 2009;10: 48–54.
5. Cowan NG, Veale JL, Gritsch HA. 9 the transplant operation and its surgical complications. Available at: http://ebookcentral.proquest.com/lib/hshsl/detail.action?docID=5472171. Accessed May 11, 2019.
6. Rosales A, Salvador JT, Urdaneta G, et al. Laparoscopic kidney transplantation. Eur Urol 2010;57:164–7.
7. Modi P, Rizvi J, Pal B, et al. Laparoscopic kidney transplantation: an initial experience. Am J Transplant 2011;11(6):1320–4.
8. Hermann M, Enseleit F, Fisler AE, et al. Cyclosporine C0-versus C2-monitoring over three years in maintenance heart transplantation. Swiss Med Wkly 2011; 141:w13149.
9. Einollahi B, Rostami Z. Does C2 level monitoring have benefit over C0 level monitoring among solid organ transplantation? Swiss Med Wkly 2012;142:w13530.
10. Lee B, Petzel R, Campara M. Appropriate timing of tacrolimus concentration measurements in the emergency department. Am J Health Syst Pharm 2016; 73(17):1297–8.
11. BC transplant. Clinical guidelines for transplant medications. Available at: http://www.transplant.bc.ca/Documents/Health%20Professionals/Clinical%20guidelines/Clinical%20Guidelines%20for%20Transplant%20Medications.pdf. Accessed March 4, 2019.

12. Rhu J, Lee KW, Park H, et al. Clinical implication of mycophenolic acid trough concentration monitoring in kidney transplant patients on a tacrolimus triple maintenance regimen: a single-center experience. Ann Transplant 2017;22:707–18.

13. Lim WH, Eris J, Kanellis J, et al. A systematic review of conversion from calcineurin inhibitor to mammalian target of rapamycin inhibitors for maintenance immunosuppression in kidney transplant recipients. Am J Transplant 2014;14: 2106–19.

14. Zaltzman JS. Is there a role for mTOR inhibitors in renal transplantation? Transplantation 2017;101(2):228–9.

15. Joffe M, Hus CY, Feldman HI, et al. Variability of creatinine measurements in clinical laboratories: results from the CRIC study. Am J Nephrol 2010;31:426–34.

16. Wiseman AC, Cooper JE. Evaluation and initial management of graft dysfunction. In: Weir M, Lerma E, editors. Kidney transplantation. New York: Springer; 2014. p. 153–8.

17. Altunbas G, Sucu M, Zengin O. Ventricular repolarization disturbances after high dose intravenous methylprednisolone theraphy. J Electrocardiol 2018;51(1): 140–4.

18. Coussement J, Scemia A, Abramowicz D, et al. Antibiotics for asymptomatic bacteriuria in kidney transplant recipients. Cochrane Database Syst Rev 2018;(2):CD011357.

19. Coussement J, Maggiore U, Manuel O, et al. Diagnosis and management of asymptomatic bacteriuria in kidney transplant recipients: a survey of current practice in Europe. Nephrol Dial Transplant 2018;33:1661–8.

20. Nicolle LE, Kalpana G, Bradley SF, Colgan R, et al. Asymptomatic Bacteriuria. Clinical Infectious Diseases 2019 [Epub ahead of print].

21. Ergin M, Dal Ü, Granit D, et al. Management of renal transplant patients in the emergency department. J Acad Emerg Med 2015;14:83–7.

22. Gołębiewska J, Dębska-Ślizień A. Chapter 3: urinary tract infections in renal transplant recipients. In: Jarzembowski T, Daca A, Dębska-Ślizień MA, editors. Urinary tract infection: the result of the strength of the pathogen, or the weakness of the host. London: InTech Open; 2018. p. 33–45.

23. Nigam LK, Vanikar AV, Patel RD, et al. Chapter 4: urinary tract infection in renal allograft recipients. In: Jarzembowski T, Daca A, Dębska-Ślizień MA, editors. Urinary tract infection: the result of the strength of the pathogen, or the weakness of the host. London: InTech Open; 2018. p. 47–64.

24. Cheungpasitporn W, Thongprayoon C, Mao MA, et al. Incidence of kidney stones in kidney transplant recipients: a systematic review and meta-analysis. World J Transplant 2016;6(4):790–7.

25. Ferreira Cassini M, Cologna AJ, Ferreira Andrade M, et al. Lithiasis in 1,313 kidney transplants: incidence, diagnosis, and management. Transplant Proc 2012; 44:2373–5.

26. Mamarelis G, Vernadiakis S, Moris D, et al. Lithiasis of the renal allograft, a rare urologic complication following renal transplantation: a single-center experience of 2045 renal transplantations. Transplant Proc 2014;46:3203–5.

27. Kamal AI, Mannon RB. Malignancies after transplantation and posttransplant lymphoproliferative disorder. In: Weir M, Lerma E, editors. Kidney transplantation. New York: Springer; 2014. p. 269–80.

28. Ghoneim MA, Shokeir AA. Emergencies following renal transplantation. In: Hohenfellner M, Santucci RA, editors. Emergencies in urology. Berlin: Springer-Verlag; 2007. p. 451–65.

29. Shahrokh H, Rasouli H, Zargar MA, et al. Spontaneous kidney allograft rupture. Transplant Proc 2005;37:3079–80.

30. Fananapazir G, Rao R, Corwin MT, et al. Sonographic evaluation of clinically significant perigraft hematomas in kidney transplant recipients. Am J Roentgenol 2015;205(4):802–6.

31. Samhan M, Al-Mousawi M. Lymphocele following renal transplantation. Saudi J Kidney Dis Transpl 2007;17(1):34–7.

32. Atray NK, Moore F, Zaman F, et al. Post transplant lymphocele: a single centre experience. Clin Transplant 2004;18(suppl 1):46–9.

33. Zagdoun E, Ficheux M, Lobbedez T, et al. Complicated lymphoceles after kidney transplantation. Transplant Proc 2010;42:4322–5.

34. Golriz M, Klauss M, Zeier M, et al. Prevention and management of lymphocele formation following kidney transplantation. Transplant Rev 2017;31:100–5.

35. Lucewicz A, Wong G, Lam VWT, et al. Management of primary symptomatic lymphocele after kidney transplantation: a systematic review. Transplantation 2011; 92:663–73.

36. Bruno S, Remuzzi G, Ruggenenti P. Transplant renal artery stenosis. J Am Soc Nephrol 2004;15(1):134–41.

37. Ayvazoglu Soy EH, Akdur A, Kirnap M, et al. Vascular complications after renal transplant: a single-center experience. Exp Clin Transplant 2017;15:79–83.

38. Hamouda M, Sharma A, Halawa A. Urine leak after kidney transplant: a review of the literature. Exp Clin Transplant 2018;16:90–5.

39. Patel P, Rebollo-Mesa I, Ryan E, et al. Prophylactic ureteric stents in renal transplant recipients: a multicenter randomized controlled trial of early versus late removal. Am J Transplant 2017;17(8):2129–38.

40. Sosin M, Lumeh W, Cooper M. Torsion of the retroperitoneal kidney: uncommon or underreported? Case Rep Transplant 2014;2014 [Article: 561506].

41. Lucewicz A, Isaacs A, Allen RD, et al. Torsion of intraperitoneal kidney transplant. ANZ J Surg 2012;82:299–302.

42. Pery R, Shaharabani E, Gazer B, et al. Laparoscopic fixation for torsion of transplanted kidney: a case report. Transplant Proc 2017;49(10):2378–80.

43. Serrano OK, Olowofela AS, Kandaswamy R, et al. Long-term graft survival after kidney allograft torsion: rapid diagnosis and surgical management key to reversibility of injury. Transplant Proc 2017;49(7):1565–9.

44. Green M. Introduction: infections in solid organ transplantation. Am J Transplant 2013;3:3–8.

45. Awan AA, Niu J, Pan JS, et al. Trends in the causes of death among kidney transplant recipients in the United States (1996-2014). Am J Nephrol 2018;48:472–81.

46. Weinrauch LA, D'Elia JA, Weir MR, et al. Infection and malignancy outweigh cardiovascular mortality in kidney transplant recipients: post hoc analysis of the FAVORIT trial. Am J Med 2018;131:165–72.

47. Hanevold CD, Kiser BA, Palmer J, et al. Vesicoureteral reflux and urinary tract infections in renal transplant recipients. Am J Dis Child 1987;141:982–4.

48. Kotton CN, Kumar D, Callendo AM, et al. The Third International Consensus Guidelines on the Management of Cytomegalovirus in Solid-Organ Transplantation. Transplantation 2018;102:900–31.

49. Azevedo LS, Pierrotti LC, Abdala E, et al. Cytomegalovirus infection in transplant patients. Clinics (Sao Paulo) 2015;70(7):515–23.

50. Ljungman P, Boeckh M, Hirsch HH, et al. Definitions of cytomegalovirus infection and disease in transplant patients for use in clinical trials. Clini Infect Dis 2017; 64(1):87–91.

51. Caillard S, Lamy FX, Quelen C, et al. Epidemiology of posttransplant lymphoproliferative disorders in adult kidney and kidney pancreas recipients: report of the French registry and analysis of subgroups of lymphomas. Am J Transplant 2012;12:682–93.
52. Green M, Michaels MG. Epstein–Barr virus infection and posttransplant lymphoproliferative disorder. Am J Transplant 2013;13:41–54.
53. Mokhlesi B, Shulzhenko O, Garimella PS, et al. Pulmonary strongyloidiasis: the varied clinical presentations. Clin Pulm Med 2004;11(1):6–13.
54. Poveda J, El-Sharkawy F, Arosemena LR, et al. *Strongyloides* colitis as a harmful mimicker of inflammatory bowel disease. Case Rep Pathol 2017;2017:2560719.
55. Aakhus S, Dahl K, Widerøe TE. Cardiovascular disease in stable renal transplant patients in Norway: morbidity and mortality during a 5-yr follow-up. Clin Transplant 2004;18(5):596–604.
56. Sarnak MJ, Levey AS, Schoolwerth AC, et al. Kidney disease as a risk factor for development of cardiovascular disease: a statement from the American Heart Association Councils on kidney in cardiovascular disease, high blood pressure research, clinical cardiology, and epidemiology and prevention. Circulation 2003;108:2154–69.
57. Gaston RS, Kasiske BL, Fieberg AM, et al. Use of cardioprotective medications in kidney transplant recipients. Am J Transplant 2009;9:1811–5.
58. Kasiske BL, Chakkera HA, Roel J. Explained and unexplained ischemic heart disease risk after renal transplantation. J Am Soc Nephrol 2000;11(9):1735–43.
59. Collins AJ. Cardiovascular mortality in end-stage renal disease. Am J Med Sci 2003;325:163–7.
60. Wali RK, Wang GS, Gottlieb SS, et al. Effect of kidney transplantation on left ventricular systolic dysfunction and congestive heart failure in patients with end-stage renal disease. J Am Coll Cardiol 2005;45:1051–60.
61. Chang G, Wu C, Pan S, et al. The diagnosis of pneumonia in renal transplant recipients using invasive and noninvasive procedures. Chest 2004;125:541–7.
62. Karacan Ö, Tutal E, Colak T, et al. Pulmonary function in renal transplant recipients and end-stage renal disease patients undergoing maintenance dialysis. Transplant Proc 2006;38:396–400.
63. Hoyo I, Linares L, Cervera C, et al. Epidemiology of pneumonia in kidney transplantation. Transplant Proc 2010;42:2938–40.
64. Gulati M, Kaur R, Jha V, et al. High-resolution CT in renal transplant patients with suspected pulmonary infections. Acta Radiol 2000;41(3):237–41.
65. Kasiske BL, Vazquez MA, Harmon WE, et al. Recommendations for the outpatient surveillance of renal transplant recipients. American Society of Transplantation. J Am Soc Nephrol 2000;11(suppl 15):S1–86.
66. Morelon E, Stern M, Israel-Biet D, et al. Characteristics of sirolimus-associated interstitial pneumonitis in renal transplant patients. Transplantation 2001;72(5):787–90.
67. Champion L, Stern M, Israël-Biet D, et al. Brief communication: sirolimus-associated pneumonitis: 24 cases in renal transplant recipients. Ann Intern Med 2006;144:505–9.
68. Shin HS, Chandraker A. Causes and management of postrenal transplant diarrhea: an underappreciated cause of transplant-associated morbidity. Curr Opin Nephrol Hypertens 2017;26:484–93.
69. Goldmannova D, Karasek d, Krystynik O, et al. New-onset diabetes mellitus after renal transplantation. Biomed Pap Med Fac Univ Palacky Olomouc Czech Repub 2016;160(2):195–200.

70. Adey DB. The prevention and treatment of coronary artery disease in kidney transplant recipients. In: Weir M, Lerma E, editors. Kidney transplantation. New York: Springer; 2014. p. 189–98.

71. Ammari Z, Pak SC, Ruzieh M, et al. Posttransplant tacrolimus-induced diabetic ketoacidosis: review of the literature. Case Rep Endocrinol 2018;2018:4606491.

72. Wright AJ, Fishman JA. Central nervous syndromes in solid organ transplant recipients. Clin Infect Dis 2014;59(7):1001–11.

73. Hasbun R, Abrahams J, Jekel J, et al. Computed tomography of the head before lumbar puncture in adults with suspected meningitis. N Engl J Med 2001;345(24):1727–33.

74. Agrawal V, Rai B, Fellows J, et al. In-hospital outcomes with thrombolytic therapy in patients with renal dysfunction presenting with acute ischaemic stroke. Nephrol Dial Transplant 2010;25:1150–7.

75. Dew MA, Rosenberger EM, Myaskovsky L, et al. Depression and anxiety as risk factors for morbidity and mortality after organ transplantation: a systematic review and meta-analysis. Transplantation 2015;100(5):988–1003.

76. Smith EP. Hematologic disorders after solid organ transplantation. Hematology Am Soc Hematol Educ Program 2010. https://doi.org/10.1182/asheducation-2010.1.281.

77. Opelz G, Döhler B. Lymphomas after solid organ transplantation a collaborative transplant study report. Am J Transplant 2003;4:222–30.

78. Heslop HE. How I treat EBV lymphoproliferation. Blood 2009;114:4002–8.

79. Abbas F, Kossi ME, Kim JJ, et al. Thrombotic microangiopathy after renal transplantation: current insights in de novo and recurrent disease. World J Transplant 2018;8(5):122–41.

80. Satoskar AA, Pelletier R, Adams P, et al. De novo thrombotic microangiopathy in renal allograft biopsies-role of antibody-mediated rejection. Am J Transplant 2010;10:1804–11.

81. Reynolds JC, Agodoa LY, Yuan CM, et al. Thrombotic microangiopathy after renal transplantation in the United States. Am J Kidney Dis 2003;42:1058–68.

82. Garg N, Rennke HG, Pavlakis M, et al. De novo thrombotic microangiopathy after kidney transplantation. Transplant Rev (Orlando) 2018;32:58–68.

83. Karthikeyan V, Parasuraman R, Shah V, et al. Outcome of plasma exchange therapy in thrombotic microangiopathy after renal transplantation. Am J Transplant 2003;3:1289–94.

84. Karras A, Thervet E, Legendre C. Hemophagocytic syndrome in renal transplant recipients: report of 17 cases and review of literature. Transplantation 2004;77(2):238–43.

85. Bia M. Evaluation and management of bone disease and fractures post transplant. Transplant Rev 2008;22:52–61.

86. Sessa A, Esposito A, Iavicoli GD, et al. Immunosuppressive agents and bone disease in renal transplant patients with hypercalcemia. Transplant Proc 2010;42(4):1148–55.

87. Naylor KL, Jamal SA, Zou G, et al. Fracture incidence in adult kidney transplant recipients. Transplantation 2016;100(1):167–75.

88. Grotz W, Breitenfeldt K, Cybulla M. Immunosuppression and skeletal disorders. Transplant Proc 2001;33:992–3.

89. Collini A, De Bartolomeis C, Barni R, et al. Calcineurin-inhibitor induced pain syndrome after organ transplantation. Kidney Int 2006;70(7):1367–70.

90. Harris AD, Fleming B, Bromberg JS, et al. Surgical site infection after renal transplantation. Infect Control Hosp Epidemiol 2015;36(4):417–23.

91. Menezes FG, Wey SB, Peres CA, et al. Risk factors for surgical site infection in kidney transplant recipients. Infect Control Hosp Epidemiol 2008;29(8):771–3.

92. Waldman M, Kopp JB. Parvovirus-B19-associated complications in renal transplant recipients. Nat Clin Pract Nephrol 2007;3(10):540–50.

93. Lee CH, Kim GH. Electrolyte and acid-base disturbances induced by calcineurin inhibitors. Electrolyte Blood Press 2007;5(2):126–30.

94. McNicholas BA, Pham MH, Carli K, et al. Treatment of hyperkalemia with a low-dose insulin protocol is effective and results in reduced hypoglycemia. Kidney Int Rep 2018;3(2):328–36.

95. Pirenne J, Lledo-Garcia E, Benedetti E, et al. Colon perforation after renal transplantation a single-institution review. Clin Transplant 1997;11(2):88–93.

96. Canet E, Zafrani L, Azoulay É. The critically ill kidney transplant recipient: a narrative review. Chest 2016;149:1546–55.

97. De Carvalho MA, Freitas FG, Silva Junior HT, et al. Mortality predictors in renal transplant recipients with severe sepsis and septic shock. PLoS One 2014;9: e111610.

98. Canet E, Osman D, Lambert J, et al. Acute respiratory failure in kidney transplant recipients: a multicenter study. Crit Care 2011;15:R91.

99. Darmon M, Canet E, Osterman M. Ten tips to manage renal transplant recipients. Intensive Care Med 2019;45(3):380–3.

Evaluation and Management of Urinary Tract Infection in the Emergency Department

Sarah B. Dubbs, MD*, Sarah K. Sommerkamp, MD, RDMS

KEYWORDS

- Urinary tract infection • Asymptomatic bacteriuria • Cystitis • Pyelonephritis
- Renal abscess • Catheter-associated urinary tract infection

KEY POINTS

- Uncomplicated cystitis, a common infection in nonpregnant women, is frequently treated with an oral antibiotic such as nitrofurantoin.
- Pyelonephritis is an infection of the upper urinary tract. Antibiotic coverage must penetrate the renal parenchyma. Patients can be treated with fluoroquinolones with or without an additional dose of intravenous cephalosporin or aminoglycoside.
- Severe infections of the urinary tract include renal and perirenal abscess and emphysematous pyelonephritis. Treatment begins with intravenous antibiotics and general resuscitation measures, but patients might require percutaneous drainage or even nephrectomy.
- Antibiotic choice should consider bacterial susceptibilities and, when unavailable, local antibiograms.
- Special populations (pregnant women, geriatric and pediatric patients, patients with spinal cord injuries, and renal transplant patients) are more complicated and require increased attentiveness in their emergency department evaluation.

INTRODUCTION

Genitourinary infections are common among emergency department patients and stem from a large spectrum of pathologic sources, causing conditions ranging from the relatively benign and easily treatable to those that threaten fertility and life.

Disclosure Statement: The authors have no relationship with a commercial company that has a direct financial interest in subject matter or materials discussed in this article or with a company making a competing product.
Department of Emergency Medicine, University of Maryland School of Medicine, 110 South Paca Street, 6th Floor, Suite 200, Baltimore, MD 21201, USA
* Corresponding author.
E-mail address: sdubbs@som.umaryland.edu

Emerg Med Clin N Am 37 (2019) 707–723
https://doi.org/10.1016/j.emc.2019.07.007
emed.theclinics.com

Many of these topics are the focus of other articles in this issue, but this article focuses on the urinary tract. It is important to note that symptoms can overlap, so the astute clinician must consider other diagnoses. Urinary tract infections (UTIs) account for about 8 million visits in outpatient settings, at a cost of $1.5 billion each year.[1,2] UTIs occur most frequently in women. They tend to be uncomplicated and can be treated with oral antibiotics; however, they can progress to involve the upper tract, leading to sepsis and other complications. When they occur in men and in special populations, treatment becomes more complex. Antibiotic resistance also complicates treatment strategies.

DEFINITIONS

The term urinary tract infection refers to an inflammatory response of the urothelium to pathogenic microorganisms within the urinary tract. Pyuria is the presence of white blood cells (WBCs) in the urine, indicating an inflammatory response. Bacteriuria is the presence of bacteria in the urine, traditionally defined as at least 10^5 cfu/mL on culture, but a positive result on dipstick is also widely accepted as functionally equivalent.

Anatomically, UTIs can be divided into lower and upper tract infections. Lower tract infections involve the bladder (cystitis) and urethra (urethritis). An upper tract infection involves the renal parenchyma and collecting system and is referred to as pyelonephritis. UTIs can be further categorized as simple or complicated. Simple UTIs, also referred to as uncomplicated UTIs, occur in young, healthy, nonpregnant women with normal anatomy.[3] Complicated UTIs are associated with involvement of the upper urinary tract; male anatomy; pregnancy; anatomic abnormalities; urolithiasis; the presence of catheters, stents, or tubes; malignancy, chemotherapy, and immunosuppression; failure of antibiotics; and hospital or health care exposure (**Box 1**).[4] They can be caused by drug-resistant organisms and are more likely to require long antibiotic courses or parenteral antibiotics. Asymptomatic bacteriuria occurs in a patient with no symptoms of UTI but significant bacteria cultured from the urine.

Box 1
Definition of complicated urinary tract infection

Male

Pregnancy

Urolithiasis

Structural abnormalities of the genitourinary tract (vesicoureteral reflux, stricture, neurogenic bladder)

Catheters or stents

Failure of antibiotics outpatient

Hospital-associated UTI

Immunocompromised

Malignancy

From Long B, Koyfman A. The emergency department diagnosis and treatment of UTI. Emerg Med Clin North Am 2018;36:685-710.

PATHOPHYSIOLOGY

In the nondiseased state, urine is sterile along the urinary tract, from the renal glomerulus to the external sphincter in males and to the bladder neck in females.[5] The main mechanism by which the tract maintains sterility is the constant unobstructed forward flow of urine, essentially flushing the system. Other mechanisms that have a significant role in preventing UTI include urine acidity, immunologic defenses, and mucosal barriers.[6]

Abnormalities in the anatomy, structure, or function of the urinary tract disrupt this flow, leading to a compromise in sterility and possibly to infection. One of the most common anatomic abnormalities predisposing patients to UTI is incompetence of the ureterovesical valve, which causes vesicoureteral reflux (VUR). VUR is present in approximately one-third of children younger than 24 months who present with febrile UTI.[7] VUR can also occur in patients with neurogenic bladder caused by spinal cord injuries and in patients who have undergone urologic surgery. Other anatomic abnormalities, including congenitally acquired urethral valves and bladder diverticulum, can predispose patients to UTI.

Structural abnormalities can impede urine flow from inside or outside the urinary tract. Calculi within the urinary tract, associated with UTI, carry significant morbidity and mortality.[8] Masses or tumors originating from the structures of the urinary tract itself or extrinsic to the tract (such as from the gastrointestinal tract or gynecologic structures) can obstruct urinary flow. For men, prostatic hypertrophy is a common cause of obstruction, as is urethral stricture. In women, fibroids, a large pregnant uterus, or, later in life, uterine prolapse or cystocele, can obstruct urinary flow.

Dysfunction in bladder emptying contributes to urinary stasis and infection. Neurogenic bladder caused by spinal cord injury is a prime example. Urinary retention can also be caused by a host of pharmacologic agents, including anticholinergics, antihistamines, antipsychotics, antidepressants, antiparkinsonian agents, sympathomimetics, and muscle relaxers.[9]

Finally, another risk factor for UTI is instrumentation anywhere along the system. Urethral catheterization is most common and has been recognized for decades as the single most important predisposing factor in nosocomial UTIs.[10] Cystoscopy or transurethral surgery of any kind, especially involving placement of stents or lysis of calculi, also puts patients at higher risk for UTI.

When urinary flow is reduced or when the urinary tract undergoes instrumentation, bacteria that colonize the area around the urethral opening can enter the collection system and ascend, causing infection. In male patients, the normal flora at the distal end of the urethra includes staphylococci, streptococci, and diphtheroid organisms. In female patients, the urethra opens into the perineum, which is colonized by *Escherichia coli* and other colonic organisms. The female urethra is short, making it easy for pathogens to ascend to the bladder.

Rarely, UTIs occur via hematogenous or lymphatic spread from adjacent infections, but these routes do not play a significant role in the most UTIs (**Fig. 1**).

The most common causative organism for UTI is *E coli*, which is responsible for more than 80% of acute community-acquired uncomplicated infections, followed by *Staphylococcus saprophyticus*, accounting for 10% to 15% of UTIs.[11] Other common community-acquired urinary pathogens include *Proteus, Klebsiella*, and *Escherichia faecalis*. Nosocomial urinary tract infections are commonly caused by *E coli, Klebsiella, Enterobacter, Citrobacter, Serratia, Pseudomonas, E faecalis, Staphylococcus,* and *Candida*.[12]

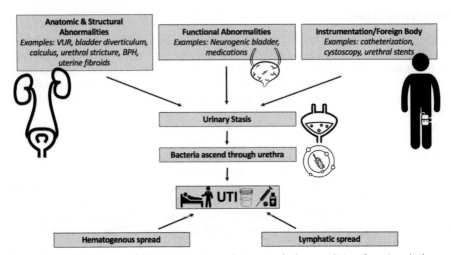

Fig. 1. Pathophysiology of UTI. Anatomic and structural abnormalities, functional abnormalities, and instrumentation or foreign bodies contribute to urinary stasis, allowing bacteria to ascend through the urethra to cause infection of the urinary tract. Rarely, UTI can be caused by hematogenous or lymphatic spread of bacteria.

CLINICAL FEATURES

A quality history and physical examination are crucial for detecting and differentiating UTIs as well as complications and life-threatening mimics.

Symptoms and Signs

Cystitis typically presents with dysuria, increased urinary frequency, odor, and suprapubic pain. Additional symptoms of fever, vomiting, and flank or back pain developing a few days after the start of the symptoms suggest pyelonephritis. As the severity of the infection progresses, the patient might experience dizziness, hypotension, and altered mental status. A thorough history will help to distinguish a UTI from its mimics (**Box 2**).[4]

Physical Examination

A genital examination should be completed most patients to allow identification of groin/genital processes that can present with similar symptoms, such as vulvovaginal candidiasis, sexually transmitted infections (STIs), torsion, and even Fournier gangrene. Tenderness to percussion at the costovertebral angle (CVA) is commonly used as an indication of pyelonephritis. Patients with renal or perinephric abscess may also display CVA tenderness on examination. UTI is a frequent cause of sepsis. The astute clinician should monitor vital signs and be observant for systemic inflammatory response syndrome (SIRS) criteria.

DIAGNOSIS
Laboratory Analysis

After the history and physical examination, laboratory testing is the third pillar in diagnosing UTI. A presumptive diagnosis is made by urinalysis and can be confirmed by urine culture. It is important to note that false-negative urinalysis and culture are possible, especially in early infection or when the quantity of bacteria or WBCs is low

---

Box 2
Common and life-threatening mimics of urinary tract infection

Bacterial vaginosis

Sexually transmitted disease/cervicitis/urethritis

Pelvic inflammatory disease and tubo-ovarian abscess

Epididymitis/orchitis

Testicular torsion/ovarian torsion

Ectopic pregnancy

Necrotizing soft tissue infection

Cholecystitis

Urolithiasis

Renal abscess, infarction, or thromboembolism

Appendicitis

Sepsis/pneumonia

Abdominal aortic aneurysm

Data from Long B, Koyfman A. The emergency department diagnosis and treatment of UTI. Emerg Med Clin North Am 2018;36:685-710.

---

or diluted. False-positive urinalysis and cultures can occur as well. Diagnostic uncertainty is caused by contamination of the specimen during collection. The presence of epithelial cells on analysis suggests a contaminated sample. The clean catch method for obtaining voided specimens is the most common method of sample collection. It involves cleaning the periurethral area with a sterile wipe and collection of mid-stream urine with the foreskin retracted in uncircumcised males or the labia fully separated in females. In patients who are unable to provide a satisfactory voided sample, urethral catheterization can be established, with either a single intermittent catheter or an indwelling catheter, if indicated. Care must be taken during catheterization, as it is possible for bacteria to be introduced into the urinary system during the placement process. Suprapubic aspiration is invasive and painful and thus is used infrequently. It is generally reserved for patients with urinary retention and inability to pass a catheter through the urethra. It is the catheterization method least likely to cause sample contamination, yielding the most accurate urinalysis and culture results.[13]

Urine dipstick testing is the most common initial step in urine laboratory testing. It can be used in combination with microscopic urine evaluation. The dipstick uses color change to indicate the presence of leukocyte esterase, nitrite, urobilinogen, protein, blood, ketones, bilirubin, and glucose and indicates a range of pH and specific gravity. In case of suspected UTI, the most useful dipstick results are leukocyte esterase and nitrite. Leukocyte esterase is a marker for WBCs in the urine; however, it does not exclude WBCs from a vaginal source, for example, Therefore, results might be falsely positive. The sensitivity of leukocyte esterase alone for UTI is between 59% and 96%. These results can also be altered by a high glucose or protein concentration, the use of glucocorticoids, and viral illness. Nitrite positivity is highly sensitive at 95% to 98%.[14] A major limitation of its use is its higher false-negative rate. False-negative results occur when the UTI is caused by non-nitrate-reducing organisms (*S saprophyticus, Pseudomonas*, or enterococci). The most specific finding is a specimen that is, positive for both leukocyte esterase and nitrite: the specificity improves to 98% to 100%, but the sensitivity declines to 35% to 84%.[14]

Microscopic evaluation should follow positive results of a urine dipstick and involves direct visualization under a microscope to count red and WBCs, bacteria, and epithelial cells. This type of evaluation helps the provider determine if the specimen is contaminated with epithelial cells (ie, was poorly collected). It also provides information about the relative number of WBCs. Hematuria and pyuria are often indicators of an inflammatory response, but bleeding from other causes (eg, vaginal bleeding or bleeding from bladder or renal masses) may cause red blood cells and WBCs to show up in the urine also. The absolute number of white cells seen in a sample with limited epithelial cells is helpful in the diagnosis of UTI. Typically, a count higher than 10 leukocytes/mm^3 correlates with bacterial concentrations of 10^5 cfu/mL, high enough to meet the definition of UTI on culture.[14]

Urine culture is not routinely requested for patients with simple UTI, and culture results are rarely available in real time to influence therapeutic decisions for a new UTI. Diagnostic and treatment decisions are made based on the presence of clinical symptoms plus a urine dip with or without microscopic evaluation. There is, however, a place for urine culture in the emergency department. In patients who are ill appearing or have a complex UTI, culture data are critical for narrowing the antibiotic regimen. The definition of positive urine culture depends on the route of collection and the presence of symptoms. A suprapubic specimen should be considered positive with essentially any bacteria present. A catheterized specimen may be considered positive as low as 10^2 cfu/mL if a single uropathogen is identified, and the patient has clear symptoms. The generally accepted definition of a positive culture in noncatheterized samples is 10^5 cfu/mL, although data support a threshold of 10^2 cfu/mL of a known uropathogen in patients who have dysuria and frequency.[15]

Diagnostic Imaging

Diagnostic imaging for UTI in adults is usually not necessary, unless there is concern about an alternative diagnosis such as the mimics discussed previously or a complication. Radiographs have the benefit of minimizing the patient's radiation exposure compared with other modalities, but they have low sensitivity for the abnormalities of the genitourinary system. In contrast, computed tomography (CT) is frequently used for evaluation of patients with a complicated UTI. It can show renal stones with or without associated hydroureter and hydronephrosis, abscess, vascular issues and other surgical mimics, necrotizing infections, abdominal aortic aneurysm, cholecystitis, or appendicitis. CT use should be limited because of the radiation exposure. Ultrasound is another diagnostic option, and it is ideal because it does not involve radiation. It is the test of choice for identifying pelvic pathology, pregnancy, torsion, and tubo-ovarian abscess (TOA). Ultrasound provides visualization of the kidneys and pathology such as hydronephrosis, abscess, and edema/stranding.

MANAGEMENT
Asymptomatic Bacteriuria

In asymptomatic bacteriuria, the patient has bacteria in the urine but no symptoms of UTI. The quantitative definition of asymptomatic bacteriuria requires a clean, midstream catch with culture results showing a quantitative count of at least 10^5 cfu/mL of a single bacterial species (in a single specimen for male patients or 2 consecutive specimens yielding the same species for female patients) or a catheterized specimen with at least 10^2 cfu/mL.[16,17] Of course, emergency medicine physicians do not routinely request urine cultures for asymptomatic patients. Patients may have had a culture obtained previously. However, frequently the results are not known during an index visit to the emergency department. The emergency physician must entertain the diagnosis of asymptomatic bacteriuria when bacteria are visualized on the microscopic portion of urinalysis. Nonpregnant patients with asymptomatic bacteriuria are typically not treated, because they often clear the bacteria without antimicrobials.[18] Pregnant women, however, are treated for 3 to 7 days to decrease the risk of preterm birth, low-weight birth, and progression to pyelonephritis.[17]

General Principles of Antimicrobial Management

The goal of treatment is to eliminate the pathogen from the urine, so antimicrobial agents are key. Two main factors are important in antimicrobial selection. First, the pathogen must be susceptible to the antimicrobial, and, second, the antimicrobial must become concentrated in the urine at a level high enough to be effective against that pathogen (above the minimal inhibitory concentration [MIC]). Fortunately, the level of many antibiotics in the urine is often hundreds of times higher than in the serum, so an inhibitory level can be achieved with oral dosing of many commonly used antimicrobial agents (except macrolides).[13] Therefore, the serum concentration of the antimicrobial is not important in cases of simple, uncomplicated cystitis. In contrast, it is critical for patients with complicating factors such as bacteremia, fever, or infections involving the renal or prostatic parenchyma. In patients with renal insufficiency, whether acute or chronic, dosage adjustments may be required for antimicrobials that are cleared primarily by the kidneys. Patients with end-stage renal failure cannot concentrate antimicrobials effectively in the urine, so eradication of urine pathogens is challenging. Finally, because urinary tract obstruction can affect antimicrobial concentration in the urine, the obstruction should always be addressed as early as possible.

Antibiotic resistance has led to difficulty in treating common illnesses such as UTIs, which is a concern for the individual being treated and for the public. The US Centers for Disease Control and Prevention (CDC) and other major organizations strongly recommend improving antibiotic stewardship.[19] The emergency physician is in a difficult position when treating bacterial infections. Urine culture results are rarely available during the emergency department evaluation, so antibiotics must be started empirically. The ideal situation is treatment that is individually tailored to the sensitivity of the pathogen that is present. When urine culture results are available, they should be used to guide treatment. When culture results are not available, the hospital antibiogram should be used to determine resistance patterns and guide antibiotic selection. There is not a standardized method of collecting information for an antibiogram, so it may be prudent to become familiar with the local antibiogram, specifically ascertaining if it includes inpatient, outpatient, and intensive care unit specimens or if it represents only outpatient or emergency department patients, who tend to have greater sensitivity to antibiotics.[20]

Uncomplicated Cystitis

The most common presentation of UTI is uncomplicated cystitis. It occurs in premenopausal, nonpregnant women who have no other anatomic genitourinary tract abnormalities. Approximately 50% of women experience uncomplicated UTI in their lifetime.[19] By definition, uncomplicated cystitis is a superficial infection of the bladder mucosa; therefore, systemic symptoms such as fever, chills, and vomiting should not be present. Patients might have suprapubic tenderness but should otherwise have an unremarkable examination.

Most uncomplicated cystitis cases are caused by E coli. The second most common cause is S saprophyticus, and the remaining but less common causes are Klebsiella, Proteus, and Enterococcus.[11]

As discussed previously, in a symptomatic patient, urinalysis showing microscopic bacteriuria and pyuria, with or without hematuria, is sufficient to make a presumptive diagnosis of UTI. Dipstick tests for bacteria (as indicated by the presence of nitrite) and WBCs (as indicated by the presence of leukocyte esterase) are more cost- and time-efficient, but they are slightly less sensitive than microscopic urine evaluation. Urine culture is not necessary in most cases of uncomplicated cystitis.

Oral antimicrobials are preferred in the treatment of uncomplicated cystitis. Nitrofurantoin is effective, well tolerated, and relatively inexpensive. Trimethoprim (TMP) and trimethoprim-sulfamethoxazole (TMP-SMX) are also well tolerated, require a short course of only 3 days, and are inexpensive. These agents are recommended as first-line therapy, as long as local E coli resistance rates are less than 20%.[21] Fluoroquinolones such as ciprofloxacin and levofloxacin are falling out of favor because of the increasing resistance to them as well as their adverse side-effect profiles. They are now used only as second-line alternatives in the treatment of uncomplicated cystitis. Fosfomycin trometamol, given in a single 3 g oral dose, is much more expensive that the aforementioned agents, but it might provide a cost savings in some situations if lack of compliance with a multiday regimen would cause recidivism due to worsening illness. Pivmecillinam is an oral antimicrobial that is available in parts of Europe, but not yet in the United States. It is an extended-spectrum penicillin with good activity against bacteria with extended-spectrum beta-lactamase (ESBL) activity and has minimal effect on intestinal and vaginal flora,[22] potentially decreasing rates of selection for antibiotic-resistant organisms. Despite their advantages, fosfomycin and pivmecillinam have decreased efficacy compared with nitrofurantoin, TMP, TMP-SMX, and fluoroquinolones.[21] Other alternative antibiotic regimens for uncomplicated UTI are penicillins and cephalosporins. Antibiotic regimens for uncomplicated cystitis are summarized in **Box 3**.

Patients with uncomplicated cystitis do not require admission to the hospital. They can be discharged home on an oral antibiotic regimen.

Pyelonephritis

Pyelonephritis is a bacterial infection of the kidney parenchyma. Most cases occur by ascension of bacteria through the urinary tract, beginning as cystitis. Few cases are caused by hematogenous spread and are associated with virulent organisms such as S aureus, P aeruginosa, Salmonella, and Candida.[23] Patients with acute pyelonephritis classically present with fever, flank pain, and vomiting associated with tenderness at the costovertebral angle and laboratory diagnosis of urinary infection. It is important to note that the urine sample might not show signs of inflammation or infection if the ureter draining the infected kidney is obstructed or if the kidney infection is outside the collecting system.

The Infectious Diseases Society of America (IDSA) recommends that urine cultures with susceptibility testing be obtained for all patients with acute pyelonephritis.[21] Blood cultures should be requested for patients who appear severely ill. Up to 25% of female patients with acute uncomplicated pyelonephritis have positive blood cultures,[24] but it is rare for the results of these cultures to alter management. Diagnostic imaging should be considered, especially if there is concern for stone or other obstruction, abscess, emphysematous pyelonephritis, mass, or other UTI mimics.

Box 3
Empiric antibiotic regimens for uncomplicated urinary tract infection

Nitrofurantoin monohydrate	100 mg	Twice daily	5 d	First line, well tolerated, inexpensive.
TMP-SMX	160 mg/800 mg	Twice daily	3 d	First line if *E coli* resistance <20%, well-tolerated, inexpensive
Fluoroquinolones				Second line: falling out of favor because of increasing resistance and adverse side-effect profiles
Ciprofloxacin	500 mg	Twice daily	7 d	
Levofloxacin	750 mg	Once daily	5 d	
Fosfomycin trometamol	3 g		Once	More expensive, slightly lower efficacy than first-line agents, but may prevent recidivism
Amoxicillin-clavulanate	500 mg/125 mg	Twice daily	3–7 d	Alternative treatment when other agents cannot be used, lower efficacy
Cephalosporins				Alternative treatment when other agents cannot be used, lower efficacy
Cefdinir	300 mg	Twice daily	7 d	
Cefaclor	500 mg	3 times daily	7 d	
Cefpodoxime	100 mg	Twice daily	7 d	
Cefuroxime	250 mg	Twice daily	7–10 d	
Pivmecillinam	400 mg	Twice daily	4–7 d	Availability limited to only some European countries

For patients with acute pyelonephritis not complicated by abscess, calculi, or other factors, the mainstay of treatment is antibiotics and supportive care. Antipyretics and antiemetics are helpful to control symptoms. Intravenous fluids may be administered if the patient is dehydrated as a result of vomiting or poor oral intake.

Antimicrobials initiated in the emergency department should include coverage against *E coli*, which accounts for the majority of cases. Coverage against more virulent or resistant organisms should be considered in patients with recurrent UTIs, indwelling urinary catheters, or a history of instrumentation. If vomiting is controlled, and the concern for bacteremia is low, outpatient treatment with oral medications is appropriate. In areas where uropathogen resistance to fluoroquinolones is less than 10%, ciprofloxacin or levofloxacin is recommended. It is common for patients to receive an intravenous dose of ceftriaxone or aminoglycoside during their emergency department stay, even if they are being discharged with a prescription for an oral fluoroquinolone. In areas where local uropathogen resistance to fluoroquinolones exceeds 10%, this parenteral regimen is actually recommended by the IDSA, to be administered in the emergency department before the patient is discharged on the fluoroquinolone. The same single-dose parenteral antibiotic regimen is recommended if TMP-SMX or beta-lactams, both second-line agents, are chosen for empiric treatment. Oral beta-lactams such as cefpodoxime are considered second-line treatment for pyelonephritis, because, even when the cultured pathogen is susceptible, treatment failure rates are high. Fosfomycin and nitrofurantoin, although effective for cystitis, are not effective for pyelonephritis, because they are mainly concentrated in the bladder.[21,25,26] Treatment choices, dosing, and duration of treatment are summarized in **Box 3**.

Indications for admission and inpatient management of patients with acute pyelonephritis include uncontrolled vomiting, signs of SIRS/sepsis, pregnancy, male anatomy, renal transplant, and other complicating factors such as the presence of calculi, ureteral stents/drains, and indwelling catheters. These patients should be initiated on intravenous antibiotics. Regimens may include fluoroquinolones, aminoglycoside with or without ampicillin, extended-spectrum cephalosporin or extended-spectrum penicillin with or without aminoglycoside, or a carbapenem. The treatment choice should be based on local resistance patterns.[21] Choices, dosing, and duration for inpatient treatment of pyelonephritis are summarized in **Box 4**.

Emphysematous Pyelonephritis

Emphysematous pyelonephritis is a urologic emergency. Gas-forming pathogens cause a severe necrotizing infection of the renal parenchyma and perirenal space. This infection typically occurs in diabetic patients, and it is hypothesized that the high glucose levels in their tissues provide a substrate and favorable environment for *E coli*, which ferments the sugar and produces carbon dioxide. Many patients with emphysematous pyelonephritis have significant renal dysfunction or urinary obstruction from calculi or papillary necrosis. This urologic emergency carries a high mortality rate, ranging from 19% to 43%.[27,28]

Patients with emphysematous pyelonephritis are at the severe end of the clinical pyelonephritis spectrum. Diagnosis is confirmed with imaging, typically CT scan of the abdomen and pelvis.

Box 4
Empiric antibiotic regimens for pyelonephritis

Outpatient Empiric Treatment

Ciprofloxacin[a]	500 mg	Oral	Twice daily	7 d
Levofloxacin[a]	750 mg	Oral	Once daily	5–7 d
Cefpodoxime	200 mg	Oral	Twice daily	10–14 d
TMP-SMX	160–800 mg (double-strength)	Oral	Twice daily	10–14 d
Ceftriaxone	1 g	Intramuscularly or intravenously	Once	
Gentamycin	5 mg/kg	Intramuscularly or intravenously	Once	
Ciprofloxacin	400 mg	Intravenously	Once	

Inpatient Empiric Treatment

Ciprofloxacin	400 mg	Intravenously	Every 12 h	
Levofloxacin	500 mg	Intravenously	Every 24 h	
Ceftriaxone	1 g	Intravenously	Every 24 h	+/− aminoglycoside (eg, gentamicin)
Gentamicin	5 mg/kg	Intravenously	Every 24 h	+/− ampicillin 2 g intravenously every 4 hours
Tobramycin	5 mg/kg	Intravenously	Every 24 h	+/− ampicillin 2 g intravenously every 4 hours
Piparacillin/ tazobactam	3.375 g	Intravenously	Every 6 h	+/− aminoglycoside (eg, gentamicin)
Meropenem	2 g	Intravenously	Every 8 h	

[a] Consider initial dose of parenteral agent if fluoroquinolone resistance is >10%, or if using second-line agent (beta-lactam such as cefpodoxime or TMP-SMX).

Prompt urology consultation, administration of intravenous broad-spectrum antibiotics, and fluid resuscitation are the keys in emergency department management of these patients. If urinary obstruction is present, percutaneous catheter drainage must be done as soon as possible, usually by an interventional radiologist. In the past, definitive treatment involved nephrectomy after resuscitation and stabilization; however, modern treatment tends toward a more conservative approach of percutaneous drainage and medical management with antibiotics.[29] In severe cases, nephrectomy may be required.

Renal Abscess and Perinephric Abscess

Renal abscesses are purulent infectious collections confined to the renal parenchyma. They occur most often in patients with renal disease or urinary obstruction and are typically caused by gram-negative organisms. Perinephric abscess results either from rupture of a cortical abscess into the perinephric space, or, less frequently, hematogenous seeding from other sites of infection. Renal abscess and perinephric abscess should be suspected in patients who are not improving after receiving appropriate antimicrobial therapy for pyelonephritis. CT is the imaging modality of choice, although larger abscesses can be visualized on ultrasound. The major advantage to CT is the ability to visualize calculi and other causes of obstruction that could have contributed to development of the abscess.

Classically, treatment of renal abscess calls for open or percutaneous drainage, but there is evidence supporting noninvasive treatment with antibiotics and observation for small abscesses (3 to 5 cm) in hemodynamically stable patients.[30–33] Antibiotic choice, as with pyelonephritis, should be directed toward gram-negative organisms, guided by local resistance patterns. *Staphylococcus* coverage may be considered if hematogenous dissemination is suspected (ie, endocarditis, skin abscess or cellulitis, or in-dwelling lines).

Small perinephric abscesses (<3 cm) can be treated nonsurgically as well.[34,35] Perinephric abscesses larger than 3 cm should be drained percutaneously or surgically as early as possible for infectious source control. Some patients will eventually require nephrectomy.

Urolithiasis

The relationship between urolithiasis and infection is complex. Traditionally, it was thought that the stones were a consequence of the infection. Certain bacteria, such as urease-producing *Proteus*, promote an environment for crystals to precipitate and form calculi. The relationship is now known to be more complex, with some infections occurring as a consequence of obstruction from the stone.[8,36,37] Whatever its origin, UTI in the setting of urolithiasis is a complex condition that warrants careful management and urologic consultation. Urinalysis results should be given special attention in patients presenting with suspected urolithiasis, looking beyond hematuria for signs of infection. Abrahamian and colleagues[38] found that a WBC count greater than 5/hpf was 86% sensitive and 79% specific for UTI confirmed by culture in the setting of nephrolithiasis. WBC count greater than 20/hpf was even more specific for UTI, at 93%. Patients in this case series were more likely to be female and to present with fever, chills, dysuria, and urinary frequency.[38] Antimicrobials should be initiated promptly. If hydronephrosis or an obstructive stone is present, intervention is necessary to mitigate worsening or life-threatening illness. Patients with UTI and a nonobstructing stone may be treated in the outpatient setting, given the availability of close outpatient follow-up with urology.[38]

Acute Bacterial Prostatitis

Acute bacterial prostatitis presents with constitutional symptoms of fever, chills, and malaise, as well as dysuria or other urinary symptoms and perineal or rectal pain. It is commonly associated with urinary retention, or it can occur after instrumentation such as cystoscopy or prostate biopsy. A digital prostate examination can reveal exquisite prostate tenderness. This manipulation of the prostate should be avoided in febrile, neutropenic, or ill-appearing patients. Imaging of the prostate is generally not necessary for the diagnosis but should be obtained if abscess or an alternative diagnosis in the differential is suspected. Treatment includes antibiotics and relief of urinary obstruction, if present, with a drainage catheter and/or alpha-blockers. Prostate abscess requires drainage, because medical management is often unsuccessful.[39,40]

Catheter-Associated Urinary Tract Infection

Catheter-associated UTIs (CAUTIs) are the fourth most common health care-associated infection.[41,42] Bacteriuria has an incidence of 10% per day of indwelling catheterization. For intermittent catheterization, bacteriuria occurs at a rate of 1% to 3% each time a patient is catheterized. The urinary catheter system provides an environment that promotes the growth of bacterial biofilms. *Pseudomonas* and *Proteus* are especially amenable to this environment, and, in addition to *E coli* and *Enterococcus,* contribute to a large percentage of CAUTIs. Most patients with bacteriuria are asymptomatic,[43] but those with active infection can present with fever, suprapubic tenderness, CVA tenderness, altered mental status, or hypotension. Therefore, only symptomatic catheter-associated bacteriuria should be treated. Criteria for CAUTI vary across the IDSA, CDC, and other guiding organizations and are heavily based on culture results, which is not helpful in the emergency department. However, studies have suggested that certain urinalysis findings indicate CAUTI, which is more helpful when making an empiric diagnosis in the emergency department. The presence of pyuria and a WBC count greater than 5/hpf has been found to have 90% specificity based on cultures with greater than 10^5 cfu/mL.[44] Another study found the presence of leukocyte esterase to have a sensitivity of 87.5% and the presence of nitrite to be 100% specific in CAUTI.[45] When CAUTI is suspected, urine cultures should be requested, and antibiotics should be started promptly. The catheter should be replaced or removed, as it is likely to be colonized with the offending microorganism, and encrustation of the biofilm can shelter the bacteria from exposure to the antimicrobial medication.

URINARY TRACT INFECTIONS IN SPECIAL POPULATIONS
Asymptomatic Bacteriuria and Urinary Tract Infection During Pregnancy

Bacteriuria in pregnant women, even when asymptomatic, has been associated with complications such as maternal sepsis, premature birth, and low birth weight and therefore should always be treated with antimicrobials. Pyelonephritis develops in up to 30% of pregnant women with untreated bacteriuria.[46,47] Aminopenicillins and cephalosporins are considered safe and generally effective in pregnant patients with asymptomatic bacteriuria. Nitrofurantoin is effective but should be avoided in patients with G6PD, as well as in the first trimester of pregnancy, because of possible linkage to birth defects. It is otherwise approved by the American College of Obstetrics and Gynecology (ACOG) for use in pregnant women in the second and third trimesters, given that they do not have G6PD. Nitrofurantoin may be used in the first trimester if no other agent is available to treat an infection.[48] ACOG notes that penicillins, erythromycin, and cephalosporins have not been found to increase the risk of birth defects and are therefore preferred agents when appropriate.[48]

Pregnant patients with pyelonephritis are at high risk for maternal and fetal complications. They require prompt obstetric consultation, parenteral antibiotics, and admission to the hospital.

Bacteriuria and Urinary Tract Infection in the Elderly

Diagnosis of UTI in the geriatric population is challenging. Traditional UTI symptoms might be absent or might not be communicated if the history is limited. Concomitant disease can mask or mimic UTI. Pyuria alone is not a good predictor of urine infection in the elderly.[49] Nitrite positivity in addition to pyuria and bacteriuria suggests active infection, although it should be understood that not all uropathogenic organisms produce nitrite. In terms of ruling out UTI, negative results for leukocyte esterase and nitrite on dipstick are reliable.[50,51] When urinalysis findings are equivocal in an elderly patient presenting with vague symptoms such as altered mental status or frequent falls, alternative diagnoses should be sought.

When evidence of a UTI warrants treatment, antibiotic choice should always be made with extra caution in the elderly population. More complicated UTIs with associated complications such as altered mental status and sepsis require parenteral antibiotics. For select patients who may be discharged home, oral antibiotics must also be chosen carefully. Nitrofurantoin, usually a first-line agent, must be avoided in patients with renal insufficiency, as decreased renal excretion causes inadequate urine concentration. This increases the possibility for toxicity, and further decreases the chance of the antibiotic to be effective, because urine levels are below the minimum inhibitory concentration. Previous data supported avoidance of nitrofurantoin in patients with creatinine clearance of less than 60 mL/min, but more recent data support using the drug in patients with creatinine clearance of 40 mL/min or higher.[52]

Urinary Tract Infection in Patients with Spinal Cord Injury

UTI is common in patients with spinal cord injury (SCI) and is the most common cause of fever in this population.[53] SCI patients have many characteristics that place them at high risk for UTI, including impaired bladder emptying, instrumentation/catheterization, decreased fluid intake, decubitus ulcers, and reduced host defenses from chronic illness. Patients with SCI usually do not experience the classic UTI symptoms of dysuria, frequency, or urgency because of their loss of sensation. They more often present with vague abdominal discomfort, spasticity, fatigue, fever, or cloudy or malodorous urine. Only 20% of UTIs in SCI patients are caused by *E coli*. Enterococci, *P mirabilis*, and *Pseudomonas* are more common in this patient population. Additionally, SCI patients are more likely to have polymicrobial UTIs.[54–56] They also demonstrate a high rate of antimicrobial resistance.[57] Typical antibiotic regimens for UTI in SCI patients include aminoglycoside plus a penicillin or a third-generation cephalosporin; however, previous culture data must be considered to screen for a history of resistant organisms.

Other Special Populations

Evaluation and management of UTI in the pediatric as well as renal transplant populations are complex as well. These topics are discussed in their respective sections of this edition of *Emergency Medicine Clinics*.

SUMMARY

UTI affects patients of all ages and is a diagnosis that an emergency physician might make multiple times per shift. The range of presentations and severity span the gamut of routine run-of-the-mill to roller-coaster resuscitation. It is essential for emergency physicians to combine a thorough history, physical examination, and selective diagnostic testing for accurate diagnosis. Fluency in the interpretation of urine tests is imperative. Appropriate antibiotic selection requires emergency physicians to be knowledgeable about the resistance patterns of uropathogens in their own hospitals and emergency departments. Special populations require adjustments in diagnosis, treatment, and antibiotic choice. A deep understanding of this subject is guaranteed to be practical and valuable in the daily clinical decision making of any emergency physician's practice.

ACKNOWLEDGMENTS

The authors would like to thank Linda J. Kesselring, MS, ELS, for copy editing this article.

REFERENCES

1. Stamm WE. Scientific and clinical challenges in the management of urinary tract infections. Am J Med 2002;113(suppl 1A):1S–4S.
2. Lingenfelter E, Drapkin Z, Fritz K, et al. ED pharmacist monitoring of provider antibiotic selection aids appropriate treatment for outpatient UTI. Am J Emerg Med 2016;34:1600–3.
3. David RD, DeBlieux PMC, Press R. Rational antibiotic treatment of outpatient genitourinary infections in a changing environment. Am J Med 2005;118(7A):7S–13S.
4. Long B, Koyfman A. The emergency department diagnosis and treatment of UTI. Emerg Med Clin North Am 2018;36:685–710.
5. Ban KM, Easter JS. Selected urologic problems. In: Marx JA, Rosen P, editors. Rosen's emergency medicine: concepts and clinical practice. 8th edition. Philadelphia: Elsevier/Saunders; 2014. p. 1326–54.
6. Abraham SN, Miao Y. The nature of immune responses to urinary tract infections. Nat Rev Immunol 2015;15(10):655–63.
7. Hoberman A, Charron M, Hickey RW, et al. Imaging studies after a first febrile urinary tract infection in young children. N Engl J Med 2003;348:195–202.
8. Borghi L, Nouvenne A, Meschi T. Nephrolithiasis and urinary tract infections: 'the chicken or the egg' dilemma? Nephrol Dial Transplant 2012;27:3982–4.
9. Serlin DC, Heidelbaugh JJ, Stoffel JT. Urinary retention in adults: evaluation and management. Am Fam Phys 2018;98(8):496–503.
10. Madsen PO, Larsen EH, Dorflinger T. Infectious complications after instrumentation of urinary tract. Urology 1985;26(1 suppl):15–7.
11. Ronald A. The etiology of urinary tract infection: traditional and emerging pathogens. Am J Med 2002;113(suppl 1A):14S–9S.
12. Guentzel MN. Escherichia, Klebsiella, Enterobacter, Serratia, Citrobacter, and Proteus. In: Baron S, editor. Medical microbiology. 4th edition. Galveston (TX): University of Texas Medical Branch at Galveston; 1996 [Chapter 26]. Available at: https://www.ncbi.nlm.nih.gov/books/NBK8035/.
13. Schaeffer AJ, Matulewicz RS, Klumpp DJ. Infections of the urinary tract. In: Wein AJ, Kavoussi LR, Partin AW, et al, editors. Campbell-Walsh urology. 11th edition. Philadelphia: Elsevier; 2016. p. 237–303.
14. Lane D, Takhar S. Diagnosis and management of UTI and pyelonephritis. Emerg Med Clin North Am 2011;29:539–52.

15. Stamm WE, Hooton TM. Management of urinary tract infections in adults. N Engl J Med 1993;329:1328–34.
16. Nicolle LE, Bradley S, Colgan R, et al, Infectious Diseases Society of America, American Society of Nephrology, American Geriatric Society. Infectious Diseases Society of America guidelines for the diagnosis and treatment of asymptomatic bacteriuria in adults. Clin Infect Dis 2005;40:643–54.
17. Colgan R, Nicolle LE, McGlone A, et al. Asymptomatic bacteriuria in adults. Am Fam Physician 2006;74:985–90.
18. Hooton TM, Scholes D, Stapleton AE, et al. A prospective study of asymptomatic bacteriuria in sexually active young women. N Engl J Med 2000;343:992–7.
19. Foxman B, Barlow R, D'Arcy H, et al. Urinary tract infection: self-reported incidence and associated costs. Ann Epidemiol 2000;10:509–15.
20. Grodin L, Conigliaro A, Lee SY, et al. Comparison of UTI antibiograms stratified by ED patient disposition. Am J Emerg Med 2017;35:1269–75.
21. Gupta K, Hooton TM, Naber KG, et al. International clinical practice guidelines for the treatment of acute uncomplicated cystitis and pyelonephritis in women: a 2010 update by the Infectious Diseases Society of America and the European Society for Microbiology and Infectious Diseases. Clin Infect Dis 2011;52:e103–20.
22. Dewar S, Reed LC, Koerner RJ. Emerging clinical role of pivmecillinam in the treatment of urinary tract infection in the context of multidrug-resistant bacteria. J Antimicrob Chemother 2014;69:303–8.
23. Bacterial urinary tract infections (UTIs). Imam T. Merck manual 2018. Available at: https://www.merckmanuals.com/professional/genitourinary-disorders/urinary-tract-infections-utis/bacterial-urinary-tract-infections-utis. Accessed January 2019.
24. Velasco M, Martinez JA, Moreno-Martinez A, et al. Blood cultures for women with uncomplicated acute pyelonephritis: are they necessary? Clin Infect Dis 2003;37:1127–30.
25. Warren JW, Abrutyn E, Hebel JR, et al. Guidelines for antimicrobial treatment of uncomplicated acute bacterial cystitis and acute pyelonephritis in women. Infectious Diseases Society of America (IDSA). Clin Infect Dis 1999;29:745–58.
26. Cronberg S, Banke S, Bergman B, et al. Fewer bacterial relapses after oral treatment with norfloxacin than with ceftibuten in acute pyelonephritis initially treated with intravenous cefuroxime. Scand J Infect Dis 2001;33:339–43.
27. Huang JJ, Tseng CC. Emphysematous pyelonephritis: clinicoradiological classification, management, prognosis, and pathogenesis. Arch Intern Med 2000;160:797–805.
28. Freiha F, Messing E, Gross D. Emphysematous pyelonephritis. J Contin Ed Urol 1979;18:9–19.
29. Lu YC, Chiang BJ, Pong YH, et al. Predictors of failure of conservative treatment among patients with emphysematous pyelonephritis. BMC Infect Dis 2014;14:418.
30. Hoverman IV, Gentry LO, Jones DW, et al. Intrarenal abscess: report of 14 cases. Arch Intern Med 1980;140:914–6.
31. Levin R, Burbige KA, Abramson S, et al. The diagnosis and management of renal inflammatory processes in children. J Urol 1984;132:718–21.
32. Shu T, Green JM, Orihuela E. Renal and perirenal abscesses in patients with otherwise anatomically normal urinary tracts. J Urol 2004;172:148–50.
33. Lee SH, Jung HJ, Mah SY, et al. Renal abscesses measuring 5 cm or less: outcome of medical treatment without therapeutic drainage. Yonsei Med J 2010;51:569–73.

34. Meng MV, Mario LA, McAninch JW. Current treatment and outcomes of perinephric abscesses. J Urol 2002;168:1337–40.
35. Siegel J, Smith A, Moldwin R. Minimally invasive treatment of renal abscess. J Urol 1996;155:52–5.
36. Melick RA, Henneman PH. Clinical and laboratory studies of 207 consecutive patients in a kidney stone clinic. N Engl J Med 1957;259:307–14.
37. Tavichakorntrakool R, Prasongwattana V, Sungkeeree S, et al. Extensive characterizations of bacteria isolated from catheterized urine and stone matrices in patients with nephrolithiasis. Nephrol Dial Transplant 2012;27:4125–30.
38. Abrahamian FM, Krishnadasan A, Mower WR, et al. Association of pyuria and clinical characteristics with the presence of urinary tract infection among patients with acute nephrolithiasis. Ann Emerg Med 2013;62(5):526–33.
39. Nickel JC. Inflammatory and pain conditions of the male genitourinary tract: prostatitis and related pain conditions, orchitis, and epididymitis. In: Wein AJ, Kavoussi LR, Partin AW, et al, editors. Campbell-Walsh urology. 11th edition. Philadelphia: Elsevier; 2016. p. 304–33.
40. Gill BC, Shoskes DA. Bacterial prostatitis. Curr Opin Infect Dis 2016;29(1): 86–91.
41. Magill SS, Edwards JR, Bamberg W, et al. Multistate point-prevalence survey of health care-associated infections, 2011. N Engl J Med 2014;370:1198–208.
42. Warren JW. Catheter-associated urinary tract infections. Infect Dis Clin North Am 1997;11:609–22.
43. Tambyah PA, Maki DG. Catheter-associated urinary tract infection is rarely symptomatic. Arch Intern Med 2000;160:678–87.
44. Tambyah PA, Maki DG. The relationship between pyuria and infection in patients with indwelling urinary catheters: a prospective study of 761 patients. Arch Intern Med 2000;160(5):673–7.
45. Lee SP, Vasilopoulos T, Gallagher TJ. Sensitivity and specificity of urinalysis samples in critically ill patients. Anaesthesiol Intensive Ther 2017;49(3):204–9.
46. Smaill FM, Vazquez JC. Antibiotics for asymptomatic bacteriuria in pregnancy. Cochrane Database Syst Rev 2015;(8):CD000490.
47. Whalley P. Bacteriuria of pregnancy. Am J Obstet Gynecol 1967;97:723–38.
48. Committee on Obstetric Practice. Committee Opinion No. 717. Sulfonamides, nitrofurantoin, and risk of birth defects. Obstet Gynecol 2017;130(3):e150–2.
49. Wagenlehner FM, Naber KG, Weidner W. Asymptomatic bacteriuria in elderly patients: significance and implications for treatment. Drugs Aging 2005;22(10): 801–7.
50. Ninan S, Walton C, Barlow G. Investigation of suspected urinary tract infection in older people. BMJ 2014;349:g4070.
51. Schulz L, Hoffman RJ, Pothof J, et al. Top ten myths regarding the diagnosis and treatment of urinary tract infections. J Emerg Med 2016;51(1):25–30.
52. Oplinger M, Andrews CO. Nitrofurantoin contraindications in patients with a creatinine clearance below 60mL/min: looking for the evidence. Ann Pharmacother 2013;47(1):106–11.
53. Beraldo PS, Neves EG, Alves CM, et al. Pyrexia in hospitalised spinal cord injury patients. Paraplegia 1993;31:186–91.
54. Edwards LE, Lock R, Powell C, et al. Post-catheterisation urethral strictures: a clinical and experimental study. Br J Urol 1983;55:53–6.
55. Monson T, Kunin CM. Evaluation of a polymer-coated indwelling catheter in prevention of infection. J Urol 1974;111:220–2.

56. Nickel JC, Olson ME, Costerton JW. In vivo coefficient of kinetic friction: study of urinary catheter biocompatibility. Urology 1987;29:501–3.
57. Patros C, Sabol M, Paniagua A, et al. Implementation and evaluation of an algorithm-based order set for the outpatient treatment of urinary tract infections in the spinal cord injury population in a VA Medical Center. J Spinal Cord Med 2018;41(2):192–8.

Sexually Transmitted Infections

Denise McCormack, MD, MPH[a],*, Kathryn Koons, MD[b]

KEYWORDS

- Sexually transmitted infections (STIs) • Sexually transmitted diseases
- Sexual assault • Postexposure prophylaxis (PEP)
- HIV pre-exposure prophylaxis (PREP)

KEY POINTS

- Gonorrhea and chlamydia are the most common sexually transmitted infections.
- Syphilis rates are increasing in the United States.
- Trichomonas is the most common parasitic sexually transmitted infection.
- SANE, SART, and SAFE are programs for the sexual assault patient.
- PEP consists of antiviral and antibiotic therapy and includes emergency contraception.

INTRODUCTION

The management of sexually transmitted infections (STIs) is primarily focused on detection, treatment, and prevention. STIs, though unlikely to be fatal in the acute phase, pose a significant public health threat to high-risk patient populations, making early detection essential. Most STIs have distinctive symptomatology, and physical examination findings lead to rapid diagnosis with clear treatment options. However, identifying patients who are at risk for STIs sometimes entails elaborate history-taking skills and lengthy discussions regarding prevention and safer sex practices. Furthermore, patients who are at high risk for contracting HIV or those who have been sexually assaulted require precise STI prevention and treatment plans with which emergency physicians (EPs) should become familiar. This article explores the most common STIs encountered in an emergency setting and discusses current recommendations for the care of 2 dynamic patient populations, patients who have been sexually assaulted and those who are candidates for HIV pre-exposure prophylaxis (PREP).

Disclosures: The authors have nothing to disclose.
[a] Department of Emergency Medicine, Albert Einstein College of Medicine, Jacobi Medical Center, 1400 Pelham Parkway South, Bronx, NY 10461, USA; [b] Jacobi-Montefiore Emergency Medicine Residency, 1400 Pelham Parkway South, Bronx, NY 10461, USA
* Corresponding author.
E-mail address: mccormad@nychhc.org

Emerg Med Clin N Am 37 (2019) 725–738
https://doi.org/10.1016/j.emc.2019.07.009
0733-8627/19/© 2019 Elsevier Inc. All rights reserved.

SEXUALLY TRANSMITTED INFECTIONS

The Centers for Disease Control and Prevention (CDC) estimate that annually there are about 2 million cases of chlamydia, gonorrhea, and syphilis in the United States.[1] The emergency department (ED) remains the forefront for identifying STIs and starting prompt treatment. Early detection is important not only for ameliorating the disease process in the patient but also for partners of those newly diagnosed. Effective detection based on examination findings and implementation of correct treatment regimens (**Table 1**) can potentially deter transmission and decrease overall STI occurrence.

The most common bacterial STIs in the United States are chlamydia and gonorrhea. Providers should also be aware of STIs such as syphilis, herpes, and trichomonas, which they are also likely to encounter in the ED. Although other STIs such as chancroid and lymphogranuloma venereum are not common in the United States, providers should also be knowledgable about these conditions.

Chlamydia

Chlamydia is the most common bacterial STI in the United States with an annual rate of 528.8 cases per 100,000 population.[1] Because of its high prevalence, the CDC recommends routine annual screening for sexually active women aged 25 years and younger and all men who have sex with men (MSM).[2] Chlamydia may be asymptomatic or can present as a range of symptoms, including dysuria, pelvic pain, vaginal

Table 1
Treatments for sexually transmitted infections

Sexually Transmitted Infections	Common Examination Findings	Recommended Treatment
Chlamydia	Dysuria Vaginal, penile, rectal discharge	Azithromycin 1000 mg once OR Doxycycline 100 mg 2×/day for 7 d
Gonorrhea	Dysuria Vaginal, penile, rectal discharge	Ceftriaxone 250 mg intramuscularly (IM) OR Cefixime 400 mg once
Primary syphilis Secondary syphilis Tertiary syphilis	Painless chancre Rash on palms and sole Condyloma lata Neurologic deficits Skin nodules "gummas"	Benzathine penicillin G 2.4 million units IM once
Genital herpes	Painful ulcerative lesions of mouth, anus, or genitalia	Acyclovir 400 mg 3×/day OR Valcyclovir 1 g 2×/day for 7–10 d
Trichomonas	Dysuria Vaginal discharge Cervical punctate hemorrhages	Metronidazole 2 g OR Tinidazole 2 g once
Chancroid	Painful genital ulcer Tender lymph nodes	Azithromycin 1 g once OR Ceftriaxone 250 mg IM
Lymphogranuloma venereum	Painful genital ulcers Inguinal lymphadenopathy Vaginal or penile lymphedema	Doxycycline 100 mg 2×/day OR Erythromycin 500 mg 4×/day for 21 d

discharge, rectal pain, or sore throat depending on the extent of infection and route of exposure. For female patients complaining of vaginal discharge or pelvic pain, EPs must suspect cervicitis or pelvic inflammatory disease (PID). In men with complaints of dysuria, a diagnosis of urethritis should be suspected, and for patients who engage in anoreceptive intercourse, rectal pain and/or discharge may be due to proctitis. Bacterial pharyngitis should be suspected when chlamydial infection is associated with sore throat. Some patients may present with systemic symptoms, such as fever and chills, especially if they have advanced PID with development of tubo-ovarian abscess.

The diagnosis is confirmed by conducting a NAAT (Nucleic Acid Amplification Test) on urine in either sex or by swabbing a sample from the cervix or vagina in women.[2,3] NAAT detects chlamydia trachomatis through amplification of RNA or DNA and is highly sensitive and specific for diagnosing the presence of infection. The test, however, is not approved for pharyngeal or rectal swabs by the Food and Drug Administration (FDA). The first-line treatment of chlamydia is azithromycin 1000 mg once or doxycycline 100 mg twice daily for 7 days, although erythromycin, levofloxacin, and ofloxacin are acceptable alternatives.[2] In addition, azithromycin is the first-line medication for chlamydia diagnosed during pregnancy. Patients should be counseled to abstain from sexual intercourse for 7 days after starting single-dose azithromycin or completing the 7-day course of doxycycline. Typically a test of cure is conducted for patients with questionable compliance and is performed 3 weeks after treatment. Patients should be tested again at 3 months to assess for reinfection by sexual partners, regardless of whether the partner was treated.[2]

Gonorrhea

Gonorrhea is the second most common bacterial STI, with an annual rate of 171.9 cases per 100,000 population.[1] The infection has a 7- to 14-day incubation period after exposure. Similarly to chlamydia, it is recommended by the CDC that annual screening for gonorrhea be done in women 25 years old and younger and all MSM.[2] Patients presenting to the ED with a localized infection may be asymptomatic, or complain of penile or vaginal discharge, pelvic pain, joint pain, sore throat, or rectal pain. Diagnoses that should be considered include urethritis, cervicitis, PID, septic arthritis, pharyngitis, and proctitis. Gonorrheal infection may also manifest as a systemic disseminated infection with findings of petechial or pustular skin lesions, polyarthralgia, tenosynovitis, perihepatitis (Fitz-Hugh-Curtis syndrome), endocarditis, or meningitis. To accurately diagnose gonorrhea, EPs can send NAAT analyses on urine samples in either sex and cervical or vaginal specimens in women.[2]

A one-time dose of ceftriaxone is recommended for gonorrhea treatment. At present, resistance to ceftriaxone is increasing and antibiotic resistance varies by region, but in the United States overall the intramuscular dose of 250 mg ceftriaxone cures up to 98% to 99% of uncomplicated infections. An oral dose of cefixime 400 mg is an alternative treatment if ceftriaxone is unavailable.[2] Disseminated infection requires intravenous ceftriaxone dosed as 1 g every 24 hours. In patients who report a penicillin allergy that did not involve Stevens-Johnson syndrome or anaphylaxis, the benefit of still giving ceftriaxone for treatment outweighs the risks. For patients who cannot tolerate ceftriaxone because of severe allergy, the CDC recommends 2 g of azithromycin administered once orally followed up by a confirmatory test of cure in 1 week.[2] Owing to high coinfection rates, patients with suspected or confirmed gonorrhea should be presumptively treated for chlamydial infection in the ED.[2,4,5] All patients should be instructed to abstain from sexual intercourse for 7 days after treatment and until all partners are treated.

Herpes Simplex Virus

Genital herpes is caused by herpes simplex virus (HSV), usually HSV-1 or HSV-2; however, not all individuals who have the virus express clinical manifestations of the infection. The HSV-2 serotype is associated with higher rates of genital outbreaks, viral shedding, and recurrence. The CDC estimates that there are 776,000 new cases of genital herpes diagnosed every year.[1] The typical presentation consists of painful genital ulcerations that may involve a single lesion or a coalescence of multiple ulcerative lesions in the mouth, anus, or genitalia in men or women. Some patients report the initial infection as the most painful and extensive. HSV can also be disseminated and present as encephalitis with altered mental status and neurologic symptoms, abdominal pain with severe hepatitis, or in the respiratory system as pneumonitis.

EPs can diagnose HSV by swabbing directly from a ruptured vesicle or mucocutaneous lesion and sending for NAAT analysis. Cell culture is not advised because it has a very low diagnostic sensitivity. HSV serologies indicate past exposure but are not specific for acute infection. Treatment should be given to all first-time outbreaks and may also be given as suppression therapy to patients with frequent recurrences and those with HIV infection.[2] HSV can be treated with acyclovir 400 mg orally 3 times a day, valcyclovir 1 g orally twice a day, or famciclovir 250 mg orally 3 times a day, all of which are given for 7 to 10 days.[2] Although valcyclovir is more convenient because of the decreased frequency of dosing, it was previously deemed to be more expensive for patients with limited insurance coverage. In pregnant patients, acyclovir is the first-line therapy for active HSV infection. For patients with disseminated HSV, intravenously antiviral therapy should be given, and admission to the hospital is warranted.[2]

Syphilis

The prevalence of syphilis has greatly increased in the United States over the past decade. More than 30,000 cases of syphilis were reported in 2017 with a rate of 9.5 cases per 100,000 population,[1] representing a 72% increase in incidence from 4 years prior. Syphilis is about 8 times more common in males and most common in the 20- to 29-year-old age range. It is caused by the spirochete *Treponema pallidum*, and transmission is thought to occur through sexual contact and exposure of genital ulcerations.

Syphilis is often called "The Great Imitator" because of the wide spectrum of presentations and symptoms seen with the infection. Primary syphilis presents as an isolated painless ulcer known as a chancre, which typically lasts 3 to 6 weeks. Secondary syphilis usually occurs 2 to 8 weeks after the initial chancre heals, and may present as a rash, typically erythematous involving the palms and soles. It can also involve wart-like skin lesions known as condyloma lata, lymphadenopathy, and mucocutaneous lesions.[1,2] Ultimately syphilis may become latent for 1 to 20 years after the secondary stage, leading to tertiary syphilis.

Tertiary syphilis may present with cardiac symptoms, skin nodules that ulcerate known as gummas, and permanent neurologic deficits. Neurosyphilis can occur during any stage of infection and may present as cranial nerve dysfunction, meningitis, stroke, or alterations in hearing or vision. Tabes dorsalis, which involves demyelination of the dorsal column nerves, can result in ataxia, decreased reflexes, abnormal proprioception, neuropathic pain, and paresis. Neurosyphilis typically occurs about 10 to 30 years after the initial infection.[1,2]

Establishing a diagnosis of syphilis will vary according to stage. In early primary syphilis, serologies will not yet be positive, and diagnosis is best made by dark-field examination of samples taken from the skin lesion or chancre. Diagnosis of secondary, latent, or tertiary syphilis requires both nontreponemal testing, such as rapid plasma reagin (RPR) or venereal disease research laboratory (VDRL), and treponemal fluorescent treponemal antibody absorbed (FTA-ABS) serologic tests to ensure adequate sensitivity and specificity.[2] Serologic tests will be falsely negative in primary syphilis and can be falsely positive in the setting of HIV, autoimmune disease, pregnancy, or other inflammatory conditions. To confirm a diagnosis of neurosyphilis, a cerebrospinal fluid sample should be sent for VDRL/RPR.

In the ED setting, screening for syphilis is typically done by sending VDRL or RPR. In the outpatient setting, VDRL/RPR titers can be trended to follow treatment response and should become negative 6 to 12 months after successful treatment.[2] However, 15% to 20% of patients will have persistently elevated titers despite successful treatment, which is referred to as exhibiting a serofast reaction. In this case, the decision to continue antibiotics is based on clinical evaluation and physician judgment.

Benzathine penicillin G is the mainstay of treatment for all stages of syphilis. Primary and secondary syphilis can be treated with a single intramuscular dose of 2.4 million units in adults.[2] Within 24 hours of starting treatment, some patients may experience fever and myalgias, known as the Jarisch-Herxheimer reaction, which is not life threatening.

Trichomonas

Trichomonas is the most prevalent parasitic STI diagnosed in the United States with an estimated prevalence of 2.3 million among women aged 14 to 49 years.[1] It is caused by a protozoan parasite called Trichomonas vaginalis. There is a disproportionately higher prevalence among African American female patients compared with Caucasian patients (13% vs 1.8%). The incubation time ranges from 3 to 28 days, and the infection may be asymptomatic in some women. Men may present with urethritis, epididymitis, or prostatitis, whereas women tend to present with vaginal discharge, dysuria, or vulvar irritation.[1,2]

On examination, women may exhibit inflamed vulvar mucosa and punctate cervical hemorrhages, described as a "strawberry cervix." The development of trichomonas is associated with a higher risk of HIV transmission and PID. NAAT is the most sensitive diagnostic test for the infection, but the diagnosis can also be made using a vaginal wet mount test or OSOM rapid test. The standard treatment is metronidazole 2 g or tinidazole 2 g once. Metronidazole 500 mg twice daily for 7 days is an acceptable alternative for treatment.[1,2]

Chancroid

Chancroid is a painful genital ulcerative condition that is caused by the bacterium Haemophilus ducreyi. The infection is typically endemic to Africa and the Caribbean, although relatively infrequent outbreaks in the United States have been reported.[1,2,6] There is no FDA-approved polymerase chain reaction test, and culture methods are unreliable; therefore, diagnosis is made based on physical examination and clinical suspicion when a patient is found to have painful genital ulcers with tender lymphadenopathy. As with other genital ulcers, chancroid increases the risk of HIV transmission, so these patients should be tested for other STIs, specifically HIV and syphilis. The first-line treatment of chancroid is azithromycin, although ceftriaxone, ciprofloxacin, and erythromycin are acceptable alternatives.[2,3] Patients should be advised that it may take up to 2 weeks for their ulcers to completely heal. Individuals with HIV/AIDS may require prolonged antibiotics because of their immunocompromised status.

Lymphogranuloma Venereum

Lymphogranuloma venereum (LGV) is predominantly prevalent in the tropics, mainly in Africa, Southeast Asia, India, the Caribbean, and South America. However, there have been occasional outbreaks in the United States, especially in high-risk populations. LGV is caused by *Chlamydia trachomatis* serovars L1, L2, and L3, and typically presents with inguinal lymphadenopathy, which is often unilateral.[2,7–9] Occasionally there is an isolated, transient genital ulcer or papule on examination. Infection transmitted by anal intercourse can result in proctocolitis, manifesting as symptoms of tenesmus, rectal discharge, fever, or constipation. If the infection extends into the lymphatic system, a late manifestation termed "esthiomene" can occur, which is elephantiasis of the female genitalia resulting from severe lymphedema. In men it can lead to penile and scrotal elephantiasis and an edematous deformed penis referred to as "saxophone" penis.[2,7–9] Examination findings for LGV classically involve inguinal edema and the appearance of second inguinal groove that is known as a groove sign. This can be complicated by ulcerations over the inguinal groove in combination with enlarged lymph nodes.

The diagnosis of LGV is made on the basis of history, examination, and swabbing open skin lesions and sending for NAAT to confirm the presence of LGV RNA or DNA. Treatment of LGV is doxycycline 100 mg twice a day or erythromycin 500 mg 4 times a day for 21 days.[2]

SEXUAL ASSAULT PATIENTS

The sexual assault victim represents a distinguishable category of ED patients. These patients not only require medical care for trauma and STI prophylaxis but also require forensics, social work, and intense psychological support. Currently the United States Department of Justice defines sexual assault as "the penetration, no matter how slight of the vagina or anus with any body part or object, or oral penetration by a sex organ of another person, without the consent of the victim." This definition is broad and encompasses a wide spectrum of unwanted sexual activity. It is estimated that nearly 18% to 19% of women and 2% to 3% of men have been the victims of sexual assault.[10–12] However, this incidence may be an underestimate because many victims often do not report their assaults for a variety of reasons including fear, shame, or stigma.

Patients who do present to the ED for sexual assault require multidisciplinary expertise and should be given an extensive amount of time for evaluation. The Sexual Assault Nurse Examiner (SANE), Sexual Assault Forensic Examiner (SAFE), and Sexual Assault Response/Resource Team (SART) are the most common specialized programs that address the medicolegal and social needs of sexual assault patients in a timely and efficient manner, in conjunction with the ED provider.[10–12] The SANE or SAFE is usually a clinician such as a nurse who is trained to perform a detailed examination focusing on sexual assault in addition to collecting key evidence using a rape kit. The SANE or SAFE belongs to a larger team commonly referred to as the SART, which includes a vast network of professionals such as social workers, patient advocates, law enforcement, and mental health providers. Depending on the region, sexual assault patients may be cared for by a SANE, SAFE, or SART, and these terms are often used interchangeably.

There are approximately 600 centers in the United States that have access to either SANE, SAFE, or SART, and most of these are associated with EDs in large medical centers.[13] Once a sexual assault victim arrives at one of these EDs, the specialized response team is made aware and arrives promptly to address the needs of the patient to ensure that they are given standardized exemplary care.

Team representatives administer superior care to sexual assault patients by coordinating care with social workers, patient advocates, and law enforcement, and providing follow-up for psychological support. In addition, they are responsible for conducting a forensic examination, rape kit collection, and sending blood and urine to the forensics laboratory using the chain-of-custody process. The protocols of SANE, SAFE, and SART are regional and state-specific but nevertheless, having these systems in place creates high standards of care for sexual assault patients nationwide. It is also important that these patients continue to be screened after discharge for depression, post-traumatic stress disorder (PTSD), pregnancy, and STIs that may have occurred because of the assault. The use of such programs nationwide facilitates follow-up of the sexual assault patient using a systematic approach that greatly extends beyond the initial ED encounter.

When a patient arrives at a facility that does not have access to a SANE, SAFE, or SART, the EP in accordance with EMTALA (Emergency Medical Treatment and Active Labor Act) should perform a medical screening examination, and arrangements can be made to transfer the patient to a designated facility with resources for sexual assault patients. Consultation regarding the initiation of PEP can be obtained through the National Clinician Postexposure Prophylaxis Hotline at (888) 448 to 4911 and any locally available resources.[11]

History

The history ascertained from the sexual assault patient varies considerably from the usual questions asked during an encounter for a medical complaint. For patients presenting to the ED after a sexual assault, it is crucial that specific questions are addressed in a compassionate and supportive manner (**Box 1**). Such questions should include information regarding the mechanism of the assault, whether objects were used to facilitate the assault, or if a drug-facilitated sexual assault (DFSA) is suspected.[14] DFSA may involve illicit drugs of abuse as well as the misuse of prescription drugs to incapacitate victims. Drugs such as ketamine, γ-hydroxybutyrate, and the potent benzodiazepine flunitrazepam, commonly referred to as "roofie," have all been associated with sexual assault.[15]

DFSA has also been reported with common over-the-counter medicine such as diphenhydramine and sleep aids that induce drowsiness and stupor. Likewise, the inconspicuous placement of Visine ophthalmic drops into a person's beverage has been implicated in DFSA. The drops contain the sedative tetrahydrozoline, which invokes symptoms ranging from somnolence to unconsciousness when ingested.[16] It

---

Box 1
History taking for sexual assault

- When did the assault take place?
- Who is the assailant? Was there more than one?
- Do you know the assailant's medical history?
- Did the assailant use objects during the assault?
- Was there oral, vaginal, or anal penetration?
- Did ejaculation take place?
- Was there an episode of amnesia, intoxication, or nakedness without explanation?
- Did you shower, change clothes, insert tampon, wipe or clean after the assault?

should be noted that the accuracy of the patient's account of events might be diminished owing to loss of memory if a DFSA has taken place. All blood and urine samples must be sent to a forensics laboratory using strict chain-of-custody protocols to ensure integrity of the specimens. In addition, because of the forensic nature of the history and examination, EPs should inquire about actions that might contaminate evidence, for example if the patient showered or changed clothing after the assault took place.

Examination

The physical examination of the sexual assault patient includes detection of injury and documentation of any type of trauma. Patients who have been sexually assaulted may arrive at the ED with significant traumatic injuries, depending on the mechanism of the assault. It is therefore important that patients be evaluated using the standardized approach for stabilization of any acute life-threatening injury. When feasible, providers should attempt to preserve forensic evidence when stabilizing medical and traumatic injuries. Once acute life-threatening injury is ruled out and/or the patient is stabilized, a thorough examination focused on detection of genitourinary trauma must take place. This entails conducting an examination that is usually performed by the SANE or SAFE in the ED within 72 to 96 hours of the assault for optimal detection of injury caused by sexual trauma. For all cases of sexual assault, consent for examination by the SANE or SAFE must be obtained. The examination focuses on the identification of not only gross trauma but also microtrauma, which may not be obvious using traditional examination techniques. When conducting an examination to detect injury, the TEARS pneumonic is recommended as a consistent method for documenting examination findings.[17]

The pneumonic represents:

- Tears, defined as any break in tissue such as a laceration, or any Tenderness
- Ecchymosis
- Abrasions
- Redness
- Swelling

In addition to using the TEARS pneumonic to provide information about sexual trauma, providers must also document the location, number, and size of injuries that are detected. Special techniques such as colposcopy, anoscopy, and application of toluidine blue dye can be used to enhance the detection of subtle injury. The use of colposcopy allows the examiner to assess a magnified view of the vagina and cervix to detect injuries that cannot be readily seen with the naked eye.[17] Anoscopy is done to assess anal trauma and aids in the collection of evidence, such as pooling of semen in the anal mucocutaneous junction. The application of toluidine blue dye is a technique used to illuminate microabrasions of the genitalia that occur from sexual trauma. The dye stains the deep portion of the epidermis and will aid in the visualization of small abrasions.[17] When toluidine blue dye is used for examination purposes, patients should be advised that after the examination is completed the dye might temporarily remain and inadvertently cause staining of the undergarments or clothing.

It must be noted that not all sexual assault patients display acute injury on the genitourinary examination. Certain characteristics such as anal trauma, assault within 24 hours of examination, and extremes of age, for example, younger than age 20 years or older than 49 years, have a higher correlation with detection of injury on examination.[17] Therefore, when performing an examination the absence of traumatic injury to the vagina and cervix does not conclusively exclude rape or sexual assault.

POSTEXPOSURE PROPHYLAXIS

It is imperative that victims of sexual assault receive postexposure prophylaxis (PEP) to cover gonorrhea, chlamydia, HIV, trichomonas, and hepatitis B. Administration of the human papilloma virus vaccine is indicated for female patients 9 to 26 years old and male patients 9 to 21 years old who are unvaccinated.[18] The recommendations for PEP in sexual assault patients are the same as those given to patients exposed to STIs arising from consensual unprotected intercourse (**Table 2**). Although it is not necessary to screen for STIs before starting prophylaxis, it is recommended that a complete blood count and complete metabolic panel be obtained to check liver and renal function when starting a patient on HIV PEP. Baseline screening for HIV, syphilis, active hepatitis B, or immunization status should also be performed, although if not readily available PEP should not be delayed for reasons of lack of testing or results.[18] Current recommendations for PEP are a 3- to 7-day regimen of tenofovir disoproxil fumarate-emtricitabine (TDF-FTC), also known as Truvada, plus raltegravir or dolutegravir, with scheduled follow-up to provide counseling and continuation of the regimen for up to 28 days. Ideally, HIV PEP should be initiated within 72 hours of the exposure to adequately limit transmission of the virus.[18]

Ceftriaxone 250 mg intramuscularly once and azithromycin 1000 mg by mouth once are adequate for the prevention of gonorrhea and chlamydia, respectively. Doxycycline 100 mg twice per day for 1 week can also be implemented against chlamydia, although it is contraindicated in pregnancy. A one-time dose of metronidazole 2 g should be administered to prevent trichomonas. Prophylaxis of hepatitis B is more complicated because it depends on the patient's immunization status. For patients who have received the vaccine and show documented immunity, no further invention is needed. However, vaccination with the hepatitis B vaccine is indicated when the perpetrator's status is unknown and the patient has never been vaccinated. When the perpetrator's status is hepatitis B positive and the sexual assault victim is unvaccinated, EPs must administer the hepatitis B vaccine plus hepatitis B Immunoglobulin.[18]

All victims of sexual assault should be offered emergency contraception (EC) in the ED. One option for EC is levonorgestrel 1.5 mg in a single dose administered in the ED.

Table 2
Postexposure prophylaxis

Infection	Prophylaxis
Chlamydia	Azithromycin 1000 mg once OR Doxycycline 100 mg 2×/day for 7 d
Gonorrhea	Ceftriaxone 250 mg intramuscularly OR Cefixime 400 mg once
Trichomonas	Metronidazole 2 g OR Tinidazole 2 g once
HIV	Tenofovir disoproxil fumarate-emtricitabine plus raltegravir or dolutegravir
Hepatitis B	Hepatitis B vaccine if patient not immunized
Pregnancy prevention	Levonorgestrel 1.5 mg once OR Ulipristal 30 mg

The single-dose regimen of levonorgestrel has the advantage of less nausea, although it is less effective in obese women and has decreased effectiveness after 72 hours.[19] Another option includes a combination of estrogen-progestin given in 2 doses 12 hours apart as 100 µg ethinyl estradiol and 0.50 mg levonorgestrel. The regimen is about 75% to 80% effective when administered within 72 hours of sexual intercourse but has the highest incidence of nausea and vomiting, which poses a significant disadvantage when compared with the other regimens.[19] The EC medication ulipristal (30 mg) has the advantage of preventing pregnancy up to 120 hours after intercourse and does not lose effectiveness in obese women. It is therefore the preferred EC for sexual assault patients when available.[20]

Follow-up appointments should be arranged through the SANE, SAFE, or SART for ongoing medical care for those who have received STI and HIV prophylaxis and EC after sexual assault. Most victims are followed up within 1 week. Importantly, victims of assault should be monitored for depression and PTSD after discharge and be provided with extensive psychosocial support as needed. ED practitioners taking care of the sexual assault patient should understand and use as many resources as possible to create a dynamic and supportive follow-up plan for all discharged sexual assault patients.

PRE-EXPOSURE PROPHYLAXIS FOR PREVENTION OF HIV

Each year in the United States there are approximately 40,000 new cases of HIV infection, making the disease a public health crisis and propelling new health initiatives focused on preventing transmission.[21] One of the most monumental health initiatives implemented to reduce the transmission of HIV among high-risk individuals has been the introduction of PREP, which was approved in 2012 by the FDA.[21,22] Before the advent of PREP, public health interventions to prevent HIV transmission were centered on safer sex practices, initiatives for HIV screening to know one's status, and needle exchange programs for those engaging in intravenous drug use (IVDU). PREP therefore remains a groundbreaking strategy to prevent the spread of HIV among individuals who are considered at high risk and often encountered in the ED for various health reasons.

PREP consists of a single daily tablet of the antiretroviral therapy tenofovir disoproxil fumarate (TDF) 300 mg plus emtricitabine 200 mg (FTC), known commercially as Truvada. The combination therapy when taken daily with high compliance has been shown to significantly decrease the chances of contracting the disease from an HIV-positive partner by almost 90% in several key studies.[21,22] The TDF-FTC regimen is dispersed in a 90-day supply, with repeat HIV testing occurring at the end of each 90-day medication cycle. The daily PREP dose is continued indefinitely as long as high-risk behavior persists. Most HIV-uninfected patients obtain a PREP prescription either from a primary care physician or specialized infectious disease clinic.

Patient Selection for Pre-exposure Prophylaxis

Although most high-risk individuals obtain PREP in the primary care setting, EPs are situated on the front line for diagnosing new cases of HIV as well as identifying patients who would benefit from using PREP, based on current guidelines and increased risk of HIV acquisition. The CDC recommends PREP be offered to 4 categories of high-risk individuals[22]:

- Adult MSM
- Heterosexual men and women who have a substantial risk of acquiring HIV
- Adults with active IVDU
- Heterosexual men and women who engage in sexual activity with partners known to be HIV-positive

In the ED, identifying these patients is not always a simple task, and many times a very detailed sexual and social history is mandatory for detecting patients who would benefit from taking daily PREP. Specific questions designed to facilitate discussion regarding sexual practices and high-risk behaviors during the patient-provider encounter are essential (**Box 2**). The answers to these questions provide a framework for determining whether an uninfected patient is at high risk for contracting HIV and whether a referral to initiate PREP therapy is needed.

In addition to asking questions in a standardized unbiased format, an EP might identify high-risk patients when they present with genitourinary symptoms including vaginal or penile discharge, pain or rash, or an asymptomatic exposure to any STI. Patients with a new diagnosis of genital herpes, chlamydia, gonorrhea, or syphilis are considered at high risk for contracting HIV and should be tested for the virus expeditiously. It is strongly suggested that these patients also be offered information about PREP.

Obtaining an adequate social history in all patients to detect active substance abuse is also essential for identifying patients with risk factors for HIV. Occasionally patients present to the ED with complaints and symptoms related to a substance abuse-related condition. During these patient encounters, it is commonplace for ED providers to address high-risk behaviors such as IVDU. The risk of HIV acquisition during IVDU is substantially high owing to the use of contaminated needles, as well as concurrent high-risk sexual practices that may take place from impaired judgment. Similar to questions that assess for high-risk sexual activity, the CDC recommends that specific questions (**Box 3**) be asked during the patient-provider encounter to ascertain prior and current IVDU activity.[21,22]

Contraindications

PREP is thought to be a well-tolerated daily medication regimen; however, there are patients who are not ideal candidates for PREP because of their underlying medical conditions. The most common mild side effects of PREP include nausea, rash, and headache. Active hepatitis B and/or C should be tested for in all patients who are candidates for PREP therapy. Initiating PREP in patients with hepatitis C is contraindicated because of the deleterious drug interactions that occur between TDF-FTC and hepatitis C antiviral regimens. These patients should be evaluated by a hepatologist to determine whether PREP would be harmful or beneficial to the patient.[23] However, since TDF-FTC single-dose daily therapy is efficacious against hepatitis B, patients with acute or chronic hepatitis B are prime candidates for receiving the PREP protocol. Studies have shown that PREP has renal toxicity and adversely affects bone health. It is thereby contraindicated in patients with osteoporosis and those with kidney disease, defined as a creatinine clearance of less than 60 mL/min.[21,22]

Box 2
Questions for assessment of high-risk sexual behavior

In the past 6 months:
- Have you had sex with men, women, or both?
- How many men or women have you had sex with?
- How many times did you have vaginal or anal sex when neither you nor your partner wore a condom?
- How many of your sex partners were HIV-positive?
- If any of your sex partners were HIV-positive, how many times did you have vaginal or anal sex without a condom?

> **Box 3**
> **Questions for assessment of substance abuse behavior**
>
> - Have you ever injected drugs that were not prescribed to you by a physician?
> - If yes, when did you last inject unprescribed drugs?
> - In the past 6 months, have you injected by using needles, syringes, or other drug preparation equipment that had already been used by another person?
> - In the past 6 months, have you been in a methadone or other medication-based treatment program?

There is currently no specific age cutoff for PREP; however, the CDC recommends PREP in adults aged 18 years and older and, likewise, daily TDF-FTC single-dose therapy is only approved by the FDA for adults. It is estimated that approximately 1.2 million adults aged 18 to 59 years have benefited from PREP therapy to date. For older adults aged 60 years and older, there are limited data to strongly support or oppose the use of PREP. In patients younger than 18 years, PREP remains controversial because of issues with parental consent as well as potential health risks of PREP, which may have a considerable impact when initiated at a younger age. It is recommended that adolescents who engage in high-risk sexual activity or IVDU be assessed for PREP on a case-by-case basis using a benefit-versus-risk approach, owing to potential side effects of renal toxicity and decreased bone mineral density. Pregnancy is not a definitive contraindication to PREP, although to date there are no well-established studies that analyze safety and risk for HIV transmission when PREP is given during pregnancy. Therefore, pregnant women are offered PREP based on an individualized assessment by their obstetricians and primary care providers.[21,22]

As public health campaigns regarding the use of PREP continue to expand regionally and nationally, routine questions and discussions surrounding PREP may become more frequent during ED encounters. It is recommended that all ED providers have a sufficient understanding of PREP therapy and the patient demographic that it most benefits. Recommending PREP to a high-risk individual should supplement routine counseling to encourage consistent condom use, referrals to substance abuse treatment centers, or local syringe programs. In addition, it should be emphasized to patients that daily PREP therapy reduces the risk of HIV transmission but does not completely eradicate the risk even with perfect compliance. Although PREP is currently not prescribed in the ED, it is suggested that ED practitioners refer high-risk individuals to local designated clinics. Further studies are needed to determine whether it is feasible for ED providers to prescribe PREP to high-risk patients as common practice. In the future, starting PREP in the ED could significantly decrease HIV prevalence and have a profound impact on high-risk communities.

SUMMARY

The growing rates of STIs continue to be a public health dilemma, and the ED remains a prime setting to combat this growing issue. Helping to identify and treat patients with signs and symptoms of STIs helps the individual patients and their partners, and may even decrease the occurrences of local epidemics. This is important for all STIs, and especially HIV and syphilis, which can have debilitating long-term impacts on patients and high-risk communities.

Prophylaxis after exposure to STIs resulting from either consensual sexual intercourse or sexual assault allows significant reduction in infectious disease transmission, namely the prevention of chlamydia, gonorrhea, trichomonas, and HIV. Furthermore, these patients have options for efficacious EC. For sexual assault patients, programs such as SANE, SAFE, and SART help patients navigate the medicolegal and psychological effects of sexual trauma. Working with these specialized programs in the ED requires patience and expertise. Most importantly, this special group of patients always requires multidisciplinary follow-up.

Lastly, the prevention of HIV transmission is a top public health priority, especially in high-risk communities such as MSM, those with active IVDU, and uninfected patients with an HIV-positive partner. HIV PREP is a novel concept with noteworthy potential. Identifying suitable candidates for HIV PREP is not always easy, and having a detailed understanding of risk factors, the medication regimen, and contraindications will facilitate the process of referring patients for PREP.

For all the aforementioned patient groups, the key components of excellent management in the emergent setting will always consist of obtaining a satisfactory history, performing an astute physical examination, and implementing the most up-to-date correct medical treatment with standard follow-up.

REFERENCES

1. Centers for Disease Control and Prevention. Sexually transmitted disease surveillance 2017. Atlanta (GA): U.S. Department of Health and Human Services; 2018.
2. Workowski KA, Bolan GA, Centers for Disease Control and Prevention. Sexually transmitted diseases treatment guidelines, 2015. MMWR Recomm Rep 2015; 64(RR-03):1–137.
3. Centers for Disease Control and Prevention. Recommendations for the laboratory-based detection of Chlamydia trachomatis and Neisseria gonorrhoeae—2014.Centers for Disease Control and Prevention. MMWR Recomm Rep 2014; 63(RR-02):1–19.
4. Dicker LW, Mosure DJ, Berman SM, et al. Gonorrhea prevalence and coinfection with chlamydia in women in the United States, 2000. Sex Transm Dis 2003;30(5):472–6.
5. Datta SD, Sternberg M, Johnson RE, et al. Gonorrhea and chlamydia in the United States among persons 14 to 39 years of age, 1999 to 2002. Ann Intern Med 2007;147(2):89–96.
6. Romero L, Huerfano C, Grillo-Ardila CF. Macrolides for treatment of Haemophilus ducreyi infection in sexually active adults. Cochrane Database Syst Rev 2017;(12):CD012492.
7. Stoner BP, Cohen SE. Lymphogranuloma venereum 2015: clinical presentation, diagnosis, and treatment. Clin Infect Dis 2015;61(suppl_8):S865–73.
8. Gupta G, Achar DR, Bhandari B. Lymphogranuloma venereum: saxophone penis with bilateral groove sign. Med J DY Patil Univ 2013;6:490–1.
9. Aggarwal K, Jain VK, Gupta S. Bilateral groove sign with penoscrotal elephantiasis. Sex Transm Infect 2002;78:458.
10. Vrees RA. Evaluation and management of female victims of sexual assault. Obstet Gynecol Surv 2017;72:39.
11. Linden JA. Clinical practice. Care of the adult patient after sexual assault. N Engl J Med 2011;365:834.
12. Ciancone AC, Wilson C, Collette R, et al. Sexual assault nurse examiner programs in the United States. Ann Emerg Med 2000;35:353.
13. Sande MK, Broderick KB, Moreira ME, et al. Sexual assault training in emergency medicine residencies: a survey of program directors. West J Emerg Med 2013; 14(5):461–6.

14. Moreno-Walton L. Chapter 293: Female and male sexual assault. In: Tintinalli JE, Stapczynski JS, Ma OJ, et al, editors. Tintinalli's emergency medicine: a comprehensive study guide. 8th edition. New York: McGraw-Hill; 2015. p. 1983–7.
15. Smith KM, Larive LL, Romanelli F. Club drugs: methylenedioxy-methamphetamine, flunitrazepam, ketamine hydrochloride, and gamma-hydroxybutyrate. Am J Health Syst Pharm 2002;59(11):1067–76.
16. Spiller HA, Rogers J, Sawyer TS, et al. Drug facilitated sexual assault using an over-the-counter ocular solution containing tetrahydrozoline (Visine). Leg Med 2007;9:192–5.
17. White C. Genital injuries in adults. Best Pract Res Clin Obstet Gynaecol 2013;27: 113–30.
18. Dominguez K, Smith DK, Vasavi T, et al, Centers for Disease Control and Prevention. Updated guidelines for antiretroviral postexposure prophylaxis after sexual, injection drug use, or other nonoccupational exposure to HIV—United States. Atlanta (GA): CDC; 2016.
19. Cheng L, Che Y, Gülmezoglu AM. Interventions for emergency contraception. Cochrane Database Syst Rev 2012;(8):CD001324.
20. Glasier AF, Cameron ST, Fine PM, et al. Ulipristal acetate versus levonorgestrel for emergency contraception: a randomised non-inferiority trial and meta-analysis. Lancet 2010;375:555.
21. Riddell J, Amico R, Mayer K. HIV preexposure prophylaxis, a review. JAMA 2018; 319(12):1261–8.
22. Centers for Disease Control and Prevention, US Public Health Service. Preexposure prophylaxis for the prevention of HIV infection in the United States—2017 update: a clinical practice guideline. Atlanta (GA): CDC; 2018.
23. AASLD/IDSA HCV Guidance Panel. Hepatitis C guidance: AASLD-IDSA recommendations for testing, managing, and treating adults infected with hepatitis C virus. Hepatology 2015;62:932–54.

Pediatric Genitourinary Infections and Other Considerations

Kathleen Stephanos, MD[a],*, Andrew F. Bragg, MD[b]

KEYWORDS

- Pediatric • Urinary tract infection • Genital trauma • Dysuria • Sexual abuse

KEY POINTS

- The clinical presentation, diagnostic workup, and management of urinary tract infections varies depending on the patient's age.
- All neonates presenting with urinary tract infection are treated as pyelonephritis and should receive broad-spectrum parenteral antibiotics while undergoing thorough infectious workup including blood cultures and inpatient observation.
- Although urologic imaging is recommended for all children presenting with a first urinary tract infection, this should not be performed during the acute infection due to a high rate of false positives.
- Although many genitourinary conditions are managed similarly in adults and children, particular consideration should be given to causes and management of prepubertal vaginal bleeding, management of the circumcised and uncircumcised penis, genital trauma, and the diagnosis of prepubertal ovarian torsion.
- Any concerning history or examination findings should prompt a complete evaluation for sexual abuse, while using caution in eliciting the history as well as with detailed documentation.

PEDIATRIC GENITOURINARY INFECTIONS
Urinary Tract Infections

Urinary tract infection (UTI) is a relatively common diagnosis among infants and children presenting to emergency departments, but the clinical presentation may be nonspecific and the appropriate management depends heavily on the patient's age. In neonates, any UTI should be managed with broad-spectrum antibiotics and inpatient admission for additional sepsis workup. Among infants and young children, all

Disclosure Statement: The authors have nothing to disclose.
[a] Department of Emergency Medicine, University of Rochester, 601 Elmwood Avenue Box 655, Rochester, NY 14642, USA; [b] Department of Pediatrics, University of Rochester, 601 Elmwood Avenue Box 655, Rochester, NY 14642, USA
* Corresponding author.
E-mail address: Kathleen_stephanos@urmc.rochester.edu

Emerg Med Clin N Am 37 (2019) 739–754
https://doi.org/10.1016/j.emc.2019.07.010
0733-8627/19/© 2019 Elsevier Inc. All rights reserved.
emed.theclinics.com

UTIs should be treated as pyelonephritis to reduce the risk of long-term renal injury. In adolescents presenting with UTI symptoms, clinicians should take a thorough social history and test for sexually transmitted infections as appropriate. When treating UTI in any age group, clinicians should consult their local antibiogram, as emerging antibiotic resistance has rendered many first-line antibiotics ineffective against common uropathogens.

Epidemiology and microbiology

Neonates UTI is a relatively common source of neonatal sepsis, and is present in 13% to 15% of term neonates (<30 days) presenting with fever.[1,2] Although there are no reliable data on preterm neonates in the outpatient setting, some intensive care unit (ICU) studies suggest that preterm neonates and those with extremely low birth weight (<1000 g) are at even higher risk for UTI.[3,4] Sex differences in this age group are not straightforward and are skewed by rates of circumcision within the population. Among febrile neonates, uncircumcised boys have the highest risk of UTI (20%), followed by girls (7%–8%), with circumcised boys having the lowest risk (2%–3%).[5]

Infants and toddlers Infants and young children presenting with fever have approximately 8% prevalence of UTI across all patients, although this varies widely by population. Girls remain at higher risk than boys, whereas uncircumcised boys are at a 4 to 10 times higher risk than their circumcised peers.[5,6] Regardless of sex, African American children have consistently been shown to have significantly lower rates of UTI than other races, although the reasons for this are not well understood.[5–7]

School age children and adolescents Pediatric UTI incidence decreases steadily with age, with school-aged children and adolescents representing the lowest-risk group.[5] Although female individuals remain at higher risk than male individuals at any age, the difference between circumcised and uncircumcised male individuals is much less pronounced after age 2[5,7] (**Table 1**). African American children continue to be at lower risk than Hispanic or White children throughout childhood.[7] A special consideration among adolescent girls is the onset of sexual activity, which increases risk for both UTI[7,8] and some UTI mimics, such as *Neisseria gonorrhoeae* and *Chlamydia trachomatis* urethritis.

Table 1 Risk factors for pediatric urinary tract infection		
Demographic	**Medical History**	**Presenting Illness**
• Younger age • Female sex • Uncircumcised boys • Non-Black race	• Premature birth • Genitourinary abnormalities • Chronic constipation • Immunocompromised • Sexually active	• Temperature max ≥39°C • Fever >48 h • No other source of fever

Data from Shaikh N, Morone NE, Bost JE, et al. Prevalence of urinary tract infection in childhood: a meta-analysis. Pediatr Infect Dis J. 2008; 27(4):302-8 and Shaikh N, Morone NE, Lopez J, et al. Does this child have a urinary tract infection? JAMA. 2007;298(24): 2895.

Microbiology The microbiology of pediatric UTI is remarkably consistent across age groups. *Escherichia coli* is by far the most prolific uropathogen, accounting for 70% to 90% of culture-proven UTIs in all age groups.[9,10] Other common uropathogens include *Klebsiella*, *Proteus*, *Enterococcus*, *Enterobacter*, and coagulase-negative Staphylococci (ie, *Staphylococcus saprophyticus*).[1,3,9,10] Fungal UTI, typically caused by *Candida* species, usually affects only premature neonates, immunocompromised children, and those with indwelling urinary catheters.[1,9] In sexually active adolescents presenting with typical UTI symptoms, clinicians also should consider urethritis caused by *N gonorrhoeae* and *C trachomatis*, which may be clinically indistinguishable from other UTIs but will not be detected by standard urine cultures.

Clinical evaluation

Neonates The diagnosis of UTI in neonates is particularly challenging, primarily because of varied and nonspecific presenting symptoms. Although fever is the most common symptom, it is present in fewer than 50% of culture-proven UTIs.[8] Other common symptoms include poor feeding, irritability, lethargy, vomiting, and tachypnea.[8,9] New onset of jaundice after the first week of life also should prompt evaluation for UTI, as 7% to 12% of new-onset neonatal jaundice is related to cholestasis secondary to UTI.[9,10] It is also important to bear in mind that positive viral testing (eg, influenza, respiratory syncytial virus) is NOT adequate to rule out UTI in a febrile or ill-appearing neonate, as a significant percentage of these children will have a concurrent bacterial infection.[11]

When evaluating potential UTI in neonates, sterile urine culture obtained by catheterization or suprapubic aspiration is considered the gold standard.[12] Although urinalysis (UA) is a useful adjunct if positive, it lacks the sensitivity to definitively rule out UTI in neonates. In one prospective study of 4100 neonates undergoing UTI evaluation, a normal UA (defined by absence of pyuria, leukocyte esterase, and nitrites) was present in 5% to 13% of culture-proven UTIs.[12]

Infants and toddlers In children younger than 2, it is important to recognize that pyelonephritis is generally indistinguishable from uncomplicated cystitis due to nonspecific symptoms and inability of very young children to describe their symptoms. Important historical elements in an infant or young child with suspected UTI include the duration of symptoms, history of vesicoureteral reflux or other urologic abnormality, new onset of back or abdominal pain, and typical urinary symptoms such as dysuria or incontinence in a toilet-trained child. Parental reporting of dark or foul-smelling urine may be weakly predictive of UTI,[13] but is not reliable to rule in or rule out the diagnosis.[14]

The decision to pursue urine testing for UTI is also more complicated in infants and young children. Because of the risks and costs of false positives and unnecessary testing/treatment, the American Academy of Pediatrics recommends against routine UA and urine culture in children with a pretest probability less than 1% to 2%.[15,16] Fortunately, there are several tools available to help with risk stratification. UTICalc (https://uticalc.pitt.edu/), developed and validated at the University of Pittsburgh,[17] uses demographic and clinical data to determine a pretest probability of UTI and, if UA results are available, to help determine whether empiric treatment should be initiated. Another option is a clinical decision tool validated by Gorelick and colleagues,[18] Shaikh and colleagues[7] (**Table 2**) which can be used to identify low-risk children who do not require testing.

As in neonates, a catheter urine culture is the gold standard for diagnosis of UTI.[16] "Clean catch" and bag samples are often used to avoid catheterization for low-risk children, but these are useful only if completely negative. Because of high rates of contamination (16%–26% for clean catch,[19–21] up to 60% for bag samples[19,22]), any positive UA or culture on these samples will need a follow-up catheter specimen, potentially resulting in increased costs and delays in care.[22]

UA in this age group is somewhat more reliable, but is not infallible. Urine nitrites and leukocyte esterase are the most specific and sensitive respectively, whereas isolated

Table 2		
Urinary tract infection (UTI) risk stratification pathway for children 2 to 24 months		
Male		**Female**
1 point each for: • Non-Black race • Temperature max $\geq$39 C • Fever >24 h		1 point each for: • Caucasian race • Age <12 mo • Temperature max $\geq$39 C • Fever >2 d • No alternate source
Circumcised	Uncircumcised	
0–2 points: $\leq$1% chance of UTI 3 points: 1%–2% chance of UTI	0 points: $\leq$2% chance of UTI	0–1 points: $\leq$1% chance of UTI 2 points: 1%–2% chance of UTI

Data from Shaikh N, Morone NE, Lopez J, et al. Does this child have a urinary tract infection? JAMA. 2007;298(24): 2895 and Gorelick MH, Hoberman A, Kearney D, et al. Validation of a decision rule identifying febrile young girls at high risk for urinary tract infection. Pediatr Emerg Care. 2003;19(3):162–164.

pyuria is a much less specific finding.[23] In all except extremely low-risk patients, "normal" urine samples should be sent for confirmatory culture because *Entero-coccus*, *Klebsiella*, and *Pseudomonas* are all known to cause UTI without pyuria or leukocyte esterase.[21] To optimize the accuracy of urine testing, specimens should be processed promptly after collection because delays can reduce the sensitivity and specificity of UA.[15] Serum inflammatory markers including erythrocyte sedimentation rate and C-reactive protein have also been studied in an attempt to differentiate pyelonephritis from lower UTI, but current evidence is weak and these should not be used to guide clinical practice.[24]

School-aged children and adolescents As children grow older, the clinical presentation of UTI becomes more predictable and more similar to the adult population. Although younger children may present with nonspecific symptoms such as vomiting or decreased appetite, older children and adolescents are far more likely to present with typical UTI symptoms. Furthermore, pyelonephritis is much easier to distinguish from cystitis in older children, as the presence of flank pain, costovertebral angle tenderness, fever, and vomiting can be reliably obtained. Still, there are a number of UTI mimics that clinicians should consider in this age group (see later in this article for differential diagnosis and **Table 3**).

Although urine culture from a catheter sample remains the gold standard for UTI diagnosis in older children, clean catch samples are widely used for uncomplicated cases. UA and urine microscopy are more reliable in this age group, and a completely negative UA (no pyuria, nitrites, or leukocyte esterase) has 99% sensitivity to rule out UTI.[7] The presence of nitrites alone is 98% specific for UTI in school-aged children, but has poor sensitivity.[25] All urine samples should still be sent for confirmatory culture, unless the patient has a completely normal UA and is considered low risk for UTI. Urine pregnancy testing should be performed on all adolescent girls, as pregnancy imparts a higher risk of pyelonephritis and may influence choice of antibiotics.

Management and disposition

Neonates All neonates with confirmed or suspected UTI are at high risk for associated bacteremia, and should be treated empirically pending urine culture results. Five percent to 20% of neonates with culture-proven UTI will have concurrent bacteremia with the same organism.[1,4,26] Although the risk of concurrent meningitis is lower (1%–

Table 3
Urinary tract infection mimics in children and adolescents

Diagnoses	Dysuria	Hematuria	Pyuria	Abdominal or Flank Pain	Fever
Viral cystitis	✓	✓	✓	✓	✓
Stevens Johnson syndrome	✓	✓	✓	—	✓
Trauma	✓	✓	—	✓	—
Pelvic inflammatory disease/ cervicitis	✓	—	(✓)	✓	✓
Genitourinary ulceration (eg, Behcet disease)	✓	✓	✓	—	(✓)
Balanitis/balanoposthitis	✓	—	✓	—	—
Vaginitis	✓	—	—	✓	—
Sterile urethritis (eg, Kawasaki disease, reactive arthritis)	✓	—	✓	—	(✓)
Constipation	✓	—	—	✓	—
Labial adhesions/urethral strictures	✓	—	—	—	—
Pinworms	✓	—	—	—	—
Dermatitis, lichen sclerosis	✓	—	—	—	—
Nephrolithiasis	—	✓	—	✓	—
Appendicitis	(✓)	—	✓	✓	✓
Colitis and terminal ileitis	—	—	✓	✓	✓

(✓) indicates a possible, less common, symptom.
Data from Mehta A, Williams V, Parajuli B. Child with Dysuria and/or Hematuria. Indian J Pediatr. 2017;84(10):792-798.

3%), it is not insignificant, and clinicians should have a low threshold to obtain cerebrospinal fluid (CSF) for cytology and culture in neonates who are febrile or otherwise ill-appearing.[4,27]

As soon as urine, blood, and CSF (if applicable) cultures have been obtained, neonates should be treated urgently with broad-spectrum parenteral antibiotics and admitted for close monitoring pending culture results. Although ampicillin and gentamicin have long been the standard regimen for neonatal sepsis, emerging ampicillin resistance has made this less effective in some regions.[28]

In neonates with recent hospital admission or prolonged neonatal ICU stays, consider substituting vancomycin for ampicillin to cover methicillin-resistant *Staphylococcus aureus*, *Enterococcus,* and coagulase-negative *Staphylococcus* species. Fluconazole also may be added for fungal coverage in premature neonates, those with indwelling urinary catheters, or if yeast is seen on urine Gram stain.

Neonates and infants presenting with UTI have been shown to have high rates of structural abnormalities of the urinary system (up to 50%), and should have imaging to evaluate for obstructive lesions or vesicoureteral reflux.[29] However, this should not be routinely performed during the acute infection because of an increased rate of false positives.[29,30] Ultrasound of the kidneys and bladder is typically used as a screening test, with voiding cystourethrogram (VCUG) reserved for follow-up of abnormal ultrasound findings or recurrent UTI.[30,31]

Infants and toddlers In children younger than 2, all UTIs should be treated as pyelonephritis due to the difficulty of clinically distinguishing pyelonephritis from cystitis and the risk of long-term harm from undertreated pyelonephritis. Studies using nuclear imaging have demonstrated pyelonephritis prevalence up to 60% among young children with febrile UTI,[29] although this is not cost-effective or practical for routine clinical use. Even more concerning, there is a significant body of research showing that delayed treatment of UTI in this age group places patients at risk for permanent renal scarring, chronic kidney disease, and hypertension.[15,30,32] Even a 48-hour delay in antibiotic administration can increase the risk of renal scarring by nearly 50%.[33]

Although infants and young children who are septic or ill-appearing will require broad-spectrum parenteral antibiotics and hospital admission, well-appearing infants older than 2 months can be safely discharged on oral antibiotics pending culture results. Close outpatient follow-up within 48 to 72 hours is necessary to assess response to treatment, and children without reliable access to follow-up should be admitted for monitoring (**Box 1**).

For outpatient treatment of pediatric UTI, narrow-spectrum antibiotics, such as cephalexin, trimethoprim-sulfamethoxazole (TMP-SMX), amoxicillin, and ampicillin, have traditionally been the first-line agents. Nitrofurantoin is not recommended, as it does not provide adequate coverage for pyelonephritis.[16] However, rising rates of antibiotic resistance have rendered these drugs less effective in many areas.[34–36] This is particularly true of ampicillin and amoxicillin, which are now effective against fewer than 40% of *Escherichia coli* isolates in some regions.[28] Although some factors can help predict antibiotic resistance (**Box 2**), clinicians should consult their institution's antibiogram when making treatment decisions.

Because of emerging drug resistance, third-generation cephalosporins, including cefpodoxime, cefdinir, and cefixime, are now recommended for empiric treatment. Ampicillin or amoxicillin may be added for *Enterococcus* coverage if the patient has a history of *Enterococcus* UTI. Fluoroquinolones are not recommended for first-line therapy unless there is high suspicion for *Pseudomonas* or another multidrug-resistant gram-negative organism.[37] Excessive use of fluoroquinolones also appears to be contributing to increasing fluoroquinolone resistance across multiple pathogens, including *Pseudomonas, Proteus,* and *E coli*.[38]

Although many clinicians routinely give a first dose of intravenous (IV) antibiotics before discharge, there is little evidence to support this practice. Multiple studies have shown no difference in time to resolution of fever, time to negative urine culture, reinfection rate, or rate of renal scarring when a first dose of IV antibiotic (usually

---

Box 1
Indications for hospital admission for febrile UTI

Age younger than 2 months

Unstable vital signs

Ill-appearing or lethargic

Unable to tolerate oral medications

Immunocompromised

Known genitourinary abnormality

Failure of outpatient treatment

Family without reliable access to transportation, telephone, or close outpatient follow-up

---

Box 2
Risk factors for antibiotic-resistant UTI

- Uncircumcised boys
- History of bowel or bladder dysfunction
- Antibiotic exposure in past 6 months
- Hispanic race

Data from Shaikh N, Hoberman A, Keren R, et al. Predictors of antimicrobial resistance among pathogens causing urinary tract infection in children. J Pediatr. 2016;171:116.

---

ceftriaxone) is given.[39–41] In children who are able to take oral medication, this practice only serves to increase treatment cost.[41]

With appropriate antibiotic treatment, approximately 90% of children will have resolution of fever within 48 hours.[42] For UTIs not responding to antibiotics, repeat urine culture may be useful to confirm antibiotic resistance patterns if the initial culture was indeterminate. Ultrasound also may be useful to evaluate for renal abscess or other structural lesions.[31,43] Most infants and children who fail to improve with appropriate outpatient antibiotics will require hospital admission.

As with neonates, all children younger than 2 with febrile UTI should have an ultrasound of the kidneys and bladder to assess for structural abnormalities that may predispose them to recurrent infections.[31] However, this should not be done until 7 to 14 days after the infection because inflammation of the renal parenchyma produces a high rate of false positives.[31,44] VCUG is generally not used as a first-line test, and should be reserved for recurrent UTI or follow-up of abnormal ultrasound results. Although VCUG often identifies low-grade vesicoureteral reflux, there is no benefit to prophylactic treatment, making the diagnosis far less meaningful.[45–47]

School-aged children and adolescents As in adults, UTI in older children and adolescents can be classified as complicated or uncomplicated (**Box 3**).

For pyelonephritis and other complicated UTI, third-generation or fourth-generation cephalosporins or ampicillin plus gentamicin are reasonable choices for empiric treatment. Oral TMP-SMX or third-generation cephalosporins (eg, cefpodoxime) can be used for outpatient treatment of pyelonephritis in otherwise healthy patients if local resistance patterns permit, but should not be used for septic or ill-appearing children. Regardless of antibiotic choice, pyelonephritis requires a longer course of treatment than cystitis, usually 10 to 14 days in total.[40]

In more complex patients, such as those with immunocompromise, GU structural anomalies, indwelling catheters, or a history of drug-resistant infections, antibiotic

---

Box 3
Features of complicated UTI

- Pyelonephritis
- History of genitourinary abnormality
- Immunocompromised
- Pregnant
- Indwelling urinary catheter
- History of multidrug-resistant infections

choice should be guided by previous culture results. These children will frequently require hospital admission for parenteral antibiotics.

For all other children with uncomplicated cystitis, choice of antibiotics is similar to adult patients. If local resistance patterns permit, narrow-spectrum antibiotics, such as TMP-SMX and cephalexin, may be used. Nitrofurantoin is widely used for uncomplicated cystitis in adolescent girls, as it covers S saprophyticus in addition to other uropathogens. Amoxicillin or ampicillin may be added for Enterococcus coverage if the patient has a history of Enterococcus UTI or if gram-positive bacteria are seen on urine Gram stain, but these are no longer effective for single-agent therapy in most areas.[28,34–36] Otherwise, broad coverage with a third-generation cephalosporin, such as cefpodoxime or cefdinir, is adequate for most uncomplicated UTIs. Uncomplicated cystitis in healthy children can generally be treated with 3 to 5 days of antibiotics, and patients should have close outpatient follow-up to assess response to treatment.

Differential diagnosis Children are often seen in the emergency department for pain with urination or decreased urine output. The causes of this are extensive and range from the aforementioned infections to mechanical causes. Commonly, constipation can result in obstruction. In urinary obstruction cases this should be excluded before further testing. Vaginitis and balanitis can produce dysuria and urinary urgency in boys and girls, respectively. Appendicitis, colitis, and terminal ileitis (as seen in Crohn disease) can all produce flank pain and fever similar to pyelonephritis, as well as pyuria secondary to ureteral irritation. Inflammatory conditions, such as Kawasaki disease, can cause noninfectious urethritis, which may present with dysuria, urinary frequency/urgency, pyuria, and/or hematuria. Finally, all adolescents should be screened for sexual activity, as N gonorrhoeae, C trachomatis, and herpes simplex virus (HSV) infections can present with sterile urethritis.[48]

Balanitis and Balanoposthitis

Balanitis, the inflammation of the glans of the penis, and balanoposthitis, inflammation of the foreskin and glans can be seen in all age groups. It is characterized by swelling, redness, and dysuria. In young children, the most common cause is candida infection, specifically Candida albicans. Rarely, bacteria can be involved, often with purulence, and is usually caused by E coli, Enterococci, S aureus, or Streptococcus pneumoniae. In sexually active individuals, sexually transmitted infections also should be considered. In addition, an atopic or irritant form exists, which is noninfectious and often due to excessive washing with soap. Initial treatment with topical antifungal is appropriate in mild to moderate infections, with low suspicion for bacterial infection in conjunction with education on appropriate hygiene practices. Balanoposthitis increases the risk for pathologic phimosis and paraphimosis in the future, particularly with delayed treatment. Close follow-up with a primary care doctor is recommended for all cases.[49]

Sexually Transmitted Infections

The treatment of sexually transmitted infections does not differ based on age. The local patterns of infection and susceptibilities should be considered for management. Although specific sexually transmitted infections in children are concerning for sexual abuse, other infections do not clearly indicate abuse. For example, human papillomavirus, presenting as warts, may occur due to self-inoculation from other areas of the body. Similarly, HSV can be found in genital regions without abuse. However, N gonorrhoeae and C trachomatis are highly suspicious for abuse, therefore identification of (or suspicion for) either should prompt investigation.[50]

Neonatal herpes simplex virus

Unlike other forms of sexually transmitted infection, HSV poses a particular concern for neonates. It is known for causing small-for-gestational age infants, but also can have significant post-delivery implications. It is typically transmitted during vaginal delivery, with the highest risk of transmission during maternal primary lesion outbreak. Although it rarely causes GU infection in an infant, its source is from the mother's GU tract. There are 3 major recognized forms of neonatal HSV: skin, eye, and mouth (SEM); central nervous system (CNS); and disseminated.

The least devastating is SEM, comprising approximately 45% of cases, and which, when identified early, has an 80% to 98% recovery with treatment using acyclovir. It typically presents at approximately 10 to 12 days of life with lesions, and ophthalmology consultation should occur early to help protect against long-term vision loss. There is a risk of rapid progression if treatment does not occur early. Full sepsis workup, including lumbar puncture with HSV polymerase chain reaction (PCR), and blood HSV PCR should be included to exclude disseminated infection in any neonate with signs of this infection. Swabs of skin and mucous membrane lesions also should be sent, to avoid false negatives from any one source.

CNS infection has a significant morbidity and mortality, with 30% normal neurologic outcome. Mortality rate is approximately 4%. Symptoms are often nonspecific with irritability, and fever, although seizures also may occur. This typically presents at 16 to 19 days of life, and up to 70% will have a skin or mucosal lesion at some point during illness. The CSF in these patients will show mononuclear pleocytosis, normal or low glucose levels, and slight protein elevation. Elevated red blood cells (RBCs) is not as common in infants as in adults, and is more often an indication of a traumatic tap, rather than a reliable indicator of HSV. Therefore, absence of elevated RBCs in CSF should not be used to decrease concern for the disease.[51]

Disseminated HSV infection can result from delayed treatment of either of the other diagnoses, but often exists on its own. Approximately 25% of cases of neonatal HSV take this form, and there is up to 85% mortality, with slight decrease when IV acyclovir is started early in infection. Symptoms include CNS involvement, myocarditis, pneumonia (this makes up 33%–54% of all early viral pneumonias in infants), liver failure, disseminated intravascular coagulation, renal injury, and necrotizing enterocolitis.[51]

Workup for each is the same, including full sepsis evaluation, CSF with HSV PCR, wound cultures (where applicable) for HSV, blood cultures, and blood or serum HSV PCR, and endotracheal aspirate for HSV (when intubated). Immediate initiation of IV acyclovir is indicated for all forms as well, with inpatient monitoring.[51]

OTHER PEDIATRIC CONSIDERATIONS

Prepubertal Vaginal Bleeding

The identification of vaginal bleeding is often very unsettling for a parent or guardian, and can result in a frantic trip with concern for internal bleeding or abuse. Fortunately, many causes are benign in nature and not related to either internal injury or abuse. In these patients, the typical adult pelvic examination is not appropriate, but external examination can be performed in a frog leg or knees-to-chest position. Vaginal examination should be performed with a gynecologist under anesthesia only.[52]

In neonates, vaginal bleeding can be a normal variant. Maternal estrogen levels begin to wane in the infant and this results in a slight sloughing of the uterine lining, which is generally self-limited and requires no additional emergent testing. Recent evidence, however, suggests it may be linked to fetal distress during pregnancy, and be an indicator of genital health issues for the child later in life. Therefore, parents should be instructed to tell the primary care doctor about this occurrence.[53] In addition, uric acid crystals can create a rust coloration to the diaper in neonates, which can appear sanguineous.[54]

Older infants and children with spotting in the underwear should have a history with particular care given to other signs of early puberty, which may require endocrine follow-up, and signs of abuse. They should also have an external examination to assess for vaginitis, which is common in children who are permitted to manage their own hygiene, as well, and children who frequently take bubble baths without fully rinsing afterward. Care should be taken to assess for trauma, foreign body, straddle injury, or signs of infection.[52]

Urethral prolapse occurs in 1 in every 2880 patients, most commonly in prepubertal girls due to lower estrogen levels, and can present with reported swelling and bleeding. Treatment is typically symptomatic, including sitz baths, estrogen cream, and pain management, with outpatient urologic follow-up. Additional treatment or immediate consultation is not needed as long as urination is possible.[52]

Occasionally an imperforate hymen, or partially imperforate hymen can present with spotting or slight bleeding, often accompanied by abdominal pain and the characteristic blue-purple hue at the introitus.

Rarely, neoplastic conditions may be identified, typically by the appearance of a mass or irregular tissue. If the patient is able to urinate, phone consultation with an oncologist and gynecologist (ideally one with pediatric specialty or experience) is appropriate. Although many new cancer diagnoses warrant admission in pediatrics, some can be discharged with urgent follow-up if otherwise stable.[52]

Infantile Circumcision

Despite controversies, the infantile male circumcision remains the most common pediatric surgery in boys, and the most common elective surgery in children, requiring no pathologic diagnosis to obtain the procedure. In the United States, estimates of circumcised male individuals range up to approximately 80% of the total male population older than 14 years.[55] The procedure, which involves removal of the prepuce, is performed by a variety of specialties (typically obstetricians, pediatricians, family practice physicians, and under special circumstances, surgeons), and by a variety of practice-level providers (eg, physicians, nurse practitioners, and physicians assistants). For a simple neonatal circumcision, the procedure involves only local anesthesia, involves clamping of the foreskin, and no suture material is required. This is starkly contrasted by older infant, child, and adult circumcision, which is done with general anesthesia, and sutures are placed.[56]

Typically this procedure occurs without incident, and results in a slight decrease in neonatal UTIs, and a decrease in certain sexually transmitted infections, most notably human immunodeficiency virus and HSV, and their transmission. In up to 3.1%, however, complications do arise, including local injury, bleeding, or infection. Of these, bleeding is the most common, and is often what is seen in the emergency department. Bleeding may be related to an undiagnosed underlying bleeding disorder. Use of a Plastibell device may have a slight increased risk of bleeding. This device is a plastic clamp left in position until it falls off due to necrosis of the underlying tissue. Infants are sent home with the device in place. Bleeding that does not respond to direct pressure may require placement of absorbable sutures, and urologic consultation. Infection is the second most common cause of emergency presentation, and although rare, should be treated as other skin infections based on local resistance patterns and covering skin flora.[56]

The Uncircumcised Pediatric Patient

Although the overall number of circumcised male individuals is high, the rate of infantile circumcision has seen a steady decline, particularly notable in recent years.[57] This results in the emergency physician seeing an increasingly higher incidence of uncircumcised infants and children. The uncircumcised neonatal male penis typically is unable to have the foreskin retracted. This is physiologic phimosis, and does not require intervention. Forceful retraction, even for a catheter placement, can result in later development of pathologic phimosis due to scarring.[56] The foreskin should be gently retracted only enough to visualize the urethral meatus. This can identify anatomic abnormalities and allow for insertion of a catheter. In one study, only 4% of infant foreskin could be retracted at birth, compared with 58% by seventh grade.[58] Look for a thickened ring along the prepuce that could indicate pathologic phimosis. This can be referred to urology, and often stretching and steroids are attempted before surgical intervention. It is important not to state that surgery will be necessary.[59]

Genitourinary Trauma

Although the overall management and care of genital traumas are often similar to adults, there is some slight variation in pediatric management. In a prepubertal child, particularly a prepubertal girl, a complete genital examination may need to be performed, and this often requires anesthesia to avoid unnecessary psychological trauma, and allow for a complete examination. Abuse should always be considered.

Hair tourniquet

A relatively common complaint in an emergency department is the hair tourniquet. They can be found on distal extremities, but also in the genital area. Although genital hair tourniquets more commonly occur in boys (approximately 25% of tourniquets), up to 6% of all hair tourniquets occur on the clitoris.[60] It occurs most often in infants between 2 and 6 months of age in association with maternal postpartum hair loss. Attempts should be made to remove the hair immediately. For tourniquets that are deep and unable to be cut by scissors, a scalpel may be used. Depilatory creams, which can be used elsewhere on the body, should be avoided in areas near mucous membranes. This should not be used in the vulva or near other mucosal tissues. If available in a timely fashion, urology, ideally pediatric urology, should be called for tourniquets that fail the preceding measures, and all patients with evidence of distal tissue ischemia. In patients without signs of ischemia, a provider should reassess patients within 24 hours.[61]

When assessing a hair tourniquet, it is necessary to obtain a thorough history. Unfortunately, hair tourniquets can be a form of abuse. Close attention should be given to patients of toilet-training age, or those older than a year. In this age, parental expectations may exceed developmental stage, resulting in frustrations over toilet training. There are reports of tourniquet use to prevent urination between toileting in boys. In this age group, incidental tourniquets are particularly unusual, because they are old enough to localize pain, and may try to remove it, which should prevent significant delay in presentation.[60]

Zipper injuries

Zipper injuries account for less than 1% of pediatric emergency department visits. Most zipper injuries occur in children or teens who are distracted or early in learning to dress themselves. A patient presenting with tissue entrapment will require release in the emergency department. Compression can improve edema. Cutting the cloth up to the zipper teeth may release the zipper. Cutting the zipper mechanism itself is the next step. In addition, mineral oil can soften the skin allowing for it to be removed more easily. If these measures fail, the patient may require local anesthetic before removal.[62]

Torsion

Although the diagnostic tools and management of both ovarian and testicular torsion are the same as those for adults, including use of ultrasound and emergency urology/gynecology or general surgery consultation (based on resources), the history may not be as clear in pediatrics. Symptoms can arise in all ages, from infancy through adulthood; however, in younger children the complaints are often vague, and sometimes the diagnosis is discovered incidentally. Referred pain, or fear of disclosure of the location of pain, may complicate the history. Intermittent crying, or concern for abdominal pain should prompt a genital examination. These cases can easily be misdiagnosed as constipation.

For ovarian torsion, most cases occur as the ovaries enlarge nearing puberty; however, earlier cases often have an associated ovarian abnormality.[63] Ovarian torsion has been identified even in the neonatal period. Pelvic ultrasound should be used with the goal of identifying both ovaries. This can be completed transabdominally, with a full bladder, on children who have never had vaginal intercourse. This is due to the variable size of pediatric ovaries, compared with an adult. In adults, a set size and volume (>4 cm and >20 mL) can be used; however, in infants and children a comparison is necessary to determine if there is ovarian enlargement. The affected ovary can appear up to 28 times the size of the normal ovary, but a size discrepancy with one ovary greater than or equal to 3 times the size of the other should cause high suspicion for torsion.[64]

Priapism

The management of priapism in children mirrors that of adults. The only additional consideration should be possible ingestion resulting in the symptoms. A careful history of possible medication exposures in the home should be elicited.[65]

Sexual Abuse

In children who are of age of consent, confirmation of consent for sexual activity should be discussed in private with the patient. Age of consent varies by location, so be sure to know your state's regulations. Those younger than set age should have social work and child protective services (CPS) involvement. CPS notification is mandatory and this should be communicated to the family in a timely fashion.[66]

Sexual abuse, or the report of abuse, is incredibly stressful for everyone involved. Often the perpetrator is a family member or a person with close connection to the family (eg, babysitter, family friend). The accusation of abuse carries with it potential to have significant implications for the family unit, and its function. Because of this, it is important to attempt some discussion with the parent or guardian in isolation from the child when possible. During the discussion with the parent or guardian, he or she should be counseled to avoid asking questions himself or herself during the interview, and that excessive emotional response from a parent or guardian can result in the child refusing to cooperate for fear of upsetting the parent, or retaliation after the interview. It also may be necessary to discuss with the parent the impact this has on their relationship with the accused, and giving some recognition of the difficulty of the situation can help gain the support of the parent for the greater good of the child. For example, if a parent's significant other is accused, this causes extreme anxiety for the parent who has an intimate relationship with someone whom they have learned to trust, and now have to choose between support of their partner or their child. Although his may seem an easy choice, it can be incredibly challenging, particularly if crucial means of survival (finances, food, shelter) are dependent on the partner. In conjunction with this, an assessment of the parent or guardian's personal safety also should be conducted.[66,67]

When asking questions, the provider should remain calm, taking care not to react negatively, or in any extreme, to what the child says, as this can limit the extent of the discussion. Do not attempt to coax a story or information from the child.[50] Use open-ended questions, and developmentally appropriate language. Ask a guardian what terminology they use with the child to describe genitals. This can help guide the conversation.[67] If they are resistant to discussion, simply move on with other history and examination. When available, a designated sexual assault provider should conduct the history and physical. In fact, many abuse specialists suggest that untrained providers refrain from any discussion about the details of the abuse with the child, and focus solely on physical symptoms and examination.[66] It is important to limit extensive documentation of the history, using quotes from the child is ideal, and leave this to a specifically trained individual, to avoid contradictory reports, which could affect reliability in court documentation. Focus in the emergency department should be on examination for injuries, documentation of these, and ensuring a medically safe disposition. Additional documentation should focus on updating social histories and medical history, including development delays.[66] It is important for the providers and the families to be aware early in the visit that this will require time, and often a lengthy stay in the department to obtain all necessary details.[66]

Families should be counseled early on that fewer than 10% of child sexual abuse cases have physical findings on examination. This does not mean that the abuse did not occur, nor does it mean ongoing investigation should be suspended.[68]

REFERENCES

1. Bonadio W, Maida G. Urinary tract infection in outpatient febrile infants younger than 30 days of age: a 10-year evaluation. Pediatr Infect Dis J 2014;33(4):342.

2. Lin DS, Huang SH, Lin CC, et al. Urinary tract infection in febrile infants younger than eight weeks of age. Pediatrics 2000;105(2):E20.

3. Eliakim A, Dolfin T, Korzets Z, et al. Urinary tract infection in premature infants: the role of imaging studies and prophylactic therapy. J Perinatol 1997;17(4):305.

4. Downey LC, Benjamin DK, Clark RH, et al. Urinary tract infection concordance with positive blood and cerebrospinal fluid cultures in the neonatal intensive care unit. J Perinatol 2013;33(4):302–6.

5. Shaikh N, Morone NE, Bost JE, et al. Prevalence of urinary tract infection in childhood: a meta-analysis. Pediatr Infect Dis J 2008;27(4):302–8.

6. Shaw KN, Gorelick M, McGowan KL, et al. Prevalence of urinary tract infection in febrile young children in the emergency department. Pediatrics 1998;102(2):16.

7. Shaikh N, Morone NE, Lopez J, et al. Does this child have a urinary tract infection? JAMA 2007;298(24):2895.

8. Hooton TM, Scholes D, Hughes JP, et al. A prospective study of risk factors for symptomatic urinary tract infection in young women. N Engl J Med 1996; 335(7):468.

9. Ismaili K, Lolin K, Damry N, et al. Febrile urinary tract infections in 0- to 3-month-old infants: a prospective follow-up study. J Pediatr 2011;158(1):91.

10. Edlin RS, Shapiro DJ, Hersh AL, et al. Antibiotic resistance patterns of outpatient pediatric urinary tract infections. J Urol 2013;190(1):222–7.

11. Byington CL, Enriquez FR, Hoff C, et al. Serious bacterial infections in febrile infants 1 to 90 days old with and without viral infections. Pediatrics 2004;113(6): 1662–6.

12. Tzimenatos L, Mahajan P, Dayan PS, et al. Accuracy of the urinalysis for urinary tract infections in infants 60 days and younger. Pediatrics 2018;141(2).

13. Gauthier M, Gouin S, Phan V, et al. Association of malodorous urine with urinary tract infection in children aged 1 to 36 months. Pediatrics 2012;129(5):885.

14. Struthers S, Scanlon J, Parker K, et al. Parental reporting of smelly urine and urinary tract infection. Arch Dis Child 2003;88(3):250.

15. Finnell SM, Carroll AE, Downs SM. Subcommittee on Urinary Tract Infection. Technical report—diagnosis and management of an initial UTI in febrile infants and young children. Pediatrics 2011;128(3):e749.

16. Subcommittee on Urinary Tract Infection, Steering Committee on Quality Improvement and Management, Roberts KB. Urinary tract infection: clinical practice guideline for the diagnosis and management of the initial UTI in febrile infants and children 2 to 24 months. Pediatrics 2011;128(3):595.

17. Hay AD. UTICalc may enhance UTI risk-estimation in young children. J Pediatr 2018;200:291–4.

18. Gorelick MH, Hoberman A, Kearney D, et al. Validation of a decision rule identifying febrile young girls at high risk for urinary tract infection. Pediatr Emerg Care 2003;19(3):162–4.

19. Tosif S, Baker A, Oakley E, et al. Contamination rates of different urine collection methods for the diagnosis of urinary tract infections in young children: an observational cohort study. J Paediatr Child Health 2012;48(8):659.

20. Labrosse M, Levy A, Autmizguine J, et al. Evaluation of a new strategy for clean-catch urine in infants. Pediatrics 2016;138(3) [pii:e20160573].

21. Shaikh N, Shope TR, Hoberman A, et al. Association between uropathogen and pyuria. Pediatrics 2016;138(1) [pii:e20160087].

22. Al-Orifi F, McGillivray D, Tange S, et al. Urine culture from bag specimens in young children: are the risks too high? J Pediatr 2000;137(2):221.

23. Gorelick MH, Shaw KN. Screening tests for urinary tract infection in children: a meta-analysis. Pediatrics 1999;104(5):e54.

24. Shaikh N, Borrell JL, Evron J, et al. Procalcitonin, C-reactive protein, and erythrocyte sedimentation rate for the diagnosis of acute pyelonephritis in children. Cochrane Database Syst Rev 2015;(1):CD009185.

25. Kunin CM, Degroot JE. Sensitivity of a nitrite indicator strip method in detecting bacteriuria in preschool girls. Pediatrics 1977;60(2):244–5.

26. Levy I, Comarsca J, Davidovits M, et al. Urinary tract infection in preterm infants: the protective role of breastfeeding. Pediatr Nephrol 2009;24(3):527.

27. Tebruegge M, Pantazidou A, Clifford V, et al. The age-related risk of co-existing meningitis in children with urinary tract infection. PLoS One 2011;6(11):e26576.

28. Byington CL, Rittichier KK, Bassett KE, et al. Serious bacterial infections in febrile infants younger than 90 days of age: the importance of ampicillin-resistant pathogens. Pediatrics 2003;111(5):964–8.

29. Hoberman A, Charron M, Hickey RW, et al. Imaging studies after a first febrile urinary tract infection in young children. N Engl J Med 2003;348(3):195–202.

30. Shaikh N, Craig JC, Rovers MM, et al. Identification of children and adolescents at risk for renal scarring after a first urinary tract infection: a meta-analysis with individual patient data. JAMA Pediatr 2014;168(10):893.

31. Wallace SS, Zhang W, Mahmood NF, et al. Renal ultrasound for infants younger than 2 months with febrile urinary tract infection. Am J Roentgenol 2015;205(4): 894–8.

32. Smellie JM, Poulton A, Prescod NP. Retrospective study of children with renal scarring associated with reflux and urinary infection. BMJ 1994;308(6938):1193.

33. Shaikh N, Mattoo TK, Keren R, et al. Early antibiotic treatment for pediatric febrile urinary tract infection and renal scarring. JAMA Pediatr 2016;170(9):848.

34. Bryce A, Hay AD, Lane IF, et al. Global prevalence of antibiotic resistance in paediatric urinary tract infections caused by *Escherichia coli* and association with routine use of antibiotics in primary care: systematic review and meta-analysis. BMJ 2016;352:i939.

35. Ladhani S, Gransden W. Increasing antibiotic resistance among urinary tract isolates. Arch Dis Child 2003;88(5):444.

36. Yakubov R, van den Akker M, Machamad K, et al. Antimicrobial resistance among uropathogens that cause childhood community-acquired urinary tract infections in central Israel. Pediatr Infect Dis J 2017;36(1):113–5.

37. Jackson MA, Schutze GE, Committee on Infectious Diseases. The use of systemic and topical fluoroquinolones. Pediatrics 2016;138(5) [pii:e20162706].

38. Pickering LK. Antimicrobial resistance among enteric pathogens. Semin Pediatr Infect Dis 2004;15(2):71.

39. Hoberman A, Wald ER, Hickey RW, et al. Oral versus initial intravenous therapy for urinary tract infections in young febrile children. Pediatrics 1999;104:79–86.

40. Strohmeier Y, Hodson EM, Willis NS, et al. Antibiotics for acute pyelonephritis in children. Cochrane Database Syst Rev 2014;(7):CD003772.

41. Neuhaus TJ, Berger C, Buechner K, et al. Randomised trial of oral versus sequential intravenous/oral cephalosporins in children with pyelonephritis. Eur J Pediatr 2008;167(9):1037.

42. Bachur R. Nonresponders: prolonged fever among infants with urinary tract infections. Pediatrics 2000;105(5):E59.

43. Cheng CH, Tsai MH, Su LH, et al. Renal abscess in children: a 10-year clinical and radiologic experience in a tertiary medical center. Pediatr Infect Dis J 2008;27(11):1025.

44. Shaikh N, Hoberman A, Keren R, et al. Predictors of antimicrobial resistance among pathogens causing urinary tract infection in children. J Pediatr 2016; 171:116.

45. Montini G, Rigon L, Zucchetta P, et al. Prophylaxis after first febrile urinary tract infection in children? A multicenter, randomized, controlled, noninferiority trial. Pediatrics 2008;122(5):1064–71.

46. Roussey-Kesler G, Gadjos V, Idres N, et al. Antibiotic prophylaxis for the prevention of recurrent urinary tract infection in children with low grade vesicoureteral reflux: results from a prospective randomized study. J Urol 2008;179(2):674–9.

47. Craig J, Simpson J, Williams G. Antibiotic prophylaxis and recurrent urinary tract infection in children. N Engl J Med 2009;361(18):1748–59.

48. Mehta A, Williams V, Parajuli B. Child with dysuria and/or hematuria. Indian J Pediatr 2017;84(10):792–8.

49. Edwards S. Balanitis and balanoposthitis: a review. Genitourin Med 1996;72(3): 155–9.

50. Herrmann B, Banaschak S, Csorba R, et al. Physical examination in child sexual abuse approaches and current evidence. Dtsch Arztebl Int 2014;111(41): 692–703.

51. Pinninti SG, Kimberlin DW. Neonatal herpes simplex virus infections. Semin Perinatol 2018;42(3):168–75.
52. McCaskill A, Inabinet CF, Tomlin K, et al. Prepubertal genital bleeding: examination and differential diagnosis in pediatric female patients. J Emerg Med 2018; 55(4):e97–100.
53. Bianchi P, Benagiano G, Brosens I. Promoting awareness of neonatal menstruation. Gynecol Endocrinol 2017;33(3):173–8.
54. Kliegman RM, Stanton B, St Geme JW III, et al. Nelson textbook of pediatrics. 20th edition. Philadelphia: Elsevier; 2015.
55. Introcaso CE, Xu F, Kilmarx PH, et al. Prevalence of circumcision among men and boys aged 14 to 59 years in the United States, National Health and Nutrition Examination Surveys 2005-2010. Sex Transm Dis 2013;40(7):521e5.
56. American Academy of Pediatrics Task Force on Circumcision. Male circumcision. Pediatrics 2012;130(3):e756–85.
57. Morris BJ, Bailis SA, Wiswell TE. Circumcision rates in the United States: rising or falling? What effect might the new affirmative pediatric policy statement have? Mayo Clin Proc 2014;89(5):677–86.
58. Chang CH, Chang SS. Foreskin development before adolescence in 2149 school-boys. Int J Urol 2006;13:968–9.
59. Dave S, Afshar K, Braga LH, et al. Canadian Urological Association guideline on the care of the normal foreskin and neonatal circumcision in Canadian infants. Can Urol Assoc J 2018;12(2):E76–99.
60. Golshevsky J, Chuen J, Tung PH. Hair-thread tourniquet syndrome. J Paediatr Child Health 2005;41(3):154–5.
61. Templet TA, Rholdon RD. Assessment, treatment, and prevention strategies for hair-thread tourniquet syndrome in infants. Nurs Womens Health 2016;20(4): 421–5.
62. Leslie SW, Taylor RS. Zipper injuries. StatPearls. Treasure Island (FL): StatPearls Publishing; 2018.
63. Cass DL. Ovarian torsion. Semin Pediatr Surg 2005;14(2):86–92.
64. Muralidharan CG, Shyam Krishna S, Jose T. Pediatric ovarian torsion: a diagnostic challenge. Radiol Bras 2018;51(4):274–5.
65. Bozkurt H, Sahin S. Olanzapine-induced priapism in a child with Asperger's Syndrome. Balkan Med J 2017;34(1):85–7.
66. Asnes AG, Leventhal JM. Managing child abuse: general principles. Pediatr Rev 2010;31(2):47–55.
67. Jenny C, Crawford-Jakubiak JE, Committee on Child Abuse and Neglect, American Academy of Pediatrics. The evaluation of children in the primary care setting when sexual abuse is suspected. Pediatrics 2013;132(2):e558–67.
68. Heger A, Ticson L, Velasquez O, et al. Children referred for possible sexual abuse: medical findings in 2384 children. Child Abuse Negl 2002;26:645–59.

The Approach to the Patient with Hematuria

George C. Willis, MD*, Semhar Z. Tewelde, MD

KEYWORDS

- Hematuria • Nephrolithiasis • Continuous bladder irrigation • Malignancy
- Clot retention

KEY POINTS

- Hematuria evaluation in the emergency department involves a workup to rule out life-threatening disease processes and to ensure subsequent close outpatient follow-up with the appropriate service.
- Although disease processes of the genitourinary tract are the most common causes of hematuria, failure to consider more rare vascular causes can be dangerous and even life-threatening.
- Although laboratory studies are inherent, diagnostic imaging in the emergency department is largely unnecessary, except to rule out life-threatening causes.

INTRODUCTION

Hematuria is a condition that frequently presents to the emergency department (ED). There are many possible causes both benign and life-threatening. A thorough history and physical focusing on identifying the possible life-threatening causes often drives the workup. Laboratory studies are the mainstay of the diagnostic workup and, sometimes, imaging is warranted. This article provides information on common and less-common causes of hematuria, diagnostic considerations, and disposition algorithms to aid patients.

BACKGROUND

The definition of hematuria is the excretion of red blood cells (RBCs) in the urine. A problem arising in the genitourinary tract anywhere from the glomerulus to the urethral meatus can result in RBCs in the urine. Hematuria is defined by the American Urological Association as greater than 3 to 5 RBCs per high-powered field under

Disclosure Statement: The authors have nothing to disclose.
Department of Emergency Medicine, University of Maryland School of Medicine, 110 South Paca Street, Sixth Floor, Suite 200, Baltimore, MD 21201, USA
* Corresponding author.
E-mail address: gwillis@som.umaryland.edu
twitter: @DocWillisMD (G.C.W.); @HeartEMed (S.Z.T.)

Emerg Med Clin N Am 37 (2019) 755–769
https://doi.org/10.1016/j.emc.2019.07.011
0733-8627/19/© 2019 Elsevier Inc. All rights reserved.

microscopy.[1-6] Macroscopic or gross hematuria is hematuria that is visible to the naked eye, whereas microscopic hematuria is only visible under microscopy.

Patients with hematuria most commonly present to primary care physicians and EDs.[7] The amount of distress caused to patients who experience hematuria, especially first-time hematuria, is often high. However, there are many patients evaluated for other chief complaints who are incidentally found to have hematuria, usually microscopic. Up to 18% of normal individuals have some form of hematuria on random screening.[3,8,9] The prevalence of microscopic hematuria in asymptomatic patients varies by age anywhere between 2% and 21%.[3,10-14]

Hematuria can result from several causes. Initially, the primary objective is to determine if it is truly blood in the urine. The term hematuria is often given to urine that is observably reddish/brown in appearance. Although this discoloration of the urine may be true hematuria, it may also be pseudohematuria, meaning a blood-like discoloration unrelated to the presence of blood. The presence of RBCs in the urine distinguishes hematuria from pseudohematuria. There are many foods and medications that can lead to a blood-colored urine sample (**Box 1**). To assist with

Box 1
Pseudohematuria (dipstick-negative) 2° medication/diet
Medications
Azathioprine
Deferoxamine
Doxorubicin
Laxatives
Phenazopyridine
Phenothiazine
Phenytoin
Pyridium
Riboflavin
Rifampin
Warfarin
Thorazine
Metronidazole
Nitrofurantoin
Diet/Dyes
Beets
Blackberries
Blueberries
B-carotene
Rhubarb
Carrots
Fava beans
Aloe
Food dyes

differentiating these 2 entities, an optimal urine sample (midstream clean-catch) with dipstick and microscopic analyses is necessary. Dipstick testing for blood relies on the peroxidase activity of hemoglobin; a positive result occurs when hemoglobin pigment oxidizes the test-strip reagent producing a color change. Therefore, a sample of blood-colored urine that is dipstick-negative for blood is pseudohematuria until proven otherwise. Disease processes that cause pseudohematuria that are dipstick-negative for blood are shown in **Box 2**. A false-negative dipstick result for blood is far more rare, but should be considered when ascorbic acid is high, such as in patients who consume daily supplemental vitamin C. In isolation, the dipstick is suboptimal in distinguishing true hematuria (intact RBCs in the urine) and pseudo-hematuria alone. For example, hemoglobinuria (lysed RBCs) and myoglobinuria (myoglobin) yield false-positive urine dipsticks for blood. Other disease processes that can yield pseudohematuria that is dipstick-positive for blood are shown in **Box 3**. Microscopic analysis revealing a lack of RBCs indicates pseudohematuria, whereas the presence of more than 3 to 5 RBC per high-powered field confirms true hematuria.

Additional pertinent history that should be obtained with regard to urine collection is the proximity to strenuous exercise, menstruation, sexual intercourse, recent instrumentation (iatrogenic or recreational), or a febrile illness, because all of these can result in transient hematuria and would not be ideal for urinalysis; follow-up urinalysis should be obtained 48 hours after refraining from these aforementioned conditions. Factitious hematuria also can occur with blood from a fingerstick mixed in the urine. If suspicion is high, a directly observed urine sample should be obtained.

CAUSES OF HEMATURIA

The causes of hematuria have been divided into 3 broad categories and are listed in **Tables 1 and 2**: renal, postrenal, hematologic, and vascular. These vary with age, sex, race, risk factor, and personal/family history. In adults, hematuria is most frequently the result of nephrolithiasis, pyelonephritis, benign prostatic hypertrophy, or malignancy, the latter especially in the elderly. In children, infection, obstruction, and malignancy should also be equally considered, but glomerular diseases by far prevail as the most common cause of hematuria in this population. In rare circumstances, hematuria heralds, or is associated with, a life-threatening vascular event.

Box 2
Pseudohematuria (dipstick-negative) 2° medical condition

Pigmenturia

Melanin

Porphyria

Hypercalciuria/hyperuricosuria (blue diaper syndrome)

Phenylketonuria/alkaptonuria

Tyrosinosis

Maple syrup urine disease

Hartnups disease

Bilirubinuria

Hepatocellular (eg, Dubin-Johnson, Rotor)

Box 3
Pseudohematuria (dipstick-positive) 2° medical condition

Hemoglobinuria

Autoimmune/microangiopathic hemolytic

Paroxysmal nocturnal/cold hemglobinuria

Drug-induced hemolytic anemia

Prosthetic valves/device

Malaria (falciparum)

Myoglobinuria

Rhabdomyolysis (crush, burn, electrical)

Heat illness (hyperthermia, vigorous exercise, prolonged seizures)

Myositis

Animal venom bite

Haff disease

Exogenous

Succinylcholine

Amphotericin B

Barbiturates

Cocaine

Codeine

Diazepam

Ethanol

Heroin

Statins

Halothane

Thiazides

Pentamidine

Methadone

Paracetamol

Antidepressants

Antipsychotics

Renal

There are many disease processes that affect the kidney that can lead to hematuria. Most glomerular diseases that cause hematuria can be diagnosed after a biopsy, and are not likely to be made in the ED, further highlighting the importance of referral for outpatient evaluation. Clinical features that may direct the provider to a more glomerular cause of hematuria are dysmorphic RBCs/red cell casts in the urine, proteinuria, lower extremity edema, hypertension, renal insufficiency, and a recent upper respiratory infection.

Inflammation and resultant infection can cause hematuria. Pyelonephritis, inflammation of the renal pelvis and kidney, is characterized by flank pain. An infectious

Table 1
Renal causes of hematuria

Origin	Cause	Disease
Trauma		Renal trauma (contusion, hematoma, laceration, rupture)
Glomerular		
	Glomerulonephritis	IgA nephropathy Membranoproliferative/mesangial Nephrotic syndrome Post-strep (other postinfectious nephritides) Rapid progressive/nephrotic
	Familial	Alport syndrome Fabry disease Nail-Patella syndrome Thin basement membrane disease
	Systemic/autoimmune	Goodpasture disease Systemic lupus erythematosus
	Vasculitis	Henoch-Schonlein purpura Periarteritis nodosa Wegeners' granulomatosis
Nonglomerular		
	Familial	Polycystic kidney disease Medullary sponge kidney
	Infectious	Pyelonephritis Tuberculosis schistosomiasis
	Neoplasm	Wilms (pediatrics) Genitourinary (renal carcinoma)

source is supported by urinalysis demonstrating pyuria (white blood cells in the urine) and/or bacteriuria (bacteria in the urine). Pyelonephritis with significant hematuria is difficult to distinguish from an infected renal calculus; therefore, if there is any suspicion for nephrolithiasis, diagnostic imaging should be obtained.[5] Treatment of obstructive pyelonephritis often requires more aggressive therapy than antibiotics alone; percutaneous nephrostomy or ureteral stent may be required.

Although hematuria is common in patients with documented nephrolithiasis, it is absent in up to 10% to 20% of patients.[15] According to 1 study, there may be a temporal correlation to when the symptoms began and presence of hematuria, suggesting that hematuria seems to abate as symptoms progress.[16]

A genitourinary malignancy must always be considered in the differential for hematuria. Renal cell carcinoma (RCC) is the most common primary renal malignancy. Smoking is a strong risk factor for RCC. In addition, the kidneys can harbor metastases from other primary malignancies, most commonly the colon, breast, lung, and head, ears, eyes, nose, and throat.[5,17]

Renal trauma is relatively common in deceleration injuries and in posterior torso injuries. The kidneys are the most commonly injured genitourinary organ in trauma, accounting for up to 24% of traumatic abdominal solid organ injuries.[5,18,19] Patients can present with gross or microscopic hematuria with or without significant back or flank pain.

It is also worth mentioning that patients with a kidney transplant are at increased risk for hematuria compared with the general population.[20,21] Infections are, by far, the most common cause of hematuria in the transplanted kidney. The incidence of

Table 2
Nonrenal causes of hematuria

Origin	Cause	Disease
Postrenal	Trauma	Urethral trauma
		Bladder trauma
		Urethral trauma
		Prostatic trauma
	Obstruction	Nephrolithiasis
		Benign prostatic hyperplasia
		Posterior ureteral valve/stricture
		Reflux nephropathy
		Foreign bodies/Foley catheter
	Infectious	Cystitis
		Prostatitis
		Epididymitis
		Urethritis
	Neoplasm	Genitourinary (ureter, bladder, prostate, urethral)
		Lymphoma/sarcoma/myeloma/metastatic
Hematologic	Coagulopathy	Inherited or acquired
		Sickle cell hemoglobinopathy
Vascular	Vascular	Arteriovenous malformation
		Renal artery (embolus, thrombus, infarct, dissection, aneurysm, malignant hypertension)
		Renal vein thrombosis
		Abdominal aortic aneurysm
		Ureteroarterial fistula

infection is much higher because of immunosuppressive medications. Opportunistic infections need to be considered in this at-risk population, and are much more likely to require admission and inpatient infectious disease consultation. Renal calculus in transplant patients can present with painless hematuria, because the kidneys are denervated during procurement.[21] Transplanted kidneys may also develop the recurrence of the glomerulopathies that affected their native kidneys, and this is among the top 3 reasons why transplanted kidneys are lost.[21,22]

Malignancies of the transplanted kidneys are also possible in this population. RCC is much higher than the general population and, surprisingly, more common in the native kidney than the transplanted kidney.[21,23] There is also an increase in prostate cancer in the first 3 years after transplant, but it reduces to that of the general population after that timeframe.[21,24] In addition, malignancies incited by viral infections, such as human papillomavirus, are more common in the transplanted patient.[21]

Postrenal

Ureter
Ureteral causes of hematuria are most commonly nephrolithiasis and trauma. Nephrolithiasis commonly causes ureteral irritation during passage of stones thus resulting in hematuria; however, it is neither a sensitive nor specific finding and may be completely absent. Isolated ureteral trauma is rare without other abdominal injury given its protected space in the retroperitoneum. Approximately 80% of ureteral injuries occur from iatrogenic injury during gynecologic, urologic, or colorectal surgeries.[5,18,25]

Bladder
Infection, trauma, and malignancy are the most common causes of bladder hematuria. Cystitis can be infectious or noninfectious, with most causes being from infections

Hemorrhagic cystitis is a very frequent cause of hematuria, especially in patients receiving radiation or those exposed to chemicals or medications. Differentiating hemorrhagic cystitis from infectious cystitis is sometimes difficult. Gross hematuria is much more rare in infectious cystitis than in noninfectious cystitis.[26] In addition, radiation-induced hemorrhagic cystitis causes much more pain and is more likely to cause gross hematuria. The biggest risk factor for radiation-induced hemorrhagic cystitis is radiation to the pelvis; however, the timeline for when the hemorrhagic cystitis occurs is variable. It can happen from days to years after the patient received the radiation therapy.[5,26,27] It is easy to assume that any hematuria postradiation therapy is radiation-induced hemorrhagic cystitis; however, in 1 study, 10% of patients who had received radiation therapy who presented with hematuria were found to have bladder cancer.[27] Therefore, the diagnosis of radiation-induced hemorrhagic cystitis is difficult to make in the ED, and other emergent causes should be investigated.

Bladder trauma is another cause of hematuria from the bladder. Pelvic fracture is the most common associated injury with bladder rupture.[18] Gross hematuria and pelvic fracture is found in 29% of patients with a bladder injury and, therefore, a patient presenting with a pelvic fracture and gross hematuria warrants imaging.[5,18,28] Other signs and symptoms that may suggest a bladder rupture include unexplained abdominal distention, oliguria or anuria, inability to void, and suprapubic pain.[18,29] Therefore, pelvic fractures that have any of these clinical signs and symptoms should also be considered for bladder rupture.

Bladder malignancy is most commonly discovered on routine follow-up for hematuria evaluation. The most common presenting complaint in 80% to 90% of patients with bladder cancer is painless gross hematuria.[5,30] The diagnosis is not usually made in the ED and, therefore, the importance of follow-up for patients presenting with hematuria is stressed.

Prostate and urethra

The most common prostatic sources of hematuria are benign prostatic hyperplasia (BPH) followed by malignancy. Patients with BPH often complain of urinary frequency from an enlarged prostate leading to urinary obstruction with sometimes overflow incontinence. Microscopic hematuria is more common compared with gross hematuria in BPH patients. Foley catheter placement in an obstructed patient from prostatic enlargement is often mistakenly thought to be the cause of hematuria; however, any microscopic or gross hematuria after insertion or manipulation of a Foley still deserves attention.[31] Urethritis and prostatitis are infections that can cause hematuria. Any blunt or penetrating trauma to the penile shaft with blood at the urethral meatus or gross hematuria is assumed to have urethral trauma until proven otherwise.

Vascular

Abdominal aortic aneurysm

Ruptured abdominal aortic aneurysm (AAA) has an overall mortality rate of 90%, but only 25% to 50% of cases actually present with the classic triad of pain, pulsatile mass, and hypotension.[32–34] AAA affects ~5% to 10% of the population over 65 years of age, and is more common in male smokers with a positive family history of aortic aneurysms.[33,35,36] A patient's symptomatology is based on the site rupture. Temporary sealing of the tear can result in a variety of ambiguous symptoms secondary to extension and compressive effects. Infrequent presentations that must be kept at the forefront for any emergency provider is flank to loin pain (eg, nephrolithiasis, testicular/groin pain, inguinal pain mimicking hernia, or limb pain/paralysis). Aorta-left renal vein fistula is uncommon but can occur when an infrarenal AAA erodes into a retro-aortic left renal vein. This syndrome is characterized by abdominal pain, hematuria, and renal insufficiency.[37,38]

Iliac artery-ureteral fistula

Even more unusual than aorta-left renal vein fistula is a ureteroarterial fistula. These are typically located at or near the junction of the iliac artery and thus can also be termed iliac artery-ureteral fistula. Clinical manifestations are variable, but intermittent hematuria with or without hydronephrosis, as well as symptomatic anemia and flank pain, have been well described.[5,39] Predisposing risk factors include any previous pelvic or vascular surgery, ureteral mobilization or indwelling stent, pelvic radiation, or known aorto-iliac aneurysm.[40]

Renal artery dissection

Renal artery dissection (RAD) is not typically isolated and often results from propagation of an aortic dissection (AD).[41,42] AD should be contemplated in any case of pain above the diaphragm (chest or back) and concomitant hematuria, pyuria, and deterioration of renal function. Renal ischemia frequently results from true lumen obliteration with AD without involvement of the renal artery itself.[43]

RAD can also occur after blunt trauma or percutaneous procedure and, although rare, even spontaneously. Spontaneous dissection has been associated with the following: connective tissues diseases (Ehlers-Danlos syndrome, Marfan syndrome, and fibromuscular dysplasia), severe atherosclerosis, and malignant hypertension.[44,45] Clinical presentation is often vague, but frequently includes hypertension, lumbar or flank pain, gross hematuria, and impaired renal function.[46]

Renal arteriovenous malformation

Renal arteriovenous malformations (AVMs) can be either congenital/cirsoid (25%) or acquired (75%).[47–49] Congenital lesions are tortuous and typically occur beneath the urothelium leading to hematuria in up to 70% of cases.[49] Conversely, acquired lesions are aneurysmal and normally have a solitary communication between artery and vein. An acquired AVM is most commonly associated with renal biopsy, but has also been known to occur with other renal procedures, trauma, malignancy, and idiopathic (3%–5%).[49,50] Clinical symptoms, hematuria, systolic hypertension, and abdominal pain, frequently do not manifest until the 4th–5th decade in life.[49]

Renal artery aneurysm/pseudoaneurysm

Some may consider the prevalence of renal artery aneurysm (0.5%) almost nominal. Moreover rupture is extremely rare, but several risk factors have been associated, such as morphology (saccular noncalcified), size (>1.5 cm), and pregnancy.[51–53] Rupture typically causes abdominal or flank pain with hematuria. Renal artery pseudoaneurysm similar to renal AVM is a well-recognized complication of renal procedures and trauma, and presents as AVM discussed above. Hematuria is commonly seen within 4 weeks of renal procedures.[54]

Renal vein thrombus

Renal vein thrombus (RVT) is the most common vascular abnormality in newborns.[55] Typically, it is bilateral and accompanied with vomiting and diarrhea. RVT occurs far less frequently in adults and, when present, is unilateral. The pathophysiology of RVT is similar to that of other venous thrombosis and is associated with 3 distinct factors: endothelial damage, stasis, and hypercoagulablity. RVT has been most associated with nephrotic syndrome, malignancy with tumor invasion, and trauma (blunt and iatrogenic).[56] Symptoms of RVT in adults are dependent on rate and extent of thrombus formation and range from nominal to those that mimic nephrolithiasis (abdominal/flank pain with hematuria).[57,58]

Renal infarct

Renal infarct (RI) is an exceedingly rare diagnosis and usually due to thromboembolism with a source of emboli most commonly arising from the heart (atrial fibrillation); this is followed by infective endocarditis, thrombi from the suprarenal aorta, RAD, hypercoagulable state, endovascular intervention, cocaine use, and sickle cell disease.[59,60] Similar to RVT, those subjects with RI present with renal colic-like symptoms, and hematuria is seen in more than 50%.

EVALUATION

When evaluating a patient in the ED for hematuria, the first and most critical step is to discern if a life-threatening cause is present. Most patients will have a benign cause and simply require outpatient follow-up with a primary care physician, urologist, or nephrologist. Physicians require a high index of suspicion based on a thorough evaluation, consisting of history and physical examination.

It is paramount to ask about pain, because pain is common among vascular causes, and because hematuria often may only be microscopic. Pain is frequently localized to the back, flank, or abdomen and described as acute in onset and severe. This must be differentiated from the similarly described pain of nephrolithiasis. Painless hematuria is much more likely to be associated with malignancy. Although an abundance of blood (secondary to malignancy) can lead to clotting and resultant urinary obstruction causing pain, specifically in the suprapubic area from bladder overdistention. Other causes of suprapubic discomfort can originate from a urinary tract infection or a distended urinary bladder secondary to BPH.

The frequency of hematuria and the portion of the urinary stream in which it occurs is significant. A single episode of brief hematuria should not be overlooked as benign because this has been linked to urologic malignancy. Hematuria at the initiation of the stream is commonly associated with a distal lesion such as urethritis, urethral stricture, or urethral laceration from a passed calculus. If it occurs toward the end of the stream it is commonly associated with more proximal lesions, such as bladder polyps or prostatitis. Hematuria throughout the entire stream usually arises from an upper genitourinary source such as a lesion in the bladder, ureter, or kidney. If hematuria occurs during a female patient's menstrual cycle, menstrual blood may be mistaken for hematuria or endometriosis implanted somewhere in the urinary tract. Therefore, it is important to ask female patients about their last menstrual cycle. The amount of hematuria is also an important inquiry. Any amount of urinary blood is likely to cause a patient distress; however, very little blood is required to alter the color of urine. Therefore, rather than asking the quantity of blood seen in the urine, a better question is the color of the urine stream (orange, pink, light red, or dark red, or dark brown-cola) and the presence or absence or clots.

History of trauma associated with hematuria may be the only sign of genitourinary tree injury and warrants further investigation/imaging. Other important clues to obtain in history include: rigorous exercise, recent drug or food ingestion, systemic symptoms (ie, fever or chills), bleeding diathesis, recent upper respiratory infection, and recent genitourinary or vascular instrumentation or surgery. Family history of pathologic conditions of vascular origin or genitourinary malignancy should heighten the provider's suspicion for these disease processes, because of any risk factors, such as smoking or environmental or occupational exposure to chemicals.

Physical examination should focus again on ruling out the more dangerous diagnoses. Abnormal vital signs should be addressed promptly. Signs of hemodynamic instability, such as tachycardia or hypotension, should also be addressed, although cautiously. Permissive hypotension is the standard in patients with a ruptured AAA and should give the provider pause before resuscitating aggressively; when resuscitating blood is preferred to dilution effects that result from crystalloids.

Physical examination, unfortunately, does not significantly assist with making a diagnosis in most situations. When present, certain findings may be suggestive of a particular causes: fever is common in infections of the genitourinary tract or systemic illness, such as endocarditis; an abdominal mass or bruit may be appreciated in vascular events; the presence of a cardiac murmur or an irregular rhythm can point toward endocarditis versus atrial fibrillation with RI; peripheral edema with hypertension indicates a glomerulonephropathy; and suprapubic pain with bladder distension likely represents an obstructive process.

DIAGNOSTIC TESTING

Laboratory studies can be helpful in the evaluation of hematuria. The urinalysis is paramount and optimally should be a midstream clean-catch urine sample or a catheterized sample to minimize contamination. Urine dipstick should be done first looking for blood which has a sensitivity of greater than 90%. Absence of blood on the urine dipstick lends to the diagnosis of pseudohematuria. Any presence of blood on the urine dipstick warrants a microscopic evaluation. Presence of blood on dipstick without the presence of RBCs suggests a myoglobinopathy and warrants other testing for conditions, such as rhabdomyolysis. Other findings on a urinalysis, such as white blood cells or RBC, imply infection and glomerular disease, respectively.

Other laboratory studies include a complete blood count to evaluate baseline hemoglobin and hematocrit, as well as a platelet count to evaluate for thrombocytopenia. A complete metabolic panel can provide insight into liver transaminases and renal indices of blood urea nitrogen and creatinine. Coagulation studies are not routinely indicated, but should be included in patients with hematuria or patients on anticoagulation. In patients with significant bleeding, a type and screen should also be obtained in case transfusion is required. A beta hCG is indicated in women of child-bearing age to evaluate for pregnancy.

Imaging should not be routinely performed in patients with hematuria. Any imaging obtained in the ED should be used to rule out emergent diagnoses. Renal sonography can evaluate for hydronephrosis. Unilateral hydronephrosis may indicate a stone or a mass that is occluding the ureter, and further imaging may be required. Any hydronephrosis, but especially bilateral hydronephrosis, warrants bladder sonography for volume assessment to evaluate for bladder outlet obstruction. Likewise, history or physical examination findings concerning urinary retention also warrant bladder sonography. Sonography is an equally useful tool for evaluating the aorta for an AAA. Despite not being sensitive for rupture, the presence of an AAA on sonography in a patient with abdominal pain or flank pain and hematuria warrants further imaging (computed tomography angiography [CTA]) to rule out rupture. CTA is, in fact, the imaging of choice if the provider is considering any of the vascular catastrophes discussed above.

Computed tomography (CT) with IV contrast is frequently performed in any trauma patient with hematuria.[18] Focused assessment with sonography in trauma can prove useful in the hemodynamically unstable patient, although it has a poor sensitivity and specificity for identifying retroperitoneal (eg, renal) injury, when a positive value indicates emergent surgical exploration. Blood at the tip of the meatus or any gross hematuria in patients with trauma requires a retrograde urethrogram and cystogram to evaluate injury to the urethra and bladder.[61] CT cystogram can also be done as it has better sensitivity and specificity for bladder injuries, but depends on availability.

Atraumatic hematuria is not as dependent on imaging. Noncontrast CT is the imaging modality of choice when evaluating nephrolithiasis, because it has good sensitivity and specificity for radiopaque stones. It can also assist with ruling out other more ominous (vascular) disease processes; however, that requires the addition of an angiographic phase to the CT. CT is also very good at evaluating for masses or suspected malignancy. Although these masses are sometimes found incidentally when evaluating for another cause, any abnormal findings should be relayed to the patient for close outpatient follow-up.

TREATMENT

Emergent management of hematuria is based on the cause of and amount of bleeding. Most patients with microscopic hematuria can be safely discharged home with close follow-up, ideally within a week. A repeat urinalysis should be performed and the outpatient provider can direct further workup. This includes trauma patients who have microscopic hematuria and negative imaging.

Gross hematuria of unknown cause that is asymptomatic can also be safely discharged with close outpatient follow-up with urology. In the elderly population, there must be screening for malignancy. All patients with gross hematuria need to be given strict return precautions and warning about the possibility of urinary retention. These patients are at much higher risk of urinary obstruction from clots in the bladder. Some recommend sending these patients home with a Foley catheter in place to prevent obstruction and a subsequent return to the ED. However, there is an increased risk of iatrogenic hematuria from the Foley catheter insertion and so the benefits need to be weighed with the risks.

Symptomatic gross hematuria will usually require a Foley catheter. A 3-way catheter can be placed for initiation of manual irrigation or continuous bladder irrigation (CBI) with normal saline to irrigate the clots out of the bladder to prevent urinary obstruction. It also prevents the formation of new clots by agitation of the contents of the bladder. Normal saline is traditionally used for irrigation. However, there is some literature that shows that the addition of tranexamic acid to the solution reduces the volume of irrigant used until transparency of urine flow.[62,63] Manual irrigation by hand is successful at clearing clots and hematuria in most circumstances. If manual irrigation is unsuccessful and severe hematuria and clots remain, CBI should be initiated. CBI requires frequent monitoring for exit port obstruction, because a clot, or any obstruction, places the patient at risk of bladder perforation. If CBI is not successful, interventional radiology may be consulted for embolization. Emergency providers may be faced with a choice of whether to reverse anticoagulation in someone who is supratherapeutic. These rare circumstances are most often limited to life-threatening hemorrhage and vascular disease processes. Rarely does hematuria result in such a profound hemorrhage in which reversal is necessary. Holding off a dose for a day is usually sufficient to return anticoagulation to optimal levels.

Urologic consultation in the ED or transfer to a center with an on-call urologist may be necessary for a small subset of patients with hematuria. Urologists can assist with initiating CBI and placement of stents and/or nephrostomy tubes in cases of obstruction due to nephrolithiasis or malignancy. In addition, they can intervene with cystoscopy in certain indications. Indications for a urologic consultation for hematuria in the ED and/or admission are found in **Box 4**.

Box 4
Indications for consultation and/or admission

- Symptomatic anemia
- Repeated catheter occlusion with clots refractory to irrigation
- Acute kidney injury
- Urinary retention
- Unstable vital signs
- Uncontrolled pain/vomiting
- Vascular cause of hematuria
- Coagulopathy
- Nephrolithiasis with associated urinary tract infection and/or acute kidney injury
- Traumatic injury

SUMMARY

Hematuria is not an infrequent occurrence in patients presenting to the ED. It is incumbent on the emergency provider to perform a thorough evaluation of the patient, including a detailed history and physical examination, as well as laboratory studies and necessary imaging. The differential diagnosis for these patients is exhaustive. Most patients will be discharged home with appropriate close outpatient follow-up. A small minority will have a condition resulting from a vascular cause, requiring angiographic imaging, thus the emergency provider must be vigilant and maintain a high index of suspicion.

REFERENCES

1. Sokolosky MC. Hematuria. Emerg Med Clin North Am 2001;19(3):621–32.
2. Sutton JM. Evaluation of hematuria in adults. JAMA 1990;263(18):2475–80.
3. Grossfeld GD, Litwin MS, Wolf JS Jr, et al. Evaluation of asymptomatic microscopic hematuria in adults: the American Urological Association best practice policy–part II: patient evaluation, cytology, voided markers, imaging, cystoscopy, nephrology evaluation, and follow-up. Urology 2001;57(4):604–10.
4. Copley JB. Isolated asymptomatic hematuria in the adult. Am J Med Sci 1986; 291(2):101–11.
5. Avellino GJ, Bose S, Wang DS. Diagnosis and management of hematuria. Surg Clin North Am 2016;96(3):503–15.
6. Yafi FA, Aprikian AG, Tanguay S, et al. Patients with microscopic and gross hematuria: practice and referral patterns among primary care physicians in a universal health care system. Can Urol Assoc J 2011;5(2):97–101.
7. Vasdev N, Kumar A, Veeratterapillay R, et al. Hematuria secondary to benign prostatic hyperplasia: retrospective analysis of 166 men identified in a single one stop hematuria clinic. Curr Urol 2013;6(3):146–9.
8. Mohr DN, Offord KP, Owen RA, et al. Asymptomatic microhematuria and urologic disease. A population-based study. JAMA 1986;256(2):224–9.
9. Mariani AJ, Mariani MC, Macchioni C, et al. The significance of adult hematuria: 1,000 hematuria evaluations including a risk-benefit and cost-effectiveness analysis. J Urol 1989;141(2):350–5.

10. Messing EM, Young TB, Hunt VB, et al. The significance of asymptomatic micro-hematuria in men 50 or more years old: findings of a home screening study using urinary dipsticks. J Urol 1987;137(5):919–22.

11. Messing EM, Young TB, Hunt VB, et al. Home screening for hematuria: results of a multiclinic study. J Urol 1992;148(2 Pt 1):289–92.

12. Messing EM, Young TB, Hunt VB, et al. Urinary tract cancers found by homescre-ening with hematuria dipsticks in healthy men over 50 years of age. Cancer 1989; 64(11):2361–7.

13. Britton JP, Dowell AC, Whelan P. Dipstick haematuria and bladder cancer in men over 60: results of a community study. BMJ 1989;299(6706):1010–2.

14. Britton JP, Dowell AC, Whelan P, et al. A community study of bladder cancer screening by the detection of occult urinary bleeding. J Urol 1992;148(3):788–90.

15. Press SM, Smith AD. Incidence of negative hematuria in patients with acute uri-nary lithiasis presenting to the emergency room with flank pain. Urology 1995; 45(5):753–7.

16. Kobayashi T, Nishizawa K, Mitsumori K, et al. Impact of date of onset on the absence of hematuria in patients with acute renal colic. J Urol 2003;170(4 Pt 1):1093–6.

17. Zhou C, Urbauer DL, Fellman BM, et al. Metastases to the kidney: a comprehen-sive analysis of 151 patients from a tertiary referral centre. BJU Int 2016;117(5): 775–82.

18. Morey AF, Brandes S, Dugi DD 3rd, et al. Urotrauma: AUA guideline. J Urol 2014; 192(2):327–35.

19. Smith J, Caldwell E, D'Amours S, et al. Abdominal trauma: a disease in evolution. ANZ J Surg 2005;75(9):790–4.

20. Previte SR, Murata GT, Olsson CA, et al. Hematuria in renal transplant recipients. Ann Surg 1978;187(2):219–22.

21. Wang Z, Vathsala A, Tiong HY. Haematuria in postrenal transplant patients. Bio-med Res Int 2015;2015:292034.

22. Hariharan S, Peddi VR, Savin VJ, et al. Recurrent and de novo renal diseases af-ter renal transplantation: a report from the renal allograft disease registry. Am J Kidney Dis 1998;31(6):928–31.

23. Master VA, Meng MV, Grossfeld GD, et al. Treatment and outcome of invasive bladder cancer in patients after renal transplantation. J Urol 2004;171(3):1085–8.

24. Dantal J, Pohanka E. Malignancies in renal transplantation: an unmet medical need. Nephrol Dial Transplant 2007;22(Suppl 1):i4–10.

25. Gross JA, Lehnert BE, Linnau KF, et al. Imaging of urinary system trauma. Radiol Clin North Am 2015;53(4):773–88, ix.

26. Haldar S, Dru C, Bhowmick NA. Mechanisms of hemorrhagic cystitis. Am J Clin Exp Urol 2014;2(3):199–208.

27. Goucher G, Saad F, Lukka H, et al. Canadian Urological Association Best Prac-tice Report: diagnosis and management of radiation-induced hemorrhagic cystitis. Can Urol Assoc J 2019;13(2):15–23.

28. Fuhrman GM, Simmons GT, Davidson BS, et al. The single indication for cystog-raphy in blunt trauma. Am Surg 1993;59(6):335–7.

29. Avey G, Blackmore CC, Wessells H, et al. Radiographic and clinical predictors of bladder rupture in blunt trauma patients with pelvic fracture. Acad Radiol 2006; 13(5):573–9.

30. Kamat AM, Hahn NM, Efstathiou JA, et al. Bladder cancer. Lancet 2016; 388(10061):2796–810.

31. Sklar DP, Diven B, Jones J. Incidence and magnitude of catheter-induced hematuria. Am J Emerg Med 1986;4(1):14–6.
32. Pearce WH, Zarins CK, Bacharach JM. Atherosclerotic Peripheral Vascular Disease Symposium II: controversies in abdominal aortic aneurysm repair. Circulation 2008;118(25):2860–3.
33. Fielding JW, Black J, Ashton F, et al. Diagnosis and management of 528 abdominal aortic aneurysms. Br Med J (Clin Res Ed) 1981;283(6287):355–9.
34. Marston WA, Ahlquist R, Johnson G Jr, et al. Misdiagnosis of ruptured abdominal aortic aneurysms. J Vasc Surg 1992;16(1):17–22.
35. Thompson RW, Curci JA, Ennis TL, et al. Pathophysiology of abdominal aortic aneurysms: insights from the elastase-induced model in mice with different genetic backgrounds. Ann N Y Acad Sci 2006;1085:59–73.
36. Lederle FA, Johnson GR, Wilson SE, et al. Prevalence and associations of abdominal aortic aneurysm detected through screening. Aneurysm Detection and Management (ADAM) Veterans Affairs Cooperative Study Group. Ann Intern Med 1997;126(6):441–9.
37. Mansour MA, Rutherford RB, Metcalf RK, et al. Spontaneous aorto-left renal vein fistula: the "abdominal pain, hematuria, silent left kidney" syndrome. Surgery 1991;109(1):101–6.
38. Meyerson SL, Haider SA, Gupta N, et al. Abdominal aortic aneurysm with aorta-left renal vein fistula with left varicocele. J Vasc Surg 2000;31(4):802–5.
39. Madoff DC, Gupta S, Toombs BD, et al. Arterioureteral fistulas: a clinical, diagnostic, and therapeutic dilemma. AJR Am J Roentgenol 2004;182(5):1241–50.
40. Kerns DB, Darcy MD, Baumann DS, et al. Autologous vein-covered stent for the endovascular management of an iliac artery-ureteral fistula: case report and review of the literature. J Vasc Surg 1996;24(4):680–6.
41. Beroniade V, Roy P, Froment D, et al. Primary renal artery dissection. Presentation of two cases and brief review of the literature. Am J Nephrol 1987;7(5):382–9.
42. Jenq CC, Chen YC, Huang JY, et al. Type B aortic dissection with early presentation mimicking acute pyelonephritis. J Nephrol 2006;19(3):341–5.
43. Slonim SM, Nyman UR, Semba CP, et al. True lumen obliteration in complicated aortic dissection: endovascular treatment. Radiology 1996;201(1):161–6.
44. Harrison EG Jr, Hunt JC, Bernatz PE. Morphology of fibromuscular dysplasia of the renal artery in renovascular hypertension. Am J Med 1967;43(1):97–112.
45. Lacombe M. Isolated spontaneous dissection of the renal artery. J Vasc Surg 2001;33(2):385–91.
46. Edwards BS, Stanson AW, Holley KE, et al. Isolated renal artery dissection, presentation, evaluation, management, and pathology. Mayo Clin Proc 1982;57(9):564–71.
47. Muraoka N, Sakai T, Kimura H, et al. Rare causes of hematuria associated with various vascular diseases involving the upper urinary tract. Radiographics 2008;28(3):855–67.
48. Ali M, Aziz W, Abbas F. Renal arteriovenous malformation: an unusual cause of recurrent haematuria. BMJ Case Rep 2013;2013 [pii:bcr2013010374].
49. Crotty KL, Orihuela E, Warren MM. Recent advances in the diagnosis and treatment of renal arteriovenous malformations and fistulas. J Urol 1993;150(5 Pt 1) 1355–9.
50. Klimberg I, Wilson J, Davis K, et al. Hemorrhage from congenital renal arteriovenous malformation in pregnancy. Urology 1984;23(4):381–4.
51. Tham G, Ekelund L, Herrlin K, et al. Renal artery aneurysms. Natural history and prognosis. Ann Surg 1983;197(3):348–52.

52. Yang JC, Hye RJ. Ruptured renal artery aneurysm during pregnancy. Ann Vasc Surg 1996;10(4):370–2.
53. Fiesseler FW, Riggs RL, Shih R. Ruptured renal artery aneurysm presenting as hematuria. Am J Emerg Med 2004;22(3):232–4.
54. Jebara VA, El Rassi I, Achouh PE, et al. Renal artery pseudoaneurysm after blunt abdominal trauma. J Vasc Surg 1998;27(2):362–5.
55. Zigman A, Yazbeck S, Emil S, et al. Renal vein thrombosis: a 10-year review. J Pediatr Surg 2000;35(11):1540–2.
56. Harrison CV, Milne MD, Steiner RE. Clinical aspects of renal vein thrombosis. Q J Med 1956;25(99):285–98.
57. Wang IK, Lee CH, Yang BY, et al. Low-molecular-weight heparin successfully treating a nephrotic patient complicated by renal and ovarian vein thrombosis and pulmonary embolism. Int J Clin Pract Suppl 2005;(147):72–5.
58. Choudhary A, Majee P, Gupta R, et al. Adult idiopathic renal vein thrombosis mimicking acute pyelonephritis. J Clin Diagn Res 2016;10(9):Pd18–9.
59. Bourgault M, Grimbert P, Verret C, et al. Acute renal infarction: a case series. Clin J Am Soc Nephrol 2013;8(3):392–8.
60. Korzets Z, Plotkin E, Bernheim J, et al. The clinical spectrum of acute renal infarction. Isr Med Assoc J 2002;4(10):781–4.
61. Elgammal MA. Straddle injuries to the bulbar urethra: management and outcome in 53 patients. Int Braz J Urol 2009;35(4):450–8.
62. Moharamzadeh P, Ojaghihaghighi S, Amjadi M, et al. Effect of tranexamic acid on gross hematuria: a pilot randomized clinical trial study. Am J Emerg Med 2017; 35(12):1922–5.
63. Yao Q, Wu M, Zhou J, et al. Treatment of persistent gross hematuria with tranexamic acid in autosomal dominant polycystic kidney disease. Kidney Blood Press Res 2017;42(1):156–64.

Female Nonobstetric Genitourinary Emergencies

Sarah Mahonski, MD[a], Kami M. Hu, MD[b],*

KEYWORDS

- Pelvic inflammatory disease • Ovarian torsion • Tubo-ovarian abscess
- Vaginal bleeding • Bartholin gland cyst

KEY POINTS

- Normal color Doppler ultrasound does not officially rule out ovarian torsion if clinical suspicion is high; emergent gynecologic consultation is still required.
- Ovarian torsion may be the initial presentation of gynecologic malignancy in older patients.
- The use of metronidazole for anaerobic coverage in pelvic inflammatory disease is an ongoing issue of debate except in cases of severe, complicated PID, such as TOA or pyosalpinx.
- Emergency management of abnormal uterine bleeding involves stabilization with appropriate blood products and IV conjugated estrogen or tranexamic acid in cases of severe ongoing hemorrhage.
- Bartholin gland cysts and abscesses are best managed by placement of a Word catheter and do not require antibiotics at discharge unless there is associated cellulitis, immunosuppression, or pregnancy.

INTRODUCTION

Abdominal pain is the most common chief complaint in the emergency department, with an estimated 23 million visits in 2013.[1] Many of the patients with these complaints are female, and the emergency provider must be well versed in the identification and management of life-threatening emergencies related to the female genitourinary system. This article provides a review of the pathophysiology, clinical presentation, and emergency department evaluation and management of must-know topics, such as ovarian torsion, pelvic inflammatory disease (PID), tubo-ovarian abscess (TOA), abnormal uterine bleeding (AUB), and Bartholin gland abscess.

Disclosures: The authors have nothing to disclose.
[a] Heritage Valley Health System, 1000 Dutch Ridge Road, Beaver, PA 15009, USA; [b] Emergency/Internal/Critical Care Medicine, University of Maryland, 110 South Paca Street, 6th Floor, Suite 200, Baltimore, MD 21201, USA
* Corresponding author.
E-mail address: khu@som.umaryland.edu
twitter: @kwhomd (K.M.H.)

Emerg Med Clin N Am 37 (2019) 771–784
https://doi.org/10.1016/j.emc.2019.07.012
0733-8627/19/Published by Elsevier Inc.

emed.theclinics.com

OVARIAN TORSION
Background

Although representing only 3% of all gynecologic emergencies,[2] ovarian torsion is a true surgical emergency that emergency physicians must be able to identify. Ovarian torsion occurs when the ovary and fallopian tube twist about the infundibulopelvic and utero-ovarian ligaments,[3] structures that contain the vascular structures supplying the ovary. The twisting leads to venous congestion, edema, and eventually compression of arterial blood flow to the ovary itself. Without prompt intervention, ischemia and necrosis ensue and future fertility is compromised.[2] More than 50% of cases are unilateral, more commonly occurring on the right, a laterality attributed to the fixed position of the sigmoid colon compared with the flexibility of the cecum.[3]

Clinical Features

Ovarian torsion classically presents with the acute onset of sharp, unilateral abdominal pain, either constant or intermittent,[3] with associated nausea and vomiting. Note, however, that patients may not reliably present with these symptoms. In one study of 101 patients with ovarian torsion, only 59% presented acutely, and 2 of the 101 patients even had symptoms for more than 150 days.[4] Fever has been reported in up to 20% of cases,[5–7] and the absence of concomitant vaginal discharge or bleeding has been shown to be associated with a higher likelihood of torsion.[8] Although abdominal tenderness is common, 30% of patients have a nontender abdomen and lack adnexal tenderness on bimanual examination.[4]

Special Populations

The young and the old

Ovarian torsion is most common in women of reproductive age but can occur in all ages; neonatal cases have been even described.[9] Approximately 20% of patients are premenarchal, with an average age of 9 years. Premenarchal patients are more likely to present after 24 hours of symptoms, and more likely to have clinical signs, such as fever or palpable mass.[10,11] Fifty percent of premenarchal patients with torsion have a normal underlying ovary, in contrast to reproductive-aged females who often exhibit torsion because of a benign ovarian mass.[3] Although no longer an issue of compromised fertility, postmenopausal patients with torsion remain at risk of other sequelae, such as adhesions and peritonitis. Postmenopausal patients also more commonly present late in the disease course, up to 48 hours after symptom onset, and may have atypical features, with one study showing more than 50% presenting with continuous dull pain. More than 50% of the patients in this study also were found to have a complex ovarian mass,[12] and ovarian torsion in this age group can be the initial presentation of ovarian cancer.

Pregnancy and assisted reproduction

Pregnancy is considered an independent risk factor for the development of ovarian torsion, with retrospective reviews reporting a pregnancy rate of 8% to 15% in patients presenting with ovarian torsion,[4,13] and a recent systematic review demonstrating an increased risk of torsion with an odds ratio of 18.[14] Torsion is more likely to occur in the first trimester when there is more space in the pelvis,[3,14,15] with most cases relating to structural pathology, such as ovarian or adnexal cysts.[11] The use of assisted reproductive technologies also increases the risk[16,17] with more recent studies showing 11% of overall torsion cases are associated with assisted reproductive technology[18] caused by enlargement of the ovaries and risk of ovarian hyperstimulation syndrome.

Evaluation

If ovarian torsion is suspected, transvaginal pelvic ultrasound (US) with Doppler looking for a decrease or absence of blood flow to the ovary is the diagnostic test of choice. Findings may also include

- An asymmetrically enlarged ovary (>4 cm in diameter)
- Hyperechoic stromal edema
- Free fluid
- Multiple peripheral follicles
- The whirlpool sign (pathognomonic)

The whirlpool sign appears as a hyperechoic structure with multiple inner hypoechoic rings (**Fig. 1**).[19] Note, however, that if torsion is highly suspected based on clinical signs and symptoms, a negative Doppler study does not rule out the diagnosis. Retrospective studies have reported cases of torsion with Doppler flow present in 1 out of 15 cases[20] and 6 out of 10 cases[21] of surgically confirmed torsion. It is therefore imperative to obtain a gynecologic consultation for potential laparoscopic evaluation if there is a high clinical index of suspicion, even with a normal Doppler study.

With undifferentiated lower abdominal pain, computed tomography (CT) scans are often performed to evaluate for nongynecologic etiologies, such as appendicitis.

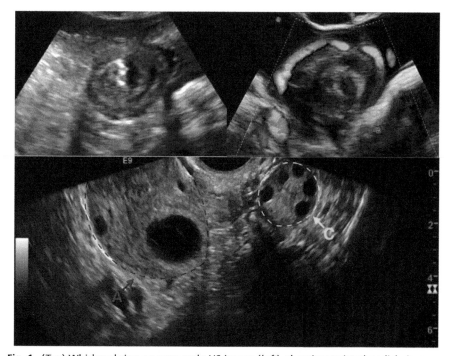

Fig. 1. (*Top*) Whirlpool sign on gray-scale US image (*left*), showing twisted pedicle in cross-section, and highlighted in color Doppler imaging (*right*). (*Bottom*) Enlarged right ovary with peripheral follicles (A) compared with normal left ovary (C). (*From* Valsky DV, Cohen SM, Hamani Y, et al. Whirlpool sign in the diagnosis of adnexal torsion with atypical clinical presentation. *Ultrasound Obstet Gynecol.* 2009;34(2):239-42 and Shyy W, Knight RS, Teismann N. Right lower quadrant abdominal pain: Do not forget about ovarian torsion on the computed tomography scan. *J Emerg Med.* 2018;55(2):e43-5.)

Although ovarian abnormalities noted on CT scan are not specific for torsion, existing evidence seems to indicate that a contrast-enhanced CT completely negative for any ovarian abnormality may virtually rule it out. In one retrospective study of 14 patients with US-confirmed torsion who had also received a contrast-enhanced CT, all had abnormalities on CT scan, including free fluid, ovarian enlargement, stranding, and tubal thickening. No patient with a normal contrast-enhanced CT had torsion confirmed on color Doppler US, leading the investigators to cite a negative predictive value of 100% for contrast-enhanced CT.[22] Another study in 2008 reviewed CT scans obtained during the diagnosis of ovarian torsion on 28 patients. All cases of surgically confirmed torsion had either an enlarged ovary, ovarian cyst, or adnexal mass on CT imaging (**Fig. 2**).[23] MRI is not recommended as an imaging modality to diagnose ovarian torsion because of the duration of the test, cost, and the availability of other diagnostic options, but a different whirlpool sign has been described in the identification of torsion on MRI (**Fig. 3**).

Management

Ovarian torsion is a surgical emergency requiring an emergent gynecologic consultation, with lower morbidity and higher chance of preserved ovarian function the sooner it is surgically addressed. In reproductive-aged females detorsion and ovarian salvage should be attempted, because there is low risk of postoperative adverse events or missed malignancy[24] and increased incidence of preserved ovarian function, even when the ovary appears necrotic.[3] In the postmenopausal woman, surgical management can differ in torsion caused by an ovarian mass. If the patient is well-appearing with well-controlled pain, outpatient management may reasonably be pursued, especially if further oncologic planning is needed.[25] These patients would need strict return precautions.

PELVIC INFLAMMATORY DISEASE
Background

PID includes a spectrum of ascending vaginal and cervical bacterial infections and includes endometritis, salpingitis, and TOA. Untreated PID can lead to systemic illness, chronic pelvic pain, ectopic pregnancy, and tubal infertility.[26] According to the National Health and Nutrition Examination Survey, 4.4% of women of reproductive age have been treated for PID in their lifetime, which estimates to 2.5 million people.[27]

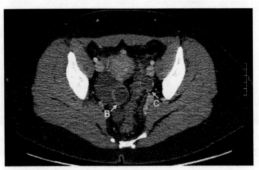

Fig. 2. Computed tomography scan with enlarged right ovary (A) with paraovarian cyst (B) and normal left ovary (C). (*From* Shyy W, Knight RS, Teismann N. Right lower quadrant abdominal pain: Do not forget about ovarian torsion on the computed tomography scan. *J Emerg Med.* 2018;55(2):e43-5; *with permission.*)

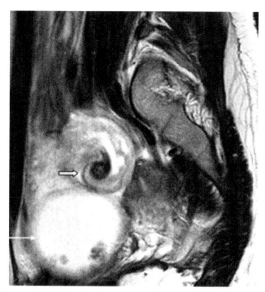

Fig. 3. T2-weighted, sagittal MRI showing the whirlpool sign indicating ovarian torsion of the right ovary (*thick arrow*). Also shown is a right ovarian cystic mass (*thin arrow*). (*From* Ghonge NP, Lall C, Aggarwal B et al. The MRI whirlpool sign in the diagnosis of ovarian torsion. *Radiol Case Rep* 2015;7(3):731; with permission.)

The gold standard for diagnosis is laparoscopy,[28] but in reality PID is a clinical diagnosis and should be considered in any female presenting with lower abdominal pain or vaginal discharge.

Clinical Features

The classic presentation of PID includes pelvic pain with purulent vaginal discharge, often shortly after menses when the cervical mucus provides less of a barrier to ascending infections.[26] Patients may also report abnormal vaginal bleeding, bleeding during intercourse, or dyspareunia. General malaise, nausea, and fever or rigors may or may not be present depending on the severity of the infection. The presence of unilateral or worsened pain on one side should raise suspicion for TOA, and associated right-upper quadrant discomfort with or without concomitant right shoulder pain is suggestive of Fitz-Hugh-Curtis syndrome, a complication of PID involving inflammation of the liver capsule and formation of perihepatic adhesions.[26,29]

Evaluation

Physical examination should be thorough and include abdominal palpation; vaginal speculum examination to evaluate for cervical friability and purulence at the cervical os; and bimanual examination for evaluation of cervical motion tenderness, uterine tenderness, and adnexal fullness, tenderness, or masses. Laboratory studies, such as an erythrocyte sedimentation rate, C-reactive protein, or white blood cell count, may be elevated, but are neither sensitive nor specific.[30] A wet mount and polymerase chain reaction testing for chlamydia and gonorrhea should be obtained, as should a bacterial Gram stain and culture of the cervical discharge, because it may identify other causative bacteria or reveal antibiotic resistance. Although PID is rare during pregnancy, particularly after the first trimester, a human chorionic gonadotropin test should also be sent because pregnancy alters antibiotic therapy selection and is an indication for hospitalization.[26]

Suspected Microbes

In acute PID, the classic pathogens include *Neisseria gonorrhoeae* (gonorrhea) and *Chlamydia trachomatis* (chlamydia). Pathogens that cause bacterial vaginosis, and streptococcus, enteric, and respiratory pathogens that have colonized the vaginal canal may also be involved,[26] and there are case reports of atypical bacteria causing PID and TOA in virgin females.[31–35] Much of the data describing the microbiology of PID come from older studies, which report gonorrhea or chlamydia as the causative organism in up to 77% of TOA isolates.[36] A more recent study showed much lower rates, with 4.4% testing positive for gonorrhea and 10% testing positive for chlamydia; co-infection was documented in 2.6% of cases.[37] The reason for this disparity is unclear, although one possibility is the increasing prevalence of *Mycoplasma genitalium* as a cause of PID.[38]

Management of Uncomplicated Pelvic Inflammatory Disease

Most cases of PID are successfully treated as an outpatient with a 14-day course of oral antibiotics, unless the patient is pregnant; seems septic; is unable to tolerate oral intake; or has a complication, such as pyosalpinx or TOA,[26] which is discussed separately later. The Centers for Disease Control and Prevention (CDC) has several recommended empiric antibiotic regimens, most recently updated in 2015, which generally involve a cephalosporin plus doxycycline (**Table 1**).[39] Of note, when cefoxitin is used, the concomitant use of probenecid is recommended to sustain its serum levels by decreasing its renal clearance and assist with the eradication of gonorrhea.[40] The use of fluoroquinolones for PID is no longer recommended because of quinolone-resistant gonorrhea; however, in the case of severe penicillin allergy levofloxacin, ofloxacin, or moxifloxacin is used cautiously in combination with metronidazole.[39] Several alternative regimens have been proposed because of the increasing prevalence of resistant gonorrhea and *M gentalium*. Similar to chlamydial species, *M genitalium* lacks peptidoglycan and therefore treatments, such as azithromycin and moxifloxacin, are effective, but it has demonstrated resistance to doxycycline with documented treatment failure rates of up to 30% to 40%.[38] Two studies evaluating the use of azithromycin in PID have demonstrated comparable rates of cure from

Table 1
Empiric antibiotic choices for pelvic inflammatory disease as recommended by the CDC for inpatient and outpatient treatment

Outpatient	Ceftriaxone 250 mg IM PLUS doxycycline 100 mg PO q 12 h	± Metronidazole 500 mg PO/IV q 12 h
	Cefoxitin 2 g IM PLUS probenecid 1 g PO PLUS doxycycline 100 mg PO q 12 h	
Inpatient	Cefotetan 2 g IV q 12 h PLUS doxycycline 100 mg PO/IV q 12 h	
	Cefoxitin 2g IV q 6 h PLUS doxycycline 100 mg PO/IV q 12 h	
	Clindamycin 900 mg IV q 8 h PLUS gentamicin 2 mg/kg IV/IM ×1 followed by 1.5 mg/kg IV/IM q 8 h	

Abbreviations: IM, intramuscular; IV, intravenous.
Data from Centers for Disease Control and Prevention. 2015 Sexually Transmitted Diseases Treatment Guidelines. https://www.cdc.gov/std/tg2015/pid.htm. Published 2015.

97% to 98% with azithromycin-based regimens when compared with doxycycline.[41,42] Note that a 2017 Cochrane Systematic Review found no significant difference in cure rates of PID between the various treatment regimens.[43]

Similarly, there is no consensus on the use of metronidazole to supplement recommended regimens. For uncomplicated PID, the CDC leaves the option of metronidazole up to the provider,[39] and the Cochrane review found no evidence to support a difference in rate of cure between groups receiving and not receiving metronidazole.[39]

Complicated or Severe Pelvic Inflammatory Disease

Severe PID is complicated by TOA or pyosalpinx, which are seen in approximately 30% of patients with PID.[44] Patients with pyosalpinx or TOA are more likely to have elevated temperatures, presence of an intrauterine device, elevated erythrocyte sedimentation rate and C-reactive protein, leukocytosis, and are more likely to require a longer hospital stay.[45] Diagnosis is primarily made by transvaginal US, the diagnostic test of choice, but may also be seen on a CT scan obtained looking for other causes.[46] These are serious conditions that generally require urgent gynecologic consultation and inpatient admission. Previously treated with hysterectomy and salpingo-oophorectomy, more contemporary management involves nonsurgical treatment with intravenous (IV) antibiotics, although approximately 25% of TOAs require surgical intervention.[47] CDC treatment guidelines are represented in **Table 1**. Of note, although the addition of metronidazole for anaerobic coverage is not mandated in simple PID, it is strongly recommended for complicated and severe PID.[39,43,48]

ABNORMAL UTERINE BLEEDING
Background

In 2012, the American College of Obstetricians and Gynecologists adopted the term AUB to describe abnormal bleeding not associated with pregnancy, including menorrhagia (heavy menstrual bleeding) and metrorrhagia (intermenstrual bleeding).[49] Although previously defined by the loss of greater than 80 mL of blood, the diagnosis of AUB is now a subjective clinical diagnosis based on patient history. The cause of AUB is broad and related to structural or nonstructural causes. The mnemonic PALM-COEIN is useful when forming a differential diagnosis and is described in **Table 2**. Common causes of AUB vary by age. Anovulation is the most common cause during adolescence, although AUB in the third and fourth decades of life is more commonly because of excessive androgens associated with obesity, polycystic

Table 2	
The PALM-COEIN pneumonic for classification of etiology of AUB	
Abnormal Uterine Bleeding	
Structural	Nonstructural
P – polyp	C – coagulopathy
A – adenomyosis	O – ovulatory dysfunction
L – leiomyoma	E – endocrine
M – malignancy	I – iatrogenic
	N – not yet classified

Adapted from Munro MG, Critchley HO, Broder MS, et al. FIGO classification system (PALM-COEIN) for causes of abnormal uterine bleeding in nongravid women of reproductive age. Int J Gynaecol Obstet. 2011 Apr;113(1):3-13. https://doi.org/10.1016/j.ijgo.2010.11.011. Epub 2011 Feb 22; with permission.

ovarian syndrome, and structural lesions.[49] After age 40, bleeding is likely to be related to menopause, but requires investigation for endometrial pathology.[50]

Evaluation

The role of the emergency physician is to identify which patients need an acute intervention for AUB, because most of the underlying causes are treated safely in the outpatient setting. History should be focused on quantifying the amount of bleeding, describing associated pain, and identifying symptoms of anemia. Useful information includes[51,52]

- Date of last menstrual period
- Frequency of sanitary napkin changes
- Presence of blood clots or the sensation of gushing blood
- Presence of anemia symptoms (dyspnea, lightheadedness, fatigue, chest pain)
- Signs of underlying coagulopathy (epistaxis, unexplained ecchymosis, gingival bleeding, family history of bleeding problem)

Physical examination should focus on signs of hemodynamic instability and blood loss, such as tachycardia, hypotension, and pallor, and include an abdominopelvic examination including speculum examination for lesions and friability and bimanual examination to assess for structural abnormalities. Any thyroid abnormalities or signs of polycystic ovarian syndrome, such as acne and hirsutism, should be noted.[49]

A complete blood count should be ordered to evaluate for anemia and potential thrombocytopenia. Coagulation studies including prothrombin time and activated partial thromboplastin time should be strongly considered, particularly in adolescents because of a higher prevalence of underlying bleeding disorder. A von Willebrand panel is ordered if available or deferred to the outpatient provider if symptoms are not severe. In patients with severe symptoms, a type and screen should be sent if a transfusion requirement is anticipated. A urine or serum pregnancy test must be obtained in all patients to exclude ectopic pregnancy. PID and sexually transmitted infections, such as chlamydia, can cause AUB and should be tested for if applicable.[49] If the history is suggestive, work-up for sepsis, liver dysfunction, hematologic malignancy, or thyroid dysfunction leading to AUB can be initiated.[53] A transvaginal US to evaluate for structural abnormality is important in adult women but can usually be deferred to the outpatient setting.[50]

Management

The mainstay of treatment of AUB in the emergency department is initial stabilization and/or outpatient referral, depending on the acuity of the patient. For acute blood loss with hemodynamic instability, transfusion of appropriate blood products is key, as is reversal of known coagulopathies or anticoagulant therapies. For patients with severe continued bleeding, IV conjugated estrogen (Premarin) or IV tranexamic acid is given while awaiting callback from the gynecologic consultant and admission to the hospital.[51,54] In more drastic scenarios, the emergency provider may consider temporization via intrauterine tamponade using a 26F Foley catheter inserted through the cervical os and infused with 30 mL of sterile water or saline, which has been previously described in the literature.[55] Although medical therapies are the preferred route, refractory cases of severe bleeding may require alternative surgical interventions, such as hysterectomy or uterine artery embolization.[56]

Providers may choose to start more stable patients who require treatment before outpatient follow-up on oral medications on discharge from the emergency department. Common medication regimens, their side effects, and contraindications are highlighted in **Table 3**.[54,57] Hormone-based medications, such as medroxyprogesterone acetate and combination oral contraceptives, are used acutely to stop AUB. Combination oral contraceptives should contain at least 30 µg of estrogen, and should be used with caution in any patient with a history of venous thromboembolism, smoking, or migraine with aura.[55] Nonsteroidal anti-inflammatory drugs are antiprostaglandin agents thought to work in AUB by counteracting the vasodilatory and angiogenic effects of prostaglandins. Mefenamic acid, naproxen, or ibuprofen are used,[54] although it should be noted that nonsteroidal anti-inflammatory drugs are also known to have antiplatelet effects and may not be appropriate for every patient. Oral iron supplementation for blood loss anemia is initiated if laboratory studies show a microcytic anemia or low ferritin levels; women taking iron should be warned about constipation. There are several other categories of treatment, such as gonadotropin-releasing hormone agonists, antigonadotropins, progesterone injectables, intrauterine devices, and endometrial ablations, which are arranged as appropriate by a gynecologist.[54] Patients with AUB should be referred to gynecology for outpatient management once deemed stable after emergency department evaluation and management.

BARTHOLIN GLAND CYST AND ABSCESS
Background

The Bartholin glands are pea-sized glands located in the lower vestibule of the vagina at the 4- and 8-o'clock position that produce mucus to lubricate the vagina and vulva.[58] Obstruction of the gland's duct can result in cyst formation and if it becomes infected, an abscess. Women with Bartholin gland cysts may be mostly asymptomatic with only discomfort on sexual stimulation. If the cyst becomes large or forms an abscess there may be tenderness and discomfort with minor activity. On examination,

Table 3
Select medications, doses, contraindications, and categories of treatments for AUB

Pharmacotherapy for Acute Abnormal Uterine Bleeding			
Drug	**Dose**	**Contraindications and Cautions**	**Category**
Tranexamic acid	10 mg/kg IV (hemodynamic instability) 1.3 g PO q 8 h or q 6 h	Color blindness, thromboembolism	Antifibrinolytic
Mefenamic acid	500 g PO q 8 h	Esophagitis, gastrointestinal bleed	Antiprostaglandin
Combined oral contraceptive	PO taper: 4 pills × 4 d, 3 pills × 3 d, 2 pills × 2 d, 1 pill × 21 d	Smoking if age >35, thromboembolism, migraine with aura, liver disease	Estrogen and progestin
Medroxyprogesterone acetate	5–10 mg q 8 h (20 mg off-label)	Thromboembolism	Progestin
Premarin	25 mg IV/IM, repeated in 6–12 hrs PRN or q 4 h ×24 hrs	Breast cancer, liver disease, thromboembolism	Conjugated estrogen
Ferrous sulfate	150–300 mg/day PO divided BID-QID	Constipation	Supplement

Data from American College of Obstetricians and Gynecologists. Committee Opinion No. 557. Obstet Gynecol. 2013;121(4):891-896.

Bartholin gland cysts are found in the lower half of the vulva and are asymmetric. They are usually round, and on palpation one might feel either a fluctuance or a tense fluid collection,[59] which is generally warm, red, and exquisitely painful if infected.

Management

Small, uninfected cysts that cause only mild discomfort are managed expectantly at home with warm compresses, sitz baths, and over-the-counter analgesics while awaiting outpatient gynecologic follow-up. The remainder of this discussion focuses on larger, more painful, or infected cysts. Historically, several different strategies have been used to treat Bartholin gland cysts and abscesses, including

- Silver nitrate ablation
- Alcohol sclerotherapy
- Excision under anesthesia
- Carbon dioxide laser therapy

These therapies are less commonly used now because they have rates of recurrence up to 20%.[60] More recently the mainstay of treatment is placement of a Word catheter, with progression to marsupialization (incision of the cyst and stitching open the edges of the incision) if Word catheter therapy fails. These methods result in lower rates of recurrence, presumably because of epithelialization of the tract. A multicenter randomized controlled trial in England and the Netherlands (WoMan trial) was published in 2017 and analyzed recurrence rates after Word catheter placement or marsupialization. This trial included 162 women and showed no significant difference between recurrence rates at 1 year, with rates ranging from 10% to 13% for cysts requiring treatment.[61] Marsupialization is a surgical procedure that may require general anesthesia, and is often reserved for implementation after Word catheter therapy has failed. Word catheter placement is, therefore, the standard of care for the emergency physician, because this is a simple procedure that is done under local anesthesia. Placement of a Word catheter is illustrated in **Fig. 4**. After placement of the catheter, patients are discharged from the emergency department with gynecology follow-up in 3 weeks. Patients should be advised that the catheter may fall out early in most women[61] and if that occurs, follow-up should be arranged sooner.

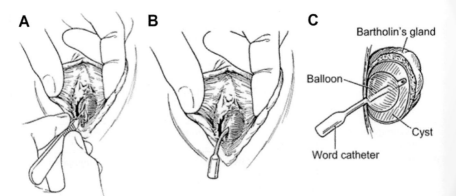

Fig. 4. Bartholin cyst drainage. (*A*) Incision of the cyst. (*B*) Insertion of Word catheter into incision. (*C*) Inflated Word catheter balloon within the cyst cavity. (*From* Campbell CJ. Incision and drainage of Bartholin's abscess. In: Rosen P, Chan TC, Vilke GM, et al. Editors. Atlas of Emergency Procedures. St Louis (MO): Mosby; 2001. p.153.)

Microbiology and Antibiotics

The organism most commonly isolated from Bartholin abscesses is *Escherichia coli*,[59,62,63] followed by *Streptococcus* species.[62] Other pathogens may include *Chlamydia, gonorrhea, Klebsiella, Pseudomonas, Bacteroides, Enterococcus,* and *Staphylococcus* species.[58,63] As with abscesses elsewhere, antibiotics are not indicated for an uncomplicated Bartholin gland abscess after drainage[64] unless there is overlying cellulitis or complicating factors, such as pregnancy or immunosuppression.[58] Typical choices may include third-generation cephalosporins, doxycycline, or amoxicillin-clavulanate.[58,62]

Special Populations

Bartholin gland cyst and abscess are more common in adolescent women and women of reproductive age. In women older than 40 years of age, the presence of a cyst should raise suspicion for other pathologies. Although they represent less than 1% of gynecologic malignancies, various carcinomas and sarcomas, and adenomas, papillomas, and endometriomas can mimic a Bartholin gland cyst,[58,65] therefore in an older population a broader differential diagnosis should be considered.

REFERENCES

1. Meltzer AC, Pines JM, Richards LM, et al. US emergency department visits for adults with abdominal and pelvic pain (2007–13): trends in demographics, resource utilization and medication usage. Am J Emerg Med 2017;35(12): 1966–9.

2. Hoffman BL, Schorge JO, Bradshaw KD, et al. Pelvic mass. In: Williams gynecology, 3e. New York: McGraw-Hill Education; 2016. Available at: http://accessmedicine. mhmedical.com/content.aspx?aid=1125285967.

3. Sasaki KJ, Miller CE. Adnexal torsion: review of the literature. J Minim Invasive Gynecol 2014;21(2):196–202.

4. Houry D, Abbott JT. Ovarian torsion: a fifteen-year review. Ann Emerg Med 2001; 38(2):156–9.

5. Pansky M, Smorgick N, Herman A, et al. Torsion of normal adnexa in postmenarchal women and risk of recurrence. Obstet Gynecol 2007;109(2 Pt 1):355–9.

6. Swenson DW, Lourenco AP, Beaudoin FL, et al. Ovarian torsion: case–control study comparing the sensitivity and specificity of ultrasonography and computed tomography for diagnosis in the emergency department. Eur J Radiol 2014;83(4): 733–8.

7. Rey-Bellet Gasser C, Gehri M, Joseph J-M, et al. Is it ovarian torsion? A systematic literature review and evaluation of prediction signs. Pediatr Emerg Care 2016; 32(4):256–61.

8. Huchon C, Panel P, Kayem G, et al. Does this woman have adnexal torsion? Hum Reprod 2012;27(8):2359–64.

9. Alrabeeah A, Galliani CA, Giacomantonio M, et al. Neonatal ovarian torsion: report of three cases and review of the literature. Pediatr Pathol 1988;8(2): 143–9. Available at: http://www.ncbi.nlm.nih.gov/pubmed/3045782. Accessed November 15, 2018.

10. Ashwal E, Hiersch L, Krissi H, et al. Characteristics and management of ovarian torsion in premenarchal compared with postmenarchal patients. Obstet Gynecol 2015;126(3):514–20.

11. Melcer Y, Sarig-Meth T, Maymon R, et al. Similar but different: a comparison of adnexal torsion in pediatric, adolescent, and pregnant and reproductive-age women. J Womens Health (Larchmt) 2016;25(4):391–6.

12. Cohen A, Solomon N, Almog B, et al. Adnexal torsion in postmenopausal women: clinical presentation and risk of ovarian malignancy. J Minim Invasive Gynecol 2017;24(1):94–7.

13. Balci O, Icen MS, Mahmoud AS, et al. Management and outcomes of adnexal torsion: a 5-year experience. Arch Gynecol Obstet 2011;284(3):643–6.

14. Asfour V, Varma R, Menon P. Clinical risk factors for ovarian torsion. J Obstet Gynaecol 2015;35(7):721–5.

15. Yen C-F, Lin S-L, Murk W, et al. Risk analysis of torsion and malignancy for adnexal masses during pregnancy. Fertil Steril 2009;91(5):1895–902.

16. Mashiach S, Bider D, Moran O, et al. Adnexal torsion of hyperstimulated ovaries in pregnancies after gonadotropin therapy. Fertil Steril 1990;53(1):76–80. Available at: http://www.ncbi.nlm.nih.gov/pubmed/2295348. Accessed November 15, 2018.

17. Govaerts I, Devreker F, Delbaere A, et al. Short-term medical complications of 1500 oocyte retrievals for in vitro fertilization and embryo transfer. Eur J Obstet Gynecol Reprod Biol 1998;77(2):239–43. Available at: http://www.ncbi.nlm.nih.gov/pubmed/9578285. Accessed November 15, 2018.

18. Romanski PA, Melamed A, Elias KM, et al. Association between peak estradiol levels and ovarian torsion among symptomatic patients receiving gonadotropin treatment. J Assist Reprod Genet 2017;34(5):627–31.

19. Ssi-Yan-Kai G, Rivain A-L, Trichot C, et al. What every radiologist should know about adnexal torsion. Emerg Radiol 2018;25(1):51–9.

20. Albayram F, Hamper UM. Ovarian and adnexal torsion: spectrum of sonographic findings with pathologic correlation. J Ultrasound Med 2001;20(10):1083–9. Available at: http://www.ncbi.nlm.nih.gov/pubmed/11587015. Accessed November 15, 2018.

21. Peña JE, Ufberg D, Cooney N, et al. Usefulness of Doppler sonography in the diagnosis of ovarian torsion. Fertil Steril 2000;73(5):1047–50. Available at: http://www.ncbi.nlm.nih.gov/pubmed/10785237. Accessed November 15, 2018.

22. Lam A, Nayyar M, Helmy M, et al. Assessing the clinical utility of color Doppler ultrasound for ovarian torsion in the setting of a negative contrast-enhanced CT scan of the abdomen and pelvis. Abdom Imaging 2015;40(8):3206–13.

23. Moore C, Meyers AB, Capotasto J, et al. Prevalence of abnormal CT findings in patients with proven ovarian torsion and a proposed triage schema. Emerg Radiol 2009;16(2):115–20.

24. Dasgupta R, Renaud E, Goldin AB, et al. Ovarian torsion in pediatric and adolescent patients: a systematic review. J Pediatr Surg 2018;53(7):1387–91.

25. Rotoli JM. Abdominal pain in the post-menopausal female: is ovarian torsion in the differential? J Emerg Med 2017;52(5):749–52.

26. Brunham RC, Gottlieb SL, Paavonen J. Pelvic inflammatory disease. N Engl J Med 2015;372(21):2039–48.

27. Kreisel K, Torrone E, Bernstein K, et al. Prevalence of pelvic inflammatory disease in sexually experienced women of reproductive age—United States, 2013–2014. MMWR Morb Mortal Wkly Rep 2017;66(3):80–3.

28. Sellors J, Mahony J, Goldsmith C, et al. The accuracy of clinical findings and laparoscopy in pelvic inflammatory disease. Am J Obstet Gynecol 1991;164(1 Pt 1):113–20. Available at: http://www.ncbi.nlm.nih.gov/pubmed/1824740. Accessed February 10, 2019.

29. You JS, Kim MJ, Chung HS, et al. Clinical features of Fitz-Hugh-Curtis syndrome in the emergency department. Yonsei Med J 2012;53(4):753–8.

30. Mitchell C, Prabhu M. Pelvic inflammatory disease. Infect Dis Clin North Am 2013; 27(4):793–809.

31. Cho H-W, Koo Y-J, Min K-J, et al. Pelvic inflammatory disease in virgin women with tubo-ovarian abscess: a single-center experience and literature review. J Pediatr Adolesc Gynecol 2017;30(2):203–8.

32. Ashrafganjooei T, Harirchi I, Iravanlo G. Tubo-ovarian abscess in a virgin girl. Iran J Reprod Med 2011;9(3):247–50. Available at: http://www.ncbi.nlm.nih.gov/pubmed/26396572. Accessed November 16, 2018.

33. Tuncer ZS, Boyraz G, Yücel SÖ, et al. Tuboovarian abscess due to colonic diverticulitis in a virgin patient with morbid obesity: a case report. Case Rep Med 2012; 2012:1–3.

34. Simpson-Camp L, Richardson EJ, Alaish SM. *Streptococcus viridans* tubo-ovarian abscess in an adolescent virgin. Pediatr Int 2012;54(5):706–9.

35. Moore MM, Cardosi RJ, Barrionuevo MJ. Tubo-ovarian abscess in an adolescent virgin female. Arch Pediatr Adolesc Med 1999;153(1):91–2. Available at: http://www.ncbi.nlm.nih.gov/pubmed/9895008. Accessed November 16, 2018.

36. Soper DE, Brockwell NJ, Dalton HP, et al. Observations concerning the microbial etiology of acute salpingitis. Am J Obstet Gynecol 1994;170(4):1008–14 [discussion: 1014–7]. Available at: http://www.ncbi.nlm.nih.gov/pubmed/8166184. Accessed November 16, 2018.

37. Burnett AM, Anderson CP, Zwank MD. Laboratory-confirmed gonorrhea and/or chlamydia rates in clinically diagnosed pelvic inflammatory disease and cervicitis. Am J Emerg Med 2012;30(7):1114–7.

38. Sethi S, Zaman K, Jain N. *Mycoplasma genitalium* infections: current treatment options and resistance issues. Infect Drug Resist 2017;10:283–92.

39. Centers for Disease Control and Prevention. 2015 sexually transmitted diseases treatment guidelines. 2015. Available at: https://www.cdc.gov/std/tg2015/pid.htm. Accessed November 20, 2018.

40. Brown GR. Cephalosporin-probenecid drug interactions. Clin Pharmacokinet 1993;24(4):289–300.

41. Savaris RF, Teixeira LM, Torres TG, et al. Comparing ceftriaxone plus azithromycin or doxycycline for pelvic inflammatory disease: a randomized controlled trial. Obstet Gynecol 2007;110(1):53–60.

42. Bevan CD, Ridgway GL, Rothermel CD. Efficacy and safety of azithromycin as monotherapy or combined with metronidazole compared with two standard multidrug regimens for the treatment of acute pelvic inflammatory disease. J Int Med Res 2003;31(1):45–54.

43. Savaris RF, Fuhrich DG, Duarte RV, et al. Antibiotic therapy for pelvic inflammatory disease. Cochrane Database Syst Rev 2017;(4):CD010285.

44. Sordia-Hernández LH, Serrano Castro LG, Sordia-Piñeyro MO, et al. Comparative study of the clinical features of patients with a tubo-ovarian abscess and patients with severe pelvic inflammatory disease. Int J Gynaecol Obstet 2016; 132(1):17–9.

45. Kim HY, Yang JI, Moon C. Comparison of severe pelvic inflammatory disease, pyosalpinx and tubo-ovarian abscess. J Obstet Gynaecol Res 2015;41(5):742–6.

46. Revzin MV, Mathur M, Dave HB, et al. Pelvic inflammatory disease: multimodality imaging approach with clinical-pathologic correlation. Radiographics 2016;36(5): 1579–96.

47. Landers DV, Sweet RL. Tubo-ovarian abscess: contemporary approach to management. Rev Infect Dis 1983;5(5):876–84. Available at: http://www.ncbi.nlm.nih.gov/pubmed/6635426. Accessed November 16, 2018.
48. Duarte R, Fuhrich D, Ross JDC. A review of antibiotic therapy for pelvic inflammatory disease. Int J Antimicrob Agents 2015;46(3):272–7.
49. Committee on Practice Bulletins—Gynecology. Practice Bulletin No. 128. Obstet Gynecol 2012;120(1):197–206.
50. Cirilli AR, Cipot SJ. Emergency evaluation and management of vaginal bleeding in the nonpregnant patient. Emerg Med Clin North Am 2012;30(4):991–1006.
51. Cheong Y, Cameron IT, Critchley HOD. Abnormal uterine bleeding. Br Med Bull 2017;123(1):103–14.
52. Mullins TLK, Miller RJ, Mullins ES. Evaluation and management of adolescents with abnormal uterine bleeding. Pediatr Ann 2015;44(9):e218–22.
53. Deligeoroglou E, Karountzos V. Abnormal uterine bleeding including coagulopathies and other menstrual disorders. Best Pract Res Clin Obstet Gynaecol 2018; 48:51–61.
54. Pinkerton JV. Pharmacological therapy for abnormal uterine bleeding. Menopause 2011;18(4):459–67.
55. American College of Obstetricians and Gynecologists. Committee opinion no. 557. Obstet Gynecol 2013;121(4):891–6.
56. Salazar GMM, Petrozza JC, Walker TG. Transcatheter endovascular techniques for management of obstetrical and gynecologic emergencies. Tech Vasc Interv Radiol 2009;12(2):139–47.
57. Ely JW, Kennedy CM, Clark EC, et al. Abnormal uterine bleeding: a management algorithm. J Am Board Fam Med 2006;19(6):590–602.
58. Lee MY, Dalpiaz A, Schwamb R, et al. Clinical pathology of Bartholin's glands: a review of the literature. Curr Urol 2014;8(1):22–5.
59. Hoffman BL, Schorge JO, Bradshaw KD, et al. Benign disorders of the lower genital tract. In: Williams gynecology. 3rd edition. New York: McGraw-Hill; 2016. Available at: https://accessmedicine-mhmedical-com.proxy-hs.researchport.umd.edu/content.aspx?bookid=1758&sectionid=118167322#1125284652. Accessed November 26, 2018.
60. Wechter ME, Wu JM, Marzano D, et al. Management of Bartholin duct cysts and abscesses. Obstet Gynecol Surv 2009;64(6):395–404.
61. Kroese J, van der Velde M, Morssink L, et al. Word catheter and marsupialisation in women with a cyst or abscess of the Bartholin gland (WoMan-trial): a randomised clinical trial. BJOG 2017;124(2):243–9.
62. Kessous R, Aricha-Tamir B, Sheizaf B, et al. Clinical and microbiological characteristics of Bartholin gland abscesses. Obstet Gynecol 2013;122(4):794–9.
63. Krissi H, Shmuely A, Aviram A, et al. Acute Bartholin's abscess: microbial spectrum, patient characteristics, clinical manifestation, and surgical outcomes. Eur J Clin Microbiol Infect Dis 2016;35(3):443–6.
64. Bora SA, Condous G. Bartholin's, vulval and perineal abscesses. Best Pract Res Clin Obstet Gynaecol 2009;23(5):661–6.
65. Heller DS, Bean S. Lesions of the Bartholin gland. J Low Genit Tract Dis 2014; 18(4):351–7.

Imaging Modalities in Genitourinary Emergencies

Julian Jakubowski, DO[a,b,*], Joshua Moskovitz, MD, MBA, MPH[c,d], Nicole J. Leonard, MD[e]

KEYWORDS

- Genitourinary imaging • Genitourinary radiographs • Genitourinary CT
- CT pyelogram • Genitourinary US • Genitourinary POCUS • Genitourinary MRI

KEY POINTS

- Kidneys ureters bladder plain radiography can be an alternative to computed tomography (CT), although it is substantially less sensitive and specific.
- Point-of-care ultrasound is an increasingly prevalent diagnostic tool with the potential to decrease exposure to ionizing radiation and time until intervention and is especially helpful in cases of suspected scrotal pathologic condition, ovarian pathologic condition, and recurrent renal colic.
- CT is the most common modality in genitourinary emergencies because it provides the most depth of evaluation and speed of acquisition.
- MRI can also be used for detailed cross-sectional examination of the genitourinary system, with superb soft tissue contrast resolution, and is especially helpful in pregnant patients with difficult to diagnose conditions. MRI can also help with equivocal CT or ultrasound evaluations.

INTRODUCTION

Emergency physicians rely on a multitude of different imaging modalities in the diagnosis of genitourinary (GU) emergencies. There are many considerations to be taken into account when deciding which imaging modality should be used first (**Table 1**), because oftentimes several diagnostic tools can be used for the same pathologic

Disclosure Statement: The authors have nothing to disclose.
[a] Department of Emergency Medicine, Emergency Medicine Residency Marietta Memorial Hospital, 401 Matthew Street, Marietta, OH 45750, USA; [b] The Ohio University Heritage College of Osteopathic Medicine, Athens, OH, USA; [c] Department of Emergency Medicine, Jacobi Medical Center, Albert Einstein College of Medicine, 1400 Pelham Parkway South, Building 6 Room 1B25, Bronx, NY 10461, USA; [d] Hofstra School of Health and Human Services, Hempstead, NY, USA; [e] Department of Emergency Medicine, Jacobi Montefiore Emergency Medicine Residency, 1400 Pelham Parkway South, Building 6, Bronx, NY 10461, USA
* Corresponding author. Department of Emergency Medicine, Emergency Medicine Residency Marietta Memorial Hospital, 401 Matthew Street, Marietta, OH 45750.
E-mail address: dr.jakubowski@gmail.com

Emerg Med Clin N Am 37 (2019) 785–809
https://doi.org/10.1016/j.emc.2019.07.013
0733-8627/19/© 2019 Elsevier Inc. All rights reserved.

emed.theclinics.com

Table 1
Initial imaging choices for genitourinary emergency diagnosis

	CT Scan	X Ray	US
Subscapular hematoma	Noncontrast		
Renal parenchymal contusion	Nephrographic phase		
Collecting duct injuries	Delayed phase		
Bladder injuries	CT cystogram		
Ureteral injuries		Retrograde urethrogram	
Testicular torsion			Testicular US
Urolithiasis	Reduced-dose noncontrast		
Priapism			Penile Doppler study
Fournier gangrene		X ray	
PID/TOA			Pelvic US
Epididymitis/orchitis			Testicular US

condition. These factors include radiation exposure, sensitivity, specificity, age of patient, availability of resources, cost, and timeliness of completion.

Plain film radiology is perhaps one of the quickest and most inexpensive modalities available with considerably less radiation exposure compared with computed tomography (CT). The role of plain film radiology is limited to urolithiasis, ureteral injury, and cases of renal injury where CT is unavailable. Ultrasound (US) has the benefit of minimizing radiation exposure to the patient. Point-of-care ultrasound (POCUS) is one of the quickest imaging modalities available and is becoming increasingly prevalent in the emergency department, but its sensitivity and specify depend on provider expertise. CT scans have a significant radiation exposure and are much more expensive compared with the previously mentioned imaging techniques. However, it allows for evaluation of multiple different systems simultaneously when the presenting complaint is vague, and the exact diagnosis is unclear. MRI has a limited role in the diagnosis of GU pathologic condition because of the fact that it is expensive, is not readily available, and takes longer to complete. However, it still plays a key role in pregnant patients who are unable to undergo other forms of imaging owing to radiation. MRI can also help with equivocal CT or US evaluations.

PLAIN FILM RADIOLOGY
Kidneys Ureters Bladder Plain Radiography

Kidneys ureters bladder plain radiography (KUB) can be used as an alternative to CT in patients with suspected urolithiasis.[1-3] The KUB is available in most emergency departments, is noninvasive, can be obtained quickly, and is less expensive than CT. KUBs, though, have lower sensitivity and specificity than a noncontrast CT. Because of their composition, most stones should be visible on plain film (radiopaque; **Fig. 1**). However, in patients with acute renal colic and no history of urolithiasis, the reported sensitivity of 45% to 58% and specificity of 60% to 77% are substantially less than other modalities.[4] The detection rate for stones less than 5 mm with KUB by itself is low, with a sensitivity of 12% or less based on size of the stone.[5] KUBs will also not provide information regarding the presence and/or degree of urinary tract obstruction. Another limitation is the decreased diagnostic utility owing to the difficulty in

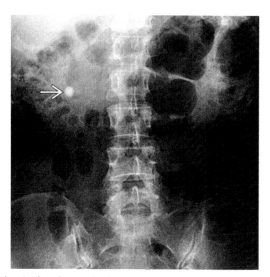

Fig. 1. Supine abdominal radiograph shows a well-defined, rounded radiopacity in the right renal region (*white solid arrow*) consistent with a renal calculus. (*From* Heller M. Urolithiasis. STATdx | Diagnostic Decision Support for Radiology. https://app.statdx.com/document/urolithiasis/6d7176d8-74a0-4d96-b7de-0d6fb51a4613?searchTerm=Urolithiasis. Accessed February 26, 2019; with permission.)

differentiating pelvic vascular calcifications (phleboliths) from stones in the pelvic ureter. Image quality can also be further degraded by patient obesity.[4]

A potential major benefit to KUB is that patients will be exposed to significantly less radiation than CT. Current estimates report patients will be exposed to approximately 0.5 to 0.9 mSv while undergoing conventional KUB.[4] As body mass index increases, this benefit is diminished owing to degraded image quality, and potential need for increased number of images acquired resulting in an increase in the effective dose. The combination of KUB and US has been proposed to improve sensitivity and specificity of the KUB. However, when studied, it did not improve compared with US alone.[5]

Intravenous Pyelogram

Intravenous pyelogram (excretory urogram, IVP) is when a series of plain film is taken after a defined period of time following an injection of contrast medium (**Fig. 2**). An IVP can establish the presence or absence of the kidneys, define the parenchyma, and outline the collecting system. Unlike the KUB, it provides limited functional and anatomic evaluations of the urogenital tract. IVP are often difficult to interpret[6] and are technically challenging to do correctly. Patients undergoing IVP would be exposed to approximately 1.3 to 3.0 mSv[4] of radiation and contrast material. Previously, IVPs were used to help evaluate for GU injury and should be considered when CT is not available.[7] Findings in a "one-shot" intravenous (IV) urogram/single-view intraoperative IVP however were found to inconsistent, unreliable, and frequently nondiagnostic.[6]

Retrograde Urethrography

After pelvic trauma, where there concern of ureteral injury exists, a retrograde urethrography should be performed to evaluate[8,9] the extent of suspected urethral injury (**Fig. 3**A). Retrograde urethrography will typically be a bedside procedure but can be done under fluoroscopy. Before the procedure, an initial KUB is obtained. Then, a small

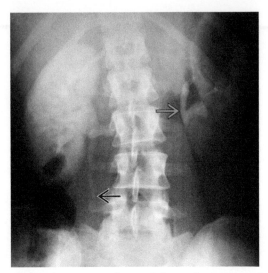

Fig. 2. Excretory urogram shows a persistent right nephrogram and delayed excretion due to a proximal ureteral stone (*black arrow*). There is a small amount of contrast within the normal left renal pelvis (*cyan arrow*). (*From* Heller M. Urolithiasis. STATdx j Diagnostic Decision Support for Radiology. https://app.statdx.com/document/urolithiasis/6d7176d8-74a0-4d96-b7de-0d6fb51a4613?searchTerm5Urolithiasis. Accessed February 26, 2019; with permission.)

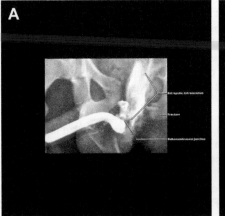
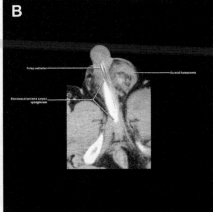

Fig. 3. (*A*) Retrograde urethrogram shows a posterior urethral injury with complete disruption of urethra at the level of the urogenital diaphragm and extravasation of contrast into the retropubic space. Posterior urethral injuries have a high association with pelvic fractures This was treated with a suprapubic catheter. A subsequent urethral stricture developed. (*B*) CT scan performed after a retrograde urethrogram in a patient with an incomplete tear of the anterior urethra shows extravasation of contrast into the corpus spongiosum. There is an associated scrotal hematoma, which is common in anterior urethral injury. ([*A, B*] *From* Penis and Urethra. STATdx | Diagnostic Decision Support for Radiology. https://app.statdx.com/document/penis-and-urethra/3b62b753-98d0-489d-a0aa-0671e7802a12?searchTerm=penis. Accessed February 26, 2019; with permission.)

piston syringe or a small Foley catheter is inserted snugly in the urethral meatus. Then, 10 to 15 mL (in children: 0.2 mL/kg)[10] of undiluted water-soluble contrast material is gently injected, and a repeat KUB is obtained. Contrast extravasation from the urethra indicates urethral injury (**Fig. 3**B). If urethral injury is detected, further instrumentation of the urethra should not occur without urologic consultation.[10]

Additional diagnoses to consider would be penile contusions, hematomas, and penile fractures. These diagnoses are often clinical diagnoses. However, cavernosography, US, or MRI can also be considered for equivocal clinical examinations.[9] Cavernosogram is an infrequently used diagnostic examination whereby radiopaque contrast is injected into the corporal body with plain film imaging used to evaluate as part of penile repair.[11]

ULTRASOUND

One of the major overall benefits of US is that it limits the patient's exposure to radiation. It is a safe and minimally noninvasive imaging modality.[12] POCUS is becoming an increasingly prevalent diagnostic tool in the emergency department. It can be used for diagnosis of many emergency conditions.[13] It is a resource that has the potential to provide quick answers, get necessary consults involved early in patient care, and decrease time until intervention. One of the biggest weaknesses of POCUS is the variability of user expertise, which affects the overall sensitivity and specificity of the test.

Renal Colic

Historically, renal US has had only fair sensitivity (37%–64%) in detecting renal stones[14] (**Figs. 4–6**), but more recent studies have shown that with modern equipment and skilled operators, that number approaches 76% to 98%, which is comparable to that of CT.[15–17] Renal US is more sensitive in identifying acute renal obstruction 74% to 85%, although not all stones result in obstruction.[14] It is also considerably less reliable in identifying the size and location of the stone, although this information may not

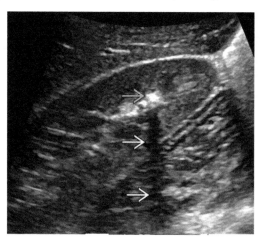

Fig. 4. Sagittal US image shows an echogenic calculus (blue arrow) within a superior pole calyx and posterior shadowing shown by a linear hypoechoic band (white arrow). In the absence of the shadowing artifact, it may be difficult to differentiate this calculus from sinus fat. (*From* Heller M. Urolithiasis. STATdx | Diagnostic Decision Support for Radiology. https://app.statdx.com/document/urolithiasis/6d7176d8-74a0-4d96-b7de-0d6fb51a4613?search Term=Urolithiasis. Accessed February 26, 2019; with permission.)

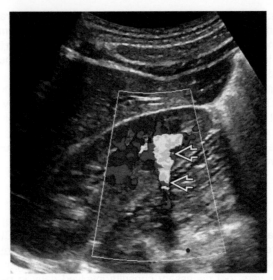

Fig. 5. Sagittal color Doppler US in the same patient reveals "twinkle" artifact (*arrow*) due to the highly refractive calculus; the "twinkle" artifact appears as a linear band or tail of disorganized, rapidly changing color posterior to the calculus. Other areas of color flow are due to blood vessels. (*From* Heller M. Urolithiasis. STATdx | Diagnostic Decision Support for Radiology. https://app.statdx.com/document/urolithiasis/6d7176d8-74a0-4d96-b7de-0d6fb51a4613?searchTerm=Urolithiasis. Accessed February 26, 2019; with permission.)

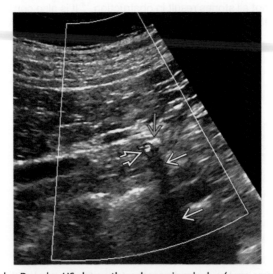

Fig. 6. Sagittal color Doppler US shows the echogenic calculus (*cyan arrow*) in the ureteral lumen; its location can be aided by shadowing (*white solid arrow*) and "twinkle" artifact (*white open arrow*), shown by the focus of disorganized color Doppler signal posterior to the calculus. (*From* Heller M. Urolithiasis. STATdx | Diagnostic Decision Support for Radiology. https://app.statdx.com/document/urolithiasis/6d7176d8-74a0-4d96-b7de-0d6fb51a4613?searchTerm=Urolithiasis. Accessed February 26, 2019; with permission.)

always be warranted. One study showed that the risk of urologic intervention in a patient with suspected renal colic and a normal renal US was very low (0.6%).[18]

In addition to attempting to visualize the stone, POCUS attempts to identify unilateral hydronephrosis as an indirect sign of obstructing ureteral stone, or bilateral hydronephrosis as a sign of bladder outlet obstruction (**Fig. 7**). Similarly, to comprehensive radiology US, POCUS scans do not always identify the location and size of the stone, but studies have suggested that a normal scan or mild hydronephrosis on POCUS indicates a smaller stone size (<5 mm)[19] whereas moderate to severe hydronephrosis implies a larger stone and therefore predicts necessity for urologic intervention. A study by Rosen and colleagues[20] showed a sensitivity and specificity of 72% and 73%, respectively, for the detection of hydronephrosis by bedside US in the emergency department. A more recent study by Gaspari and Horst[21] reported a sensitivity of 87% and specificity of 85%.

Renal Trauma

Patients with suspected GU trauma may receive a focused assessment with sonography in trauma (FAST) during their initial evaluation. A positive FAST examination with the right clinical picture (hematuria, flank pain) could predict renal injury. Subscapular hematoma can also potentially be seen on bedside US. A FAST examination cannot however definitively exclude renal injury.[7,9] US cannot clearly delineate parenchymal lacerations, vascular injuries, or collecting system injuries, nor can it accurately detect urinary extravasation.[22]

Bladder

US also facilitates bladder assessment. Traditionally, bladder scanners have been used to assess bladder fullness in emergency departments. Although convenient, they cannot reliably differentiate between the bladder and other cystic pelvic structures, which may lead to falsely elevated bladder volumes.[23–25]

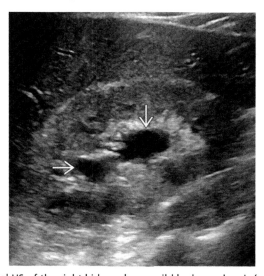

ig. 7. Longitudinal US of the right kidney shows mild hydronephrosis (*arrows*) in a patient resenting with right flank pain. (*From* Furlan A. Hydronephrosis. STATdx | Diagnostic Decision Support for Radiology. https://app.statdx.com/document/hydronephrosis/8d3a1e74-f55-4682-92e6-1728fec24964?searchTerm=hydronephrosis. Accessed February 26, 2019; with permission.)

US/POCUS is a rapid and noninvasive method to evaluate bladder fullness.[26] Bladder volume can be calculated by obtaining measurements in the midtransverse plane and midsagittal plane. These calculated volumes are within 10% to 20% of the actual bladder volume.[27–29] A distended bladder after an attempt to void indicates urinary retention and the need for emergent urinary catheterization. Measuring bladder wall thickness may also predict bladder outlet obstruction with greater accuracy than free uroflowmetry, postvoid residual urine, and prostate volume,[30] whereas a collapsed bladder rules out retention and prompts further evaluation for alternative diagnosis.

In addition, the bladder provides an acoustic window for the pelvis. Consequently, the need for a full bladder often delays comprehensive transabdominal pelvic US performed by the department of radiology. POCUS assessment of bladder decreases these delays by assessing patient readiness for transabdominal pelvic US more quickly than patient sensation of bladder fullness.[26]

Scrotal Pathologic Condition

Scrotal/testicular pain is a common emergency department complaint. The test of choice to evaluate for testicular torsion in a patient with acute scrotal pain remains US with Doppler.[31,32] Color Doppler and other grayscale/B-mode US findings of architecture of the testis have been used to predict viability/likelihood for testicular salvage (**Figs. 8** and **9**). Parenchymal heterogeneity of the testicular echotexture and loss of testicular arterial blood flow by Doppler (**Fig. 10**) were reported to be 100% predictive of testicular loss at exploration.[33,34]

False negatives on grayscale/B-mode US are more likely to happen early after the onset of symptoms. The torsed testis may appear normal for the first 4 to 6 hours.[35] It may then become swollen and hypoechoic. It can take up to 12 hours before a heterogeneous structural pattern can be observed. Furthermore, absence of identifiable

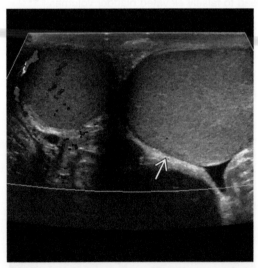

Fig. 8. Color Doppler US performed on a young man with acute scrotal pain shows no flow within a relatively enlarged left testis (*arrow*). Doppler parameters should be optimized to detect slow flow, and comparison to the contralateral (asymptomatic) testis is critical. (*From* Bhatt S, Tublin M. Testicular Torsion. STATdx | Diagnostic Decision Support for Radiology https://app.statdx.com/document/testicular-torsion/3f76d681-f5d4-4821-9301-cb33b7df9c60? searchTerm=torsion. Accessed February 26, 2019; with permission.)

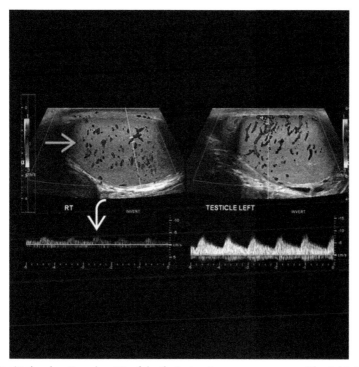

Fig. 9. Sagittal color Doppler US of both testes in a young man with right testicular pain shows an asymmetric blood flow with reduced flow to the right testis (*cyan arrow*), as seen on color flow and spectral waveform (*white arrow*). This was surgically confirmed to be partial (180') right testicular torsion. (*From* Bhatt S, Tublin M. Testicular Torsion. STATdx | Diagnostic Decision Support for Radiology. https://app.statdx.com/document/testicular-torsion/3f76d681-f5d4-4821-9301-cb33b7df9c60?searchTerm=torsion. Accessed February 26, 2019; with permission.)

intratesticular flow with Doppler US was only 86% to 94% sensitivity, but nearly 100% specificity, and 97% accurate for the diagnosis of testicular torsion.[36,37] The degree of torsion likely explains the 6% to 14% of patients with torsion who have a false negative Doppler evaluation. Low-degree torsion of the spermatic cord causes only closure of the veins and lymphatics within the spermatic cord, whereas the arteries still remain patent so that arterial flow signals are still visible within the affected testis.[38,39] Also, in cases of torsion-detorsion, blood flow may actually be increased (compensatory hyperemia) and mistaken for the alternate diagnosis of epididymitis.[40] In addition, the epididymis will remain perfused despite color Doppler flow being absent in the rest of the affected testis because of its different blood supply.[38] Other signs of testicular torsion include visualization of a torsion knot or whirlpool pattern of concentric layers (spiral twist of spermatic cord cranial to testis and epididymis; **Fig. 11**).[41] Absent or high-resistance waveforms on Doppler and increased resistive indices with decreased, absent, or reversed diastolic flow suggest vascular occlusion.[35,38,42] Contrast-enhanced US is a newer modality that has the potential to provide improved sensitivity in detecting flow and improved characterization of acute testicular segmental infarction.[43,44]

Because of case reports of false negative US results, clinicians need to be mindful in their use of color flow to exclude the diagnosis of testicular torsion.[36,42,45–49] US

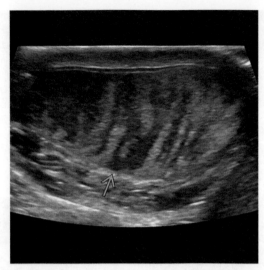

Fig. 10. Sagittal grayscale US of right testis shows an enlarged, heterogeneous right testis (*arrow*) with a striated appearance suggestive of partial infarcts. The patient had a history of partial testicular torsion. (*From* Bhatt S, Tublin M. Testicular Torsion. STATdx | Diagnostic Decision Support for Radiology. https://app.statdx.com/document/testicular-torsion/3f76d681-f5d4-4821-9301-cb33b7df9c60?searchTerm=torsion. Accessed February 26, 2019; with permission.)

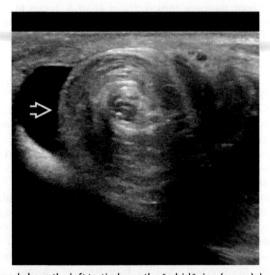

Fig. 11. US performed above the left testis shows the "whirl" sign (*arrow*) due to twisting of the spermatic cord. Direct visualization of the twisted cord may increase examination accuracy, particularly in cases of partial torsion. (*From* Bhatt S, Tublin M. Testicular Torsion. STATdx | Diagnostic Decision Support for Radiology. https://app.statdx.com/document/testicular-torsion/3f76d681-f5d4-4821-9301-cb33b7df9c60?searchTerm=torsion. Accessed February 26, 2019; with permission.)

results need to viewed in context of the history of present illness, physical examination, and whether the patient was symptomatic or whether symptoms dissipated before the examination. POCUS has shown 95% sensitivity and 94% specificity in the differentiation of emergent surgical versus other acute scrotal pain cause.[50]

Clinicians need to be vigilant because testicular torsion is commonly misdiagnosed as epididymitis.[51] Epididymitis and orchitis are more common causes of acute scrotal pain in adults and adolescent boys.[52] Epididymitis is more common than orchitis.[51] With epididymitis, the epididymis will appear enlarged on US with associated increased flow/hyperemic on color Doppler (**Fig. 12**). It can be increased or decreased in echogenicity,[31] whereas with orchitis, the testis will appear enlarged and hyperemic and will have a mottled echotexture with hypoechoic regions.[39] Epididymoorchitis can also be present with a combination of the above findings.

Fournier gangrene

The diagnosis of Fournier gangrene is an emergent urogenital condition that requires prompt surgical intervention and is usually a clinical diagnosis. When it is suspected, imaging should not delay surgical consultation. POCUS can be helpful when the diagnosis and clinical findings are ambiguous, and/or to assess degree of extension at the bedside. Findings would include diffuse scrotal edema and reverberation artifacts/"dirty" shadowing that represents gas within the scrotal wall[53–56] (**Fig. 13**). These "dirty shadows" may even be seen before clinical crepitus.[54,55] There may also be peritesticular fluid. The testes and epididymides are often normal in size and echo architecture.[55] The scrotal contents can also be examined to help differentiate an incarcerated inguinoscrotal hernia from Fournier gangrene. If a hernia is visualized, Doppler imaging can be used to assess for ischemia.

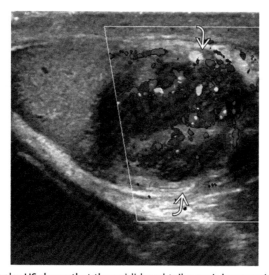

Fig. 12. Color Doppler US shows that the epididymal tail mass is hyperemic (*arrows*). The patient ultimately reported a recent history of treated sexually transmitted disease. Clinical symptoms and vascularity improved after a course of antibiotics. The clinical history and Doppler appearance are classic for early, uncomplicated epididymitis. (*From* Tublin M, Bhatt , Desai A. Epididymitis. STATdx | Diagnostic Decision Support for Radiology. https://app. tatdx.com/document/epididymitis/35bc8dc6-3b73-4394-978f-bb36ab66c0d1? earchTerm=Epididymitis. Accessed February 26, 2019; with permission.)

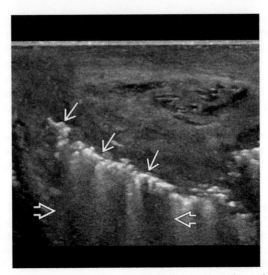

Fig. 13. Transverse US performed on a 54-year-old diabetic man with a 2-day history of scrotal pain and erythema shows posterior scrotal wall echogenicity (*solid arrows*) and "dirty" posterior shadowing (*open arrows*), a characteristic appearance of soft tissue gas. (*From* Tublin M. Fournier Gangrene. STATdx | Diagnostic Decision Support for Radiology. https://app.statdx.com/document/fournier-gangrene/8aad8e09-33d0-4967-b4d8-4051c7a2ea18?searchTerm=Fournier%27s%20gangrene. Accessed February 26, 2019; with permission.)

Tuboovarian abscess Pelvic infection is the most frequent gynecologic cause of emergency department visits, and tuboovarian abscess (TOA) occurs in up to 15% of women with pelvic inflammatory disease (PID).[57] Transvaginal US is often first line in evaluating high-risk patients when TOA is highly suspected given its good sensitivity and specificity (56% to 93% and 86% to 98%, respectively) and lack of radiation exposure.[58–60] On US, a TOA appears as a heteroechogenic mass with septations or as the loss of delineation between ovary and fallopian tube by edematous tissue[61] (**Fig. 14**). US can also be useful in this setting to simultaneously evaluate for ovarian torsion, which may mimic TOA.

Priapism Priapism is another urologic surgical emergency. Determining if priapism is ischemic or nonischemic is usually determined through cavernous blood gas analysis. However, penile Doppler study can be a useful adjunct.[62,63] In the ischemic subgroup, the cavernosal blood flow will be absent with a low-velocity trace to suggest high resistance (**Fig. 15**). The sinusoids will be engorged and noncompressible[64] (**Figs. 16 and 17**). In the nonischemic subgroup, normal or elevated arterial velocities will be noted with high diastolic flow. The sinusoids will also appear engorged but are often compressible because of the lack of thrombus.[65] This study has a sensitivity that nears 100% in identifying posttraumatic arteriocavernosal fistulas, with color Doppler showing turbulent flow within the fistula.[66]

COMPUTED TOMOGRAPHY SCAN

The "as low as reasonably achievable" (ALARA) principle has long been the guiding principle governing medical imaging. The National Academy of Science's most recent report on the Biological Effects of Ionizing Radiation VII indicates that a single lifetime

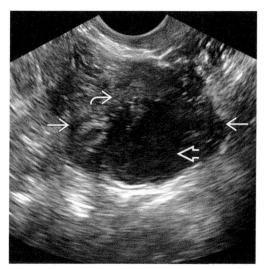

Fig. 14. Transvaginal US shows a left adnexal mass (*solid arrow*) with solid (*curved arrow*) and cystic (*open arrows*) components in this patient with TOA. Note posterior acoustic enhancement. A normal ovary could not be identified. (*From* Rezvani M. Tubo-Ovarian Abscess. STATdx | Diagnostic Decision Support for Radiology. https://app.statdx.com/document/tubo-ovarian-abscess/54fca316-58e4-4171-bcb0-4cde1ed52e0e?searchTerm=TOA. Accessed February 26, 2019; with permission.)

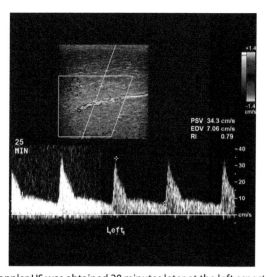

Fig. 15. Sagittal Doppler US was obtained 20 minutes later at the left aspect of the penile base and shows that the end-diastolic velocity has only decreased to 7 cm/s, consistent with venous insufficiency. (*From* Heller M. Erectile Dysfunction. STATdx | Diagnostic Decision Support for Radiology. https://app.statdx.com/document/erectile-dysfunction/18c50e10-c5be-48fd-8c50-4e4d1a7b061f?searchTerm=Penile%20Doppler%20Study. Accessed February 25, 2019; with permission.)

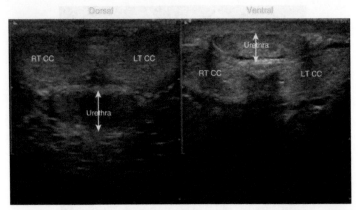

Fig. 16. Transverse view of the phallus with the transducer placed on either the dorsal or the ventral surface. Note the compression of the urethra and corporal spongiosum compression in the ventral projection with minimal pressure applied to the phallus. CC, corpora cavernosa; LT, left; RT, right. (*From* Campbell M, Walsh P, Wein A, Kavoussi L. *Campbell-Walsh Urology*. Philadelphia, PA: Elsevier; 2016; with permission.)

dose of 10 mSv is associated with a lifetime-attributable risk for developing a solid cancer or leukemia of 1 in 1000.[67] The International Commission on Radiological Protection (ICRP) recommends an average effective dose limit of 20 mSv per year over 5 years.[68] The ICRP also cautions that the effective dose should not exceed 50 mSv in any single year.[67] In accordance with ALARA, health care professionals have a responsibility to minimize radiation exposure if a reasonable alternative is possible.

With this in mind, CT is readily accessible in most departments and enables clinicians to quickly obtain detailed images of the abdomen and pelvis. CT is imaging modality of choice for many disease processes (eg, acute nonlocalized abdominal pain,[69] urolithiasis,[70] hematuria[71]). The clinician's most likely suspected pathologic condition will determine the need for contrast enhancement or not (eg, renal colic does not need enhancement). Discussion with either radiologist or CT technologist is suggested to

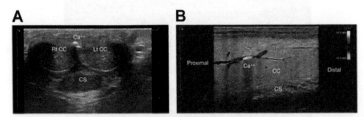

Fig. 17. (*A*) In the transverse plane, scanning from the dorsal surface of the midshaft of the penis, the CC are paired structures seen dorsally, whereas the corpus spongiosum (CS) is seen ventrally in the midline. A calcification (Ca^{++}) is seen between the 2 CC with posterior shadowing. (*B*) In the parasagittal plane, the CC is dorsal with the relatively hypoechoic CS seen ventrally. Within the CC, the cavernosal artery is shown with a calcification (Ca^{++}) in the wall of the artery and posterior shadowing. Lt, left; Rt, right. (*From* Campbell M, Walsh P, Wein A, Kavoussi L. *Campbell-Walsh Urology*. Philadelphia, PA: Elsevier; 2016; with permission.)

determine need and/or to facilitate specific protocols (eg, ordering CT with contrast vs CT Urogram). CTs, however, have a substantially greater doses of ionizing radiation compared with other modalities,[69,72] and they may not always be the best choice for an individual patient. CT comprises the single largest source of medical exposure to ionizing radiation in the US population.[73] CT is also significantly more expensive than US or plain film radiography.[74,75] The lifetime risk of radiation and the cost should prompt clinicians to at least consider alternative imaging in all patients.

Genitourinary Trauma

Because up to 10% of traumas have an associated injury to the GU tract,[76] current guidelines recommend IV contrast-enhanced abdominal/pelvic CT with delayed imaging for stable trauma patients with suspected GU injury.[8,9] Use of delayed imaging once contrast is in the collecting system is crucial for assessing for subtle urothelial abnormalities.[77]

The kidneys are the most commonly injured portion of the GU system.[76] CT can quickly and accurately identify and grade injuries. It will also establish the presence of the contralateral kidney and demonstrate concurrent injuries to other organs. Standard whole-body imaging protocols used in trauma typically do not include multiphase imaging of the GU system.[78] When an isolated GU injury is suspected, a multiphase CT protocol should be considered rather than standard CT protocol. Multiphase CT[8] includes precontrast images that can identify subcapsular hematomas that may otherwise be obscured on postcontrast sequences. Arterial phase images provide assessment for vascular injury and presence of active extravasation of contrast. Nephrographic phase images demonstrate parenchymal contusions and lacerations. Delayed phase imaging reliably identifies collecting system/ureteric injury.

The American Association for the Surgery of Trauma (AAST) Kidney Injuries Scale[79] is commonly used to help guide management of these injuries. It has 5 grades, and there is a good correlation with CT appearances.[9] Grade IV and V injuries have a greater incidence of required surgical exploration.[6,80,81] Conversely, ureteral injuries only comprise 1%[6] of injuries. A CT Urogram provides detailed upper tract imaging. It includes unenhanced axial CT of the kidneys, enhanced CT of the abdomen and pelvis with corticomedullary phase, nephrographic phase, and excretory phase imaging of the abdomen and pelvis.[77] A CT Urogram protocol should be used to evaluate for ureteral injuries. The AAST Urethral Injury Severity Scale is also commonly used to help guide management of urethral injuries.[82] It also has 5 grades that are defined by degree of transection and length of devitalized Urethral. The AAST Urethral Injury Severity Scale, however, does not correlate with CT findings. CT cannot distinguish between grades 2 or 3 injuries nor can it identify ureteral contusion. Extravasation of contrast medium on CT scans (or in IVP) is the hallmark sign of ureteral trauma.[83] In complete transection of the ureter, the distal portion does not opacify, whereas in partial ureteral injury, there will be contrast distally. Other findings suggestive of injury include periureteral fat stranding or periureteral fluid.[22]

CT cystogram or a plain film retrograde cystography[8,9] should be used to evaluate or bladder injuries. Identification of bony fragments in the bladder, bladder neck injuries, and other abdominal injuries are better visualized with CT cystography.[84,85]

Renal Colic

Emergency department visit rates for urolithiasis increased from 178 to 340 visits per 100,000 individuals from 1992 to 2009.[86] Noncontrast CT of the abdomen and pelvis with reduced-dose techniques uses newer protocols to decrease radiation. Consequently, noncontrast CT of the abdomen and pelvis with reduced-dose techniques is currently thought to be the preferred imaging study for most patients.[3,87,88] CT has the greatest sensitivity of 95% to 98% and specificity of 96% to 100%[89] for urolithiasis of all imaging modalities for the diagnosis of renal colic. Reduced-dose techniques reduce patient radiation exposure by as much as 70% (from 100 mAs down to 30 mAs), which results in similar detection of renal calculi.[90] Not only does CT imaging have the benefit of identifying the presence and location of calculi but it is also more accurate in measuring the stone size.[14,91–94] CT can also help select the best candidate for shock wave lithotripsyversus ureteroscopy.[88] As many as 14% of patients with suspected urolithiasis who have CT imaging are ultimately diagnosed with an alternate diagnosis, such as appendicitis.[95]

Although CTs have superior diagnostic characteristics (**Fig. 18**), they also expose patients to greater amounts of ionizing radiation. Another consideration is that renal colic is also often recurrent. Patients with a history of recurrent symptomatic urolithiasis are at increased risk for serial CT examinations with potentially high cumulative effective doses of ionizing radiation.[1,2] A multicenter retrospective study of stone clinic patients indicated that 20% of patients received greater than 50 mSv threshold in the first year of follow-up.[1]

Fournier gangrene

Subcutaneous emphysema is a characteristic finding in Fournier gangrene.[55] When the clinical examination suggests crepitus/soft tissue gas, the first study recommended for confirmation is X ray.[96] CT, however, can help in the evaluation of both the superficial and the deep fascia (in contrast to X rays). Contrast-enhanced CT, however, can provide early diagnosis, assessment of the extent of the disease, and differentiation between necrotic and viable tissue.[55,97,98] Despite Subcutaneous emphysema being a hallmark feature, the high sensitivity and specificity in detection of abnormal gas collection on CT, subcutaneous emphysema is rarely seen in CT in early disease[99] (**Fig. 19**).

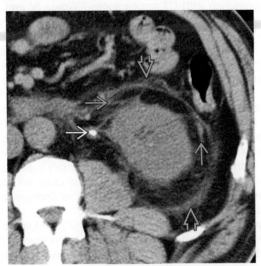

Fig. 18. Axial non-enhanced computed tomography (NECT) shows a proximal ureteral stone (*white arrow*) with a "rim" of soft tissue, which represents the ureteral wall. Note the moderate degree of perinephric stranding (*cyan solid arrow*) and fascial thickening (*cyan open arrow*). (*From* Heller M. Urolithiasis. STATdx | Diagnostic Decision Support for Radiology. https://app.statdx.com/document/urolithiasis/6d7176d8-74a0-4d96-b7de-0d6fb51a4613?searchTerm=Urolithiasis. Accessed February 26, 2019; with permission.)

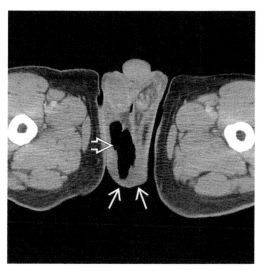

Fig. 19. Axial contrast-enhanced computed tomography (CECT) shows scrotal wall edema (*solid arrows*) and extensive gas (*open arrow*). Fournier gangrene is a surgical emergency. This patient was successfully treated with broad-spectrum antibiotics, partial scrotectomy, and ultimately, flap reconstruction. (*From* Tublin M. Fournier Gangrene. STATdx | Diagnostic Decision Support for Radiology. https://app.statdx.com/document/fournier-gangrene/ 8aad8e09-33d0-4967-b4d8-4051c7a2ea18?searchTerm=Fournier%27s%20gangrene. Accessed February 26, 2019; with permission.)

Tuboovarian abscess In female patients with unclear cause of lower abdominal or pelvic pain or in those with inconclusive US findings, CT with IV contrast has shown utility. It is helpful in identifying the extent of PID and its complications as well as diagnosing other pathologic conditions that may mimic PID, such as appendicitis.[100] The most common finding for TOA on CT with IV contrast in cases of TOA is a multilocular septate cystic mass in the adnexa with a thick uniformly enhancing wall.[101] Sensitivity of CT with IV contrast in patients with inconclusive US scans is 78% to 100%.[100]

Priapism CT angiography can also be a quick, noninvasive test to evaluate for arteriolar-sinusoidal fistula in most nonischemic priapism. CT has little role in the evaluation of ischemic priapism. CT as a whole is a secondary test after penile Doppler study.[102]

MRI

MRI in the emergency department has classically been reserved for evaluation of neurologic and/or neurosurgical emergencies. MRI can also be used for detailed cross-sectional examination for of the GU system. It has superb soft tissue contrast resolution. MRI uses very high-powered electromagnetic field and does not expose patients to ionizing radiation. Because of the use of electromagnetic fields, not all patients are candidates for its imaging (eg, certain pacemakers, defibrillators, and metal foreign bodies) because of the risk for harm to the patient and/or the MRI itself. MRI is associated with greater cost and is not as readily available, and imaging acquisition takes longer when compared with other Emergency department modalities. Because of inherent characteristics of MRI, there may be the need for sedation in some patients. There is also concern that patients with poor renal function who receive IV gadolinium-based contrast agents are at risk of development of nephrogenic systemic fibrosis.[103]

Renal Colic

MRI can be used in suspected urolithiasis. However, unlike CT, it does not allow the visualization of the stones directly, only the indirect signs of their presence.[104] Unenhanced magnetic resonance urography (T2-weighted) can assess for the presence, degree, and level of urinary tract obstruction, but has low sensitivity and specificity in identifying stones.[105] Mass effect from a gravid uterus, as an example, could result in an obstructive uropathy. Gadolinium-enhanced imaging of the kidneys and urinary tract does provide a more comprehensive study. However, because of animal studies and theoretic concern for teratogenicity, gadolinium use should be limited to situations in which the benefits clearly outweigh the possible risks.[106] Notwithstanding this limitation, MRI urography has an established accuracy rate of 92.8% for stone and 100% in other causes of obstructive uropathy.[107] MRI, however, is less accessible and more time consuming and costly than the other modalities available to emergency departments.[108] Because of these limitations, US should be considered before MRI.

Scrotal Pathologic Condition

Although sonography is the imaging modality of choice in the initial assessment of scrotal lesions, it is sometimes inconclusive. Dynamic contrast-enhanced (DCE) subtracted MRI in combination with T2- and T2*-weighted images is useful in the diagnosis of testicular torsion and in the detection of testicular necrosis.[109] DCE-MR was reported to 100% sensitive in diagnosing complete torsion by showing a decrease or lack of testicular perfusion.[110] With cases of Fournier gangrene, MRI is superior to US and CT when imaging soft tissues, even without contrast.[111] MRI can detect the extent of inflammatory changes in patients with necrotizing soft tissue skin infections and is superior to US and X ray.[55] Because of its greater soft tissue resolution, it can better define the depth needed for debridement than CT.[55]

Priapism

The role of MRI in a case of priapism is mainly to detect the presence and quantity of the cavernosal infarct in the ischemic groups in order to determine if evacuation and prosthesis are required.[112] This modality can also be useful in detecting metastasis that may cause malignant priapism.

Tuboovarian Abscess

TOA will appear as a hypointense pelvic mass on MRI T1-weighted images with heterogeneous high-signal intensity on T2-weighted images.[113] Because of the presence of granulation tissue and hemorrhage, a hyperintense rim along the inner wall of the abscess cavity can be seen on T1-weighted MRI.[114] With the addition of diffusion-weighted imaging, MRI has a sensitivity of 91.2% and specificity of 98.4% for PID.[115]

NUCLEAR MEDICINE

The use of nuclear medicine in emergency practice is limited. Scrotal scintigraphy using ^{99m}Tc-pertechnetate (Tc-99m) is a nuclear medicine functional imaging technique that may be used to help differentiate acute epididymitis from testicular torsion. Tc-99m was found to have a positive predictive value of 75%, a sensitivity of 90%, and specificity of 95% in differentiating torsion from epididymitis.[116]

SUMMARY

Numerous factors need to be taken into consideration when deciding which imaging modality should be used in the evaluation of GU emergencies. In addition to sensitivity and specificity, clinicians need to consider the availability of the imaging modalities, cost, timeliness of completion, potential radiation exposure, and the likelihood for additional imaging in the future before using an imaging study for an individual patient. CT as an example may be the best study for the evaluation of renal colic, but it may not be the best choice for the individual patient who has already had 6 CTs for kidney stones this year. For this patient, US, which is an inferior modality, may still be the more appropriate choice.

REFERENCES

1. Ferrandino M, Bagrodia A, Pierre S, et al. Radiation exposure in the acute and short-term management of urolithiasis at 2 academic centers. J Urol 2009; 181(2):668–73.
2. Fahmy N, Elkoushy M, Andonian S. Effective radiation exposure in evaluation and follow-up of patients with urolithiasis. Urology 2012;79(1):43–7.
3. Sudah M, Türk C, Petřík A, et al. EAU guidelines on diagnosis and conservative management of urolithiasis. Eur Urol 2016;69:468–74.
4. Mandeville J, Gnessin E, Lingeman J. Imaging evaluation in the patient with renal stone disease. Semin Nephrol 2011;31(3):254–8.
5. Kanno T, Kubota M, Funada S, et al. The utility of the kidneys-ureters-bladder radiograph as the sole imaging modality and its combination with ultrasonography for the detection of renal stones. Urology 2017;104:40–4.
6. Bjurlin M, Fantus R. Current surgical therapy: chapter retroperitoneal injuries: kidney and ureter. 12th edition. Philadelphia: Elsevier; 2017. p. 1200–9.
7. ACR Appropriateness Criteria® clinical condition: renal trauma. American College of Radiology. Available at: https://acsearch.acr.org/docs/69373/Narrative/. Accessed January 28, 2019.
8. Clinical guidelines: urotrauma. American Urological Association. Available at: https://www.auanet.org/guidelines/urotrauma-(2014-amended-2017. Accessed January 27, 2019.
9. Urogenital trauma guidelines. European Association of Urology. Available at: https://uroweb.org/guideline/urological-trauma/#4. Accessed January 28, 2019.
10. Roberts J, Custalow C, Thomsen T. Roberts and Hedges' clinical procedures in emergency medicine and acute care. 7th edition. Philadelphia: Elsevier; 2019. p. 1141–85.e2. Chapter 55 Urologic Procedures.
11. Kavoussi P. Campbell-walsh urology. In: Chapter 21: surgical, radiographic, and endoscopic anatomy of the male reproductive system. Philadelphia: Elsevier; 2016. p. 498–515.
12. Byrne MW, Kimberly HH, Noble V. Emergency renal ultrasonography. EM Clinical Essentials 2012;2:998–1002.
13. Ultrasound guidelines: emergency, point-of-care, and clinical ultrasound guidelines in medicine. American College of Emergency Physicans (ACEP); 2016. Available at: https://www.acep.org/globalassets/new-pdfs/policy-statements/ultrasound-guidelines—emergency-point-of-care-and-clinical-ultrasound-guidelines-in-medicine.pdf. Accessed January 26, 2019.
14. Lin EP, Bhatt S, Dogra VS, et al. Sonography of urolithiasis and hydronephrosis. Ultrasound Clin 2007;2:1–16.

15. Patlas M, Farkas A, Fisher D, et al. Ultrasound vs CT for the detection of ureteric stones in patients with renal colic. Br J Radiol 2001;74:901–4.

16. Ripolles T, Agramunt M, Errando J, et al. Suspected ureteral colic: plain film and sonography vs unenhanced helical CT. A prospective study in 66 patients. Eur Radiol 2004;14:129–36.

17. Park SJ, Yi BH, Lee HK, et al. Evaluation of patients with suspected ureteral calculi using sonography as an initial diagnostic tool. J Ultrasound Med 2008; 27:1441–50.

18. Edmonds ML, Yan JW, Sedran RJ, et al. The utility of renal ultrasonography in the diagnosis of renal colic in emergency department patients. CJEM 2010; 12:201–6.

19. Goertz JK, Lotterman S. Can the degree of hydronephrosis on ultrasound depict kidney stone size? Am J Emerg Med 2010;28:813–6.

20. Rosen CL, Brown DF, Sagarin MJ, et al. Ultrasonography by emergency physicians in patients with suspected ureteral colic. J Emerg Med 1998;16:865–70.

21. Gaspari RJ, Horst K. Emergency ultrasound and urinalysis in the evaluation of flank pain. Acad Emerg Med 2005;12:1180–4.

22. Dane B, Baxter A, Bernstein M. Imaging genitourinary trauma. Radiol Clin North Am 2017;55(2):321–35.

23. Cooperberg M, Chambers S, Rutherford T, et al. Cystic pelvic pathology presenting as falsely elevated postvoid residual urine measured by portable ultrasound bladder scanning: report of 3 cases and review of the literature. Urology 2000;55(4):590.

24. Elsamra S, Gordon Z, Ellsworth P. The pitfalls of BladderScan™ PVR in evaluating bladder volume in adolescent females. J Pediatr Urol 2011;7(1):95–7.

25. Choe J, Lee J, Lee K. Accuracy and precision of a new portable ultrasound scanner, the BME-150A, in residual urine volume measurement: a comparison with the BladderScan BVI 3000. Int Urogynecol J Pelvic Floor Dysfunct 2006; 18(6):641–4.

26. Dessie A, Steele D, Liu A, et al. Point-of-care ultrasound assessment of bladder fullness for female patients awaiting radiology-performed transabdominal pelvic ultrasound in a pediatric emergency department: a randomized controlled trial. Ann Emerg Med 2018;72(5):571–80.

27. Simforoosh N, Dadkhah F, Hosseini S, et al. Accuracy of residual urine measurement in men: comparison between real-time ultrasonography and catheterization. J Urol 1997;158(1):59–61.

28. Ghani K, Pilcher J, Rowland D, et al. Portable ultrasonography and bladder volume accuracy—a comparative study using three-dimensional ultrasonography. Urology 2008;72(1):24–8.

29. Park Y, Ku J, Oh S. Accuracy of post-void residual urine volume measurement using a portable ultrasound bladder scanner with real-time pre-scan imaging. Neurourol Urodyn 2011;30(3):335–8.

30. Oelke M, Höfner K, Jonas U, et al. Diagnostic accuracy of noninvasive tests to evaluate bladder outlet obstruction in men: detrusor wall thickness, uroflowmetry, postvoid residual urine, and prostate volume. Eur Urol 2007;52(3):827–35.

31. ACR Appropriateness Criteria® acute onset of scrotal pain-without trauma without antecedent mass. Acsearch.acr.org. 2018. Available at: https://acsearch.acr.org/docs/69363/Narrative/. Accessed January 24, 2019.

32. DaJusta D, Granberg C, Villanueva C, et al. Contemporary review of testicular torsion: new concepts, emerging technologies and potential therapeutics. J Pediatr Urol 2013;9(6):723–30.

33. Baker L, Sigman D, Mathews R, et al. An analysis of clinical outcomes using color Doppler testicular ultrasound for testicular torsion. Pediatrics 2000;105(3): 604–7.

34. Kaye J, Shapiro E, Levitt S, et al. Parenchymal echo texture predicts testicular salvage after torsion: potential impact on the need for emergent exploration. J Urol 2008;180(4s):1733–6.

35. Bertolotto M, Cantisani V, Valentino M, et al. Pitfalls in imaging for acute scrotal pathology. Semin Roentgenol 2016;51(1):60–9.

36. Burks D, Markey B, Burkhard T, et al. Suspected testicular torsion and ischemia: evaluation with color Doppler sonography. Radiology 1990;175(3):815–21.

37. Yagil Y, Naroditsky I, Milhem J, et al. Role of Doppler ultrasonography in the triage of acute scrotum in the emergency department. J Ultrasound Med 2010;29(1):11–21.

38. Lin E, Bhatt S, Rubens D, et al. Testicular torsion: twists and turns. Semin Ultrasound CT MR 2007;28(4):317–28.

39. Weatherspoon K, Polansky S, Catanzano T. Ultrasound emergencies of the male pelvis. Semin Ultrasound CT MR 2017;38(4):327–44.

40. Coley B. The acute pediatric scrotum. Ultrasound Clin 2006;1(3):485–96.

41. Esposito F, Di Serafino M, Mercogliano C, et al. The "whirlpool sign", a US finding in partial torsion of the spermatic cord: 4 cases. J Ultrasound 2014; 17(4):313–5.

42. Dohle G, Schröder F. Ultrasonographic assessment of the scrotum. Lancet 2001;357(9257):721–2.

43. Coley B, Frush D, Babcock D, et al. Acute testicular torsion: comparison of unenhanced and contrast-enhanced power Doppler US, color Doppler US, and radionuclide imaging. Radiology 1996;199(2):441–6.

44. Bertolotto M, Derchi L, Sidhu P, et al. Acute segmental testicular infarction at contrast-enhanced ultrasound: early features and changes during follow-up. AJR Am J Roentgenol 2011;196(4):834–41.

45. Ingram S, Hollman A, Azmy A. Testicular torsion: missed diagnosis on colour Doppler sonography. Pediatr Radiol 1993;23(6):483–4.

46. Holcomb G. Testicular torsion: pitfalls of color doppler sonography. J Pediatr Surg 1994;29(3):470.

47. Yazbeck S, Patriquin H. Accuracy of Doppler sonography in the evaluation of acute conditions of the scrotum in children. J Pediatr Surg 1994;29(9):1270–2.

48. Allen T, Elder J. Shortcomings of color Doppler sonography in diagnosis of testicular torsion. J Urol 1995;154(4):1508–10.

49. Kalfa N, Veyrac C, Lopez M, et al. Multicenter assessment of ultrasound of the spermatic cord in children with acute scrotum. J Urol 2007;177(1):297–301.

50. Blaivas M, Sierzenski P, Lambert M. Emergency evaluation of patients presenting with acute scrotum using bedside ultrasonography. Acad Emerg Med 2001; 8(1):90–3.

51. Trojian T, Lishnak T, Heiman D. Epididymitis and orchitis: an overview. Am Fam Physician 2009;79(7):583–7.

52. Pilatz A, Wagenlehner F, Bschleipfer T, et al. Acute epididymitis in ultrasound: results of a prospective study with baseline and follow-up investigations in 134 patients. Eur J Radiol 2013;82(12):e762–8.

53. Begley M, Shawker T, Robertson C, et al. Fournier gangrene: diagnosis with scrotal US. Radiology 1988;169(2):387–9.

54. Bahner D, Kube E, Stawicki S. Ultrasound in the diagnosis of Fournier's gangrene. Int J Crit Illn Inj Sci 2012;2(2):104.

55. Shyam D, Rapsang A. Fournier's gangrene. Surgeon 2013;11(4):222–32.
56. Di Serafino M, Gullotto C, Gregorini C, et al. A clinical case of Fournier's gangrene: imaging ultrasound. J Ultrasound 2014;17(4):303–6.
57. Curtis KM, Hillis SD, Kieke BA Jr, et al. Visits to emergency departments for gynecologic disorders in the United States, 1992-1994. Obstet Gynecol 1998; 91(6):1007–12.
58. Tukeva TA, Aronen HJ, Karjalainen PT, et al. MR imaging in pelvic inflammatory disease: comparison with laparoscopy and US. Radiology 1999;210(1):209–16.
59. Taylor KJ, Wasson JF, De Graaff C, et al. Accuracy of grey-scale ultrasound diagnosis of abdominal and pelvic abscesses in 220 patients. Lancet 1978; 1(8055):83–4.
60. Patten RM, Vincent LM, Wolner-Hanssen P, et al. Pelvic inflammatory disease: endovaginal sonography with laparoscopic correlation. J Ultrasound Med 1990;9(12):681–9.
61. Varras M, Polyzos D, Perouli E, et al. Tubo-ovarian abscesses: spectrum of sonographic findings with surgical and pathological correlations. Clin Exp Obstet Gynecol 2003;30(2–3):117–21.
62. Montague DK, Jarow J, Broderick GA, et al. American Urological Association guideline on the management of priapism. J Urol 2003;170:1318–24.
63. Guidelines on priapism. European Association of Urology. Available at: https://uroweb.org/wp-content/uploads/15_Priapism_LR-page-18-corrected-29-July-2014.pdf. Accessed January 31, 2019.
64. Halls J, Bydawell G, Patel U. Erectile dysfunction: the role of penile Doppler ultrasound in diagnosis. Abdom Imaging 2009;34:712–25.
65. Wilkins CJ, Sriprasad S, Sidhu PS. Colour Doppler ultrasound of the penis. Clin Radiol 2003;58:514–23.
66. Bastuba MD, Saenz de Tejada I, Dinlenc CZ, et al. Arterial priapism: diagnosis, treatment and long-term followup. J Urol 1994;151:1231–7.
67. Beir VII: health risks from exposure to low levels of ionizing radiation. The National Academy of Science. 2005. Available at: http://dels.nas.edu/resources/static-assets/materials-based-on-reports/reports-in-brief/beir_vii_final.pdf. Accessed January 21, 2019.
68. Valentin J. 2007 the recommendations of the International Commission on Radiological Protection. Annals of ICRP Publication, vol. 37. ICRP Publication; 2007. 103.
69. ACR Appropriateness Criteria® acute nonlocalized abdominal pain. American College of Radiology. Available at: https://acsearch.acr.org/docs/69467/Narrative/. Accessed January 26, 2019.
70. ACR Appropriateness Criteria® acute onset flank pain—suspicion of stone disease (Urolithiasis). Acsearch.acr.org. 2015. Available at: https://acsearch.acr.org/docs/69362/Narrative/. Accessed January 27, 2019.
71. ACR Appropriateness Criteria® clinical condition: hematuria variant3: all patients except those described in variant 1 or 2. American College of Radiology. 2014. Available at: https://acsearch.acr.org/docs/69490/Narrative/. Accessed January 27, 2019.
72. Hirshfeld J, Ferrari V, Bengel F, et al. 2018 ACC/HRS/NASCI/SCAI/SCCT expert consensus document on optimal use of ionizing radiation in cardiovascular imaging: best practices for safety and effectiveness. J Am Coll Cardiol 2018; 71(24):e283–351.
73. Brenner D. Radiation injury: Chapter 20 radiation injury. 25th edition. Philadelphia: Saunders; 2016. p. 82–6.e1.

74. Turkcuer I, Serinken M, Karcioglu O, et al. Hospital cost analysis of management of patients with renal colic in the emergency department. Urol Res 2010;38: 29–33.
75. Grisi G, Stacul F, Cuttin R, et al. Cost analysis of different protocols for imaging a patient with acute flank pain. Eur Radiol 2000;10:1620–7.
76. Shewakramani S, Reed K. Genitourinary trauma. Emerg Med Clin North Am 2011;29(3):501–18.
77. Wymer D, Wymer D. Nephrology secrets. 4th edition. St Louis (MO): Elsevier/Mosby; 2018. p. 30–6. CHAPTER 4 Kidney imaging techniques.
78. Sierink J, Treskes K, Edwards M, et al. Immediate total-body CT scanning versus conventional imaging and selective CT scanning in patients with severe trauma (REACT-2): a randomised controlled trial. Lancet 2016;388(10045):673–83.
79. Injury Scoring Scales–The American Association for the Surgery of Trauma. The American Association for the Surgery of Trauma. Available at: http://www.aast.org/library/traumatools/injuryscoringscales.aspx#kidney. Accessed January 27, 2019.
80. Santucci R, McAninch J. Diagnosis and management of renal trauma: past, present, and future. J Am Coll Surg 2000;191(4):443–51.
81. Santucci R, Wessells H, Bartsch G, et al. Evaluation and management of renal injuries: consensus statement of the renal trauma subcommittee. BJU Int 2004; 93(7):937–54.
82. Injury scoring scales The American Association for the Surgery of Trauma. The American Association for the Surgery of Trauma. Available at: http://www.aast.org/library/traumatools/injuryscoringscales.aspx#ureter. Accessed January 27, 2019.
83. Serafetinides E, Kitrey N, Djakovic N, et al. Review of the current management of upper urinary tract injuries by the EAU trauma guidelines panel. Eur Urol 2015; 67(5):930–6.
84. Figler B, Edward Hoffler C, Reisman W, et al. Multi-disciplinary update on pelvic fracture associated bladder and urethral injuries. Injury 2012;43(8):1242–9.
85. Matlock K, Tyroch A, Ziad K, et al. Blunt traumatic bladder rupture: a 10-year perspective. Am Surg 2013;79(6):589–93 (5).
86. Fwu C, Eggers P, Kimmel P, et al. Emergency department visits, use of imaging, and drugs for urolithiasis have increased in the United States. Kidney Int 2013; 83(3):479–86.
87. ACR Appropriateness Criteria® clinical condition: acute onset flank pain—suspicion of stone disease (urolithiasis). Acsearch.acr.org. 2015. Available at: https://acsearch.acr.org/docs/69362/Narrative/. Accessed January 27, 2019.
88. Assimos MDD, Krambeck MDA, Miller MDN, et al. Surgical management of stones: AUA/Endourology Society Guideline. Auanet.org. 2016. Available at: https://www.auanet.org/guidelines/stone-disease-surgical-. Accessed January 10, 2019.
89. Kothari K, Hines J. CT imaging of emergent renal conditions. Semin Ultrasound CT MR 2018;39(2):129–44.
90. Heneghan J, McGuire K, Leder R, et al. Helical CT for nephrolithiasis and ureterolithiasis: comparison of conventional and reduced radiation-dose techniques. Radiology 2003;229(2):575–80.
91. Sheafor DH, Hertzberg BS, Freed KS, et al. Nonenhanced helical CT and US in the emergency evaluation of patients with renal colic: prospective comparison. Radiology 2000;217:792–7.

92. Catalano O, Nunziata A, Altei F, et al. Suspected ureteral colic: primary helical CT versus selective helical CT after unenhanced radiography and sonography. AJR Am J Roentgenol 2002;178:379–87.
93. Fowler KA, Locken JA, Duchesne JH, et al. US for detecting renal calculi with nonenhanced CT as a reference standard. Radiology 2002;222:109–13.
94. Ray AA, Ghiculete D, Pace KT, et al. Limitations to ultrasound in the detection and measurement of urinary tract calculi. Urology 2010;76:295–300.
95. Kambadakone A, Andrabi Y, Patino M, et al. Advances in CT imaging for urolithiasis. Indian J Urol 2015;31(3):185.
96. ACR Appropriateness Criteria® Variant 8: clinical examination suggesting crepitus. Suspected so ft-tissue gas. First study. American College of Radiology. 2016. Available at: https://acsearch.acr.org/docs/3094201/Narrative/. Accessed January 26, 2019.
97. Wysoki M, Santora T, Shah R, et al. Necrotizing fasciitis: CT characteristics. Radiology 1997;203(3):859–63.
98. Levenson R, Singh A, Novelline R. Fournier gangrene: role of imaging. Radiographics 2008;28(2):519–28.
99. Sherman J, Solliday M, Paraiso E, et al. Early CT findings of Fournier's gangrene in a healthy male. Clin Imaging 1998;22(6):425–7.
100. Gagliardi PD, Hoffer PB, Rosenfield AT. Correlative imaging in abdominal infection: an algorithmic approach using nuclear medicine, ultrasound, and computed tomography. Semin Nucl Med 1988;18(4):320–34.
101. Hiller N, Appelbaum L, Simanovsky N, et al. CT features of adnexal torsion. AJR Am J Roentgenol 2007;189(1):124–9.
102. Suzuki K, Nishizawa S, Muraishi O, et al. Post-traumatic high flow priapism: demonstrable findings of penile enhanced computed tomography. Int J Urol 2001;8:648–51.
103. Kitajima K, Maeda T, Watanabe S, et al. Recent topics related to nephrogenic systemic fibrosis associated with gadolinium-based contrast agents. Int J Urol 2012;19(9):806–11.
104. Villa L, Giusti G, Knoll T, et al. Imaging for urinary stones: update in 2015. Eur Urol Focus 2016;2(2):122–9.
105. Kalb B, Sharma P, Ogan K, et al. Acute abdominal pain: is there a potential role for MRI in the setting of the emergency department in a patient with renal calculi? J Magn Reson Imaging 2010;32(5):1011.
106. Guidelines for diagnostic imaging during pregnancy and lactation - ACOG. Acog.org. Available at: https://www.acog.org/Clinical-Guidance-and-Publications/Committee-Opinions/Committee-on-Obstetric-Practice/Guidelines-for-Diagnostic-Imaging-During-Pregnancy-and-Lactation. Accessed January 21, 2019.
107. Karabacakoglu A, Karakose S, Ince O, et al. Diagnostic value of diuretic-enhanced excretory MR urography in patients with obstructive uropathy. Eur J Radiol 2004;52(3):320–7.
108. Gottlieb M, Long B, Koyfman A. The evaluation and management of urolithiasis in the ED: a review of the literature. Am J Emerg Med 2018;36(4):699–706.
109. Tsili A, Giannakis D, Sylakos A, et al. MR imaging of scrotum. Magn Reson Imaging Clin N Am 2014;22(2):217–38.
110. Watanabe Y, Nagayama M, Okumura A, et al. MR imaging of testicular torsion features of testicular hemorrhagic necrosis and clinical outcomes. J Magn Reson Imaging 2007;26(1):100–8.
111. Pooler B, Repplinger M, Reeder S, et al. MRI of the nontraumatic acute abdomen. Gastroenterol Clin North Am 2018;47(3):667–90.

112. Kirkham AP, Illing RO, Minhas S, et al. MR imaging of nonmalignant penile lesions. Radiographics 2008;28:837–53.
113. Coutinho A, Krishnaraj A, Pires C, et al. Pelvic applications of diffusion magnetic resonance images. Magn Reson Imaging Clin N Am 2011;19(1):133–57.
114. Kim S, Kim S, Yang D, et al. Unusual causes of tubo-ovarian abscess: CT and MR imaging findings. Radiographics 2004;24(6):1575–89.
115. Li W, Zhang Y, Cui Y, et al. Pelvic inflammatory disease: evaluation of diagnostic accuracy with conventional MR with added diffusion-weighted imaging. Abdom Imaging 2013;38(1):193–200.
116. Jawa Z, Okoye O. Differentiating acute epididymitis from testicular torsion using scrotal scintigraphy. Sahel Medical Journal 2017;20(3):89.

Genitourinary Procedures

Michael P. Jones, MD*, Kumelachew Mekuria, MD

KEYWORDS

- Genitourinary • Procedure • Intervention • Complication

KEY POINTS

- Knowledge of critical procedures is important to prevent severe complications.
- The emergency provider must know key genitourinary procedures to avoid severe life- or limb-threatening outcomes.
- A strong knowledge of pelvic anatomy is important to understanding these key interventions and avoiding complications.

INTRODUCTION

Emergency medicine providers may encounter serious GU conditions that need rapid diagnosis and early intervention to avoid severe life- and limb-threatening complications. A fundamental knowledge of several key procedural interventions is incredibly important to optimal patient outcomes. The most important procedures to be familiar with are:

- Priapism drainage
- Paraphimosis reduction
- Removal of retained foreign bodies
- Suprapubic aspiration or catheter placement
- Continuous bladder irrigation
- Urinary catheter placement
- Manual detorsion of the testes

CONTENT

Priapism Drainage

Priapism is a painful condition that can lead to erectile dysfunction and irreversible ischemic damage of the penis if not treated within 4 hours. Although intervention after 72 hours of an erectile state may resolve the unwanted erection and discomfort, it has little to no benefit in preserving potency.

Priapism can be a result of either an ischemic or nonischemic process. Ischemic priapism is caused by venous outflow obstruction and stasis, mostly seen in patients with

Department of Emergency Medicine, Jacobi Medical Center, 1400 Pelham Parkway South, Suite 1B-25, Bronx, NY 10461, USA
* Corresponding author.
E-mail address: michael.jones@nychhc.org

Emerg Med Clin N Am 37 (2019) 811–819
https://doi.org/10.1016/j.emc.2019.07.014   emed.theclinics.com

hematologic disorders (eg, sickle cell anemia and leukemia), as well as a result of pre-scription medications (eg, antidepressants). Unlike ischemic priapism, nonischemic priapism is not considered an emergent disorder. It is an abnormality of arterial flow and may resolve spontaneously. The subsequent focus will be on ischemic priapism and management in the emergency department setting.

Once priapism is identified and deemed to be ischemic, emergent intervention is required. The goal of intervention is to achieve detumescence via corpora cavernosal aspiration and administration of a sympathomimetic agent. The aspiration is per-formed in order to evacuate the viscous and hypoxic blood, and the sympathomimetic agent (injected intracavernously) will cause vasoconstriction. Because of its selectivity for alpha-adrenergic receptors and its limited cardiovascular effects, phenylephrine is the preferred sympathomimetic agent.

Before starting the procedure, the physician needs to determine that the patient does not have any contraindications to the procedure. That is, the mechanism of pri-apism must be ischemic; there can be no overlying cellulitis, and the patient must not have an uncontrolled bleeding disorder.

Preparation includes obtaining sterile gloves, drapes, basin (for collection), gauze, 1% lidocaine for local anesthesia, 2 30 mL syringes, and needles (18 gauge, 25 gauge and butterfly). The patient should be placed on a cardiac-monitor in a supine position.

First, one should administer a penile block using 1% lidocaine for pain control. Next, oneshould prepare a dilute solution of phenylephrine by mixing 1 mL of a 10 mg/mL phenylephrine in 99 mL of normal saline (a final concentration of 100 mg/mL).

Then, one should insert a butterfly needle into the lateral aspect of either corporal cavernosum to aspirate blood and inject 1 to 2 mL of the dilute phenylephrine intraca-vernously. Finally, one should repeat injection every 2 minutes until detumescence is achieved or a total of 10 mL diluted solution of phenylephrine is injected.

If phenylephrine and butterfly aspiration fail to achieve detumescence, the caver-nosa should be irrigated with normal saline, and a second butterfly needle can be placed on the opposite side of the corporal cavernosa to increase the rate of aspira-tion. If this all fails, emergent evaluation by a urologist is required with possible surgical intervention.[1-4]

Paraphimosis Reduction

Paraphimosis is a urologic emergency characterized by the inability to reduce the fore-skin over the glans penis, leading to constriction of penile tissue proximally, and swelling distally (**Fig. 1**). It is a condition of uncircumcised or partially circumcised males, and is most often caused iatrogenically following a penile examination, urethral catheterization (when the practitioner is unable to return the retracted foreskin to its normal position), or cystoscopy. Health care providers should be educated in prevention by stressing the importance of returning the prepuce to cover the glans after penile manipulation.

Treatment of paraphimosis is directed toward reducing penile edema and subse-quent reduction of the paraphimosis. Before attempting reduction, it is important to achieve adequate pain control either with use of a dorsal penile nerve block, as described previously, or with topical or oral analgesic medications. When the pain is well-controlled, the physician should immediately attempt to reduce the edema through either mechanical compression, pharmacologic therapy, or a dorsal slit.

Reducing Penile Edema

First, one should use a gloved hand to apply circumferential pressure to the distal aspect of the penis. In addition to mechanical compression, an ice pack can be inter mittently applied after wrapping the penis with plastics.

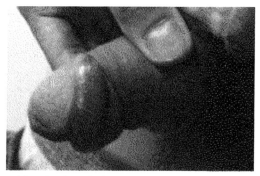

Fig. 1. Photo of Paraphimosis of penis. (*From* Morteza K, Yen G. Dorsal Slit for Phimosis. *In* Pfenninger JL, Fowler, GC (eds). *Pfenninger and Fowler's Procedures for Primary Care, 3e.* Philadelphia, PA: Mosby Elsevier, 2011; with permission.)

If this technique fails to improve the edema, a circumferential compressive elastic dressing can be applied around the penis from the glans to the base. It is important to periodically monitor the penis for the resolution of swelling, as the patient may no longer complain of pain after receiving adequate pain control.

Granulated sugar can also be applied directly to the surface of the edematous preputce and glans to create an osmotic gradient, promoting the transfer of fluid and reduction in swelling. Alternatively, a hyaluronidase injection can be used to decrease swelling by enhancing the diffusion of fluid trapped between tissue planes.

Reducing the Paraphimosis

First, one should place the thumbs of both hands on the glans while wrapping the fingers behind the prepuce. Then, with the thumbs, one should apply a gentle and steady pressure to the glans while simultaneously applying countertraction to the foreskin with the fingers. This procedure should help mobilize the constricting band of tissue over the glans, restoring the prepuce to its normal position.

If manual reduction (**Fig. 2**) fails, a dorsal slit (**Fig. 3**) should be done. First, one should ensure adequate analgesia as noted previously. Next, one should drape the penis in a sterile fashion. Then, one should use 2 hemostat forceps to crush the foreskin at a 12 o'clock position perpendicular to the corona for approximately 2 minutes.

After 2 minutes, the prepuce between the hemostat forceps should be incised, releasing the constricting band of tissue. Absorbable sutures should be used to approximate the edges of the incision.

Note: In the subset of patients with paraphimosis who also have an indwelling urethral catheter, the catheter should be removed before manipulating the penis. If necessary, the catheter can be replaced after the successful reduction of paraphimosis.

After resolution of the acute episode, a circumcision should be performed to prevent recurrence of paraphimosis.[5–7]

Retained Foreign Body

Penile shaft entrapment is a condition that requires urgent intervention and treatment. Most cases of penile entrapment are caused by attempts at maintaining prolonged erections during sexual intercourse with the use of rings, bottles, and pipes. When the entrapping object is thin and nonmetallic, there is little difficulty in removing the object. However, metal objects, bottles, and rigid or firm rings present a bigger challenge and can potentially lead to severe vascular obstruction. These cases require emergent release and decompression to prevent gangrene, necrosis, and amputation of the penis.

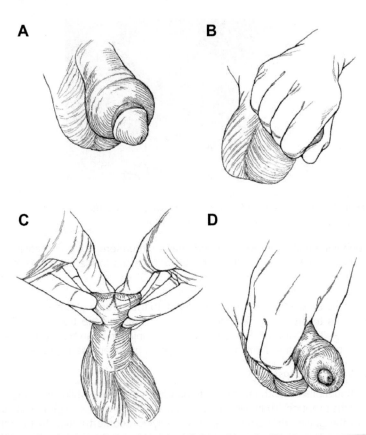

Fig. 2. Manual reduction of paraphimosis. (*A*) Paraphimosis. (*B*) Manual compression. (*C*) Manual reduction. (*D*) Reduced paraphimosis. (*From* Rosen, P, Chan, TC., Vilke, GM., Sternbach, GL. Atlas of emergency procedures. St. Louis, MO: Mosby, 2001; with permission.)

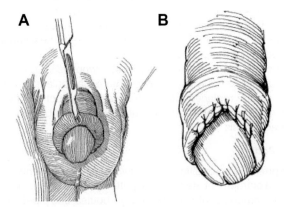

Fig. 3. Dorsal slit. (*A*) Dorsal slit incision. (*B*) Completed dorsal slit procedure. (*From* Wan J. Kraft K. Circumcision and Dorsal Slit or Preputioplasty Circumcision. In Smith JA, Howards SS, Preminger GM, Hinman F, (eds). *Hinman's Atlas of Urologic Surgery*. Philadelphia: Elsevier/Saunders, 2012.)

There are different degrees of penile entrapment ranging from edema of the distal penis (grade 1) to gangrenous necrosis and complete amputation of the distal penis (grade 5). The difficulty of resolving the entrapment depends on the degree to which the penis is entrapped, the object involved, and the level of the resulting edema.

One way of releasing an entrapped penis is to use a motor operated blade (such as micromotor) to cut away the entrapping material. Because of the proximity of penile tissue to the entrapping object and the heat generated in the process of cutting, this can be a delicate process.[8–10]

Releasing an entrapped penis involves several steps:

1. Ensure adequate analgesia and anxiolysis in the patient.
2. To prevent tissue injury secondary to heat, cool the metal blade by continuous application of normal saline to the penile tissue and the blade.
3. Avoid cutting the penile tissue by making 2 different cuts on the entrapping material during removal and breaking the material at the very end using hemostats.[8–10]

Suprapubic Aspiration/Catheterization

Suprapubic aspiration (**Fig. 4**) is indicated in the setting of a suspected lower urinary tract infection when one cannot obtain a urine sample, either by voiding or urethral catheterization, or in cases of urinary obstruction when a urethral catheter cannot be placed. This procedure is contraindicated if there is overlaying cellulitis at the site of needle insertion.

Equipment needed for the procedure includes:

Sterile container for urinalysis and urine culture
A 10 mL syringe
Long (approximately 10 cm) 22-gauge needle for aspiration
Lidocaine 1% or 2% (with or without epinephrine)
Sterile drape

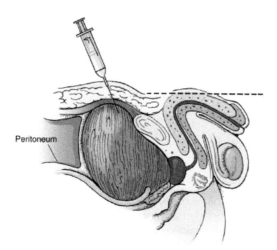

Peritoneum

Fig. 4. Suprapubic aspiration. The peritoneum is pushed cephalad by the filled bladder during suprapubic aspiration in an adult. Direct the needle slightly caudal. (*From* Urologic Procedures. In Roberts JR, Hedges JR. In Custalow CB., Roberts JR., Thomsen, T W, et al. (eds). Roberts and Hedges' clinical procedures in emergency medicine, 5e. Philadelphia, PA: Elsevier/Saunders, 2013.)

Antiseptic solution

The aspiration procedure involves

Positioning the patient supine on a stretcher at a height comfortable to the provider performing the procedure

Using ultrasound to identify the bladder, or, if ultrasound is unavailable, anatomic landmarks to palpate the bladder anterior and proximal to the suprapubic bone. If the bladder cannot be clearly identified, consider intravenous hydration in the event that it is not contraindicated by patient's medical history.

Preparing and draping the suprapubic region in a sterile fashion

Administering 3 to 5 cc lidocaine transdermally approximately 5 cm above the pubic symphysis

With the obturator in place, inserting a 22-gauge needle through the skin at the same insertion point. Direct the needle slightly posterior and inferior. A measurement of 5 cm is approximately the depth at which the needle is expected to enter the abdominal bladder. If available, ultrasound can be used to confirm the needle placement.

Removing the obturator, connecting a sterile syringe, and aspirating urine from the bladder

Transferring the urine to UA and culture tubes

A long-term catheter that can be left in place following similar instructions[11–13]

CONTINUOUS BLADDER IRRIGATION

Continuous bladder irrigation (CBI) is used to maintain the patency of indwelling catheters, minimize clot formation, and provide additional comfort to the patient. It is indicated in the setting of a urinary catheter outflow obstruction, typically the result of a blood clot. Continuous irrigation with normal saline allows the restoration of urinary free flow and will maintain catheter patency. Furthermore, infection is always a concern with indwelling catheters. Using CBI to maintain catheter patency helps minimize the incidence of urinary tract infections (UTIs).

Prepare the following prior to the start of the procedure:

Normal saline for the purpose of irrigation (have extra bags available in case further irrigation needed)

A 3-way urinary catheter

Continuous bladder irrigation set and closed urinary drainage bag with antireflux valve

Intravenous pole

Sterile and nonsterile gloves

Antiseptic solution

To perform the procedure:

Position the patient in a supine or upright/tilted position for easy access to the catheter. Maintain patient comfort as much as possible.

Hang irrigation flasks on the intravenous pole.

Prime the irrigation set while maintaining sterility. Open only one of the irrigation flask clamps when priming to prevent fluid running from one flask to another.

After priming the irrigation set, ensure that all clamps are once again closed.

Wear personal protective devices, especially a facial mask with a shield.

Prepare the urinary catheter irrigation and ports by cleaning with an antiseptic solution.

While maintaining sterility, connect the irrigation set to the irrigation lumen of the catheter.

Ensure urine is draining freely before commencing continuous irrigation.

Unclamp the irrigation flask used to prime the irrigation set and set the rate of administration by adjusting the roller clamp.

The goal of bladder irrigation is to produce rose-colored urine that is completely free of clot. The rate of irrigation should be adjusted to obtain the aforementioned goal and does not need to run at a set rate throughout irrigation. Continue to empty and hang new bags of normal saline until consistent rose-colored urine free of clot is seen.[14–16]

URINARY CATHETER PLACEMENT, DIFFICULTY PASSING

Urinary catheter placement is a common emergency department procedure predominantly handled by nursing. Most urinary catheters can be inserted without difficulty; however, in more challenging instances, most providers attempt to use a reinforced catheter tip, such as a Coudé tip. Continuous attempts at placing a difficult urinary catheter (or any type of reinforced catheter), often using considerable force, increase the risk of false passage in patients with urethral stricture, and lead to further urologic complications.

When a patient has risk factors for difficult urinary catheter placement, such as with urethral stricture or BPH, ensure adequate pain control (topical anesthetics such as 2% xylocaine jelly) and sufficient lubrication of the urethra and the catheter. When reinforced catheters fail to work, consider a glidewire-assisted technique rather than attempting to use force placement of the catheter.

Glidewire-Assisted Technique

One should first submerge the glidewire in sterile water to keep it moist during use.

The soft, floppy end of the glidewire should then be inserted into the urethral meatus. In the absence of false passages, the glidewire will often advance into the bladder without difficulty, even in the setting of severe strictures.

Using a surgical blade, one should slit the urinary catheter tip to expose the lumen (or use a premade catheter/wire kit), taking extra precaution to avoid damaging the balloon.

After ensuring the balloon integrity, one should insert the stiff end of the glidewire into the slit tip of a regular urinary catheter (16 Fr or 18 Fr). If a smaller and stiffer catheter is needed because of the level of stricture, a 12 Fr or 14 Fr should be considered.

Once ready, one may advance the catheter over the glidewire all the way into the bladder. A series of rigid dilating catheters may also be utilized; however, extreme caution must be taken to not develop a false lumen.[17–21]

MANUAL DETORSION OF TESTES

The tunica vaginalis, a serous membrane composed of both a parietal layer and a visceral layer, comes together to surround the testes, attaching posteriorly to the scrotal wall. These 2 layers of the tunica vaginalis create a potential space in which the testicles may rotate around the spermatic cord, termed testicular torsion. When this occurs, the venous return is obstructed, leading to edema, and, without immediate correction, arterial occlusion, ischemia, infarction, and ultimately, infertility. It is a true urologic emergency that needs to be promptly addressed.[22,23]

Testicular torsion can be diagnosed clinically, although ultrasound is used to further confirm the findings. If torsion is suspected, do not delay treatment to confirm the diagnosis. Although the definitive treatment for testicular torsion is surgical intervention, it may not be readily available, and the providing physician should attempt

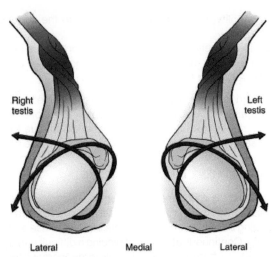

Right   Left
testis   testis

Lateral   Medial   Lateral

Fig. 5. Detorsing testes. (*From* Fowler, GC. *In* Pfenninger JL, Fowler, GC (eds). *Pfenninger and Fowler's Procedures for Primary Care, 2e.* Philadelphia, PA: Mosby Elsevier, 2019, with permission.)

manual detorsion (**Fig. 5**). This maneuver temporarily restores blood flow to the testicle. The procedure is painful, so one should consider intravenous sedation or analgesia prior to attempting.[22,23]

Manual Detorsion

Adequate analgesia and/or sedation should be provided to patient. The patient should be positioned supine.

The testicle should be grasped gently and rotated away from the midline (as though opening a book). Torsions may be caused by complete rotation, so more than one such rotation may be required to detorse the testicle. A successful detorsion will be marked by sudden and dramatic pain relief.

In a small minority of torsions, the testicle has rotated around the cord away from the midline. If this is the case, it will be difficult to further rotate away from the midline, at which point the physician should attempt to untwist in the other direction.[22,23]

SUMMARY

Genitourinary emergencies can require immediate life- and limb-salvaging interventions. An adequate knowledge of these interventions is paramount for the effective emergency physician.

REFERENCES

1. Jeffrey Bassett J. Diagnostic and therapeutic options for the management of ischemic and nonischemic priapism. Rev Urol 2010;12(1):56–63.
2. Montague DK, Jarow J, Broderick GA, et al. American Urological Association guideline on the management of priapism. J Urol 2003;170:1318–24.
3. Berger R, Billups K, Brock G, et al. Report of the American Foundation for Urologic Disease (AFUD) Thought Leader Panel for evaluation and treatment of priapism. Int J Impot Res 2001;13(suppl. 5):S39–43.

4. Auanet.org. 2019. American Urological Association. [online]. Available at: https://www.auanet.org/guidelines/male-sexual-dysfunction-priapism-(2003-reviewed-for-currency-2010). Accessed March 1, 2019.

5. Choe J. Paraphimosis: current treatment options. 2019. Available at: https://www.aafp.org/afp/2000/1215/p2623.html.

6. Olson C. Emergency treatment of paraphimosis. Can Fam Physician 1998;44:1253–41257.

7. Hollowood AD, Sibley GN. Non-painful paraphimosis causing partial amputation. Br J Urol 1997;80:958.

8. Paonam S, Kshetrimayum N, Rana I. Penile strangulation by iron metal ring: a novel and effective method of management. Urol Ann 2017;9(1):74.

9. Noh J, Kang TW, Heo T, et al. Penile strangulation treated with the modified string method. Urology 2004;64:591.

10. Santucci RA, Deng D, Carney J. Removal of metal penile foreign body with a widely available emergency-medical-services-provided air-driven grinder. Urology 2004;63:1183–4.

11. David Ponka F. Suprapubic bladder aspiration. 2019. Available at: https://www.ncbi.nlm.nih.gov/pmc/articles/PMC3555656/.

12. Ozkan B, Kaya O, Akdak R, et al. Suprapubic bladder aspiration with or without ultrasound guidance. Clin Pediatr 2000;39(10):625–6.

13. O'Callaghan C, McDougall PN. Successful suprapubic aspiration of urine. Arch Dis Child 1987;62(10):1072–3.

14. Scholtes S. Management of clot retention following urological surgery. Nurs Times 2002;98(8):48–50.

15. Ng C. Assessment and intervention knowledge of nurses in managing catheter patency in continuous bladder irrigation following TURP. Urol Nurs 2001;21(2):97–8, 101-7, 110-1.

16. Lockwood C, Page T, Nurs H, et al. Management of short-term indwelling urethral catheters to prevent urinary tract infections. JBI Libr Syst Rev 2004;2(8):1–36.

17. Rei K, Chiou W. Glidewire-assisted Foley catheter placement: a simple and safe technique for difficult male catheterization. 2019. Available at: https://www.ncbi.nlm.nih.gov/pmc/articles/PMC2692169/.

18. Clinical Practice Guidelines Task Force. Society of Urologic Nurses and Associates. Male urethral catheterization. Urol Nurs 2006;26:315.

19. Villanueva C, Hemstreet GP III. Difficult male urethral catheterization: a review of different approaches. Int Braz J Urol 2008;34:401–11.

20. Liss MA, Leifer S, Sakakine G, et al. The Liss maneuver: a nonendoscopic technique for difficult Foley catheterization. J Endourol 2009 Aug;23(8):1227–30.

21. Aci.health.nsw.gov.au. 2019 [online]. Available at: https://www.aci.health.nsw.gov.au/__data/assets/pdf_file/0007/165589/Bladder-Irrigation-Toolkit.pdf. Accessed March 1, 2019.

22. Yancey L. Testicular torsion. 2019 [online] Saem.org. Available at: https://www.saem.org/cdem/education/online-education/m4-curriculum/group-m4-genitourinary/testicular-torsion. Accessed March 1, 2019.

23. Silverman M, Schneider RE. Urologic procedures. In: Roberts JR, Hedges JR, editors. Roberts: clinical procedures in emergency medicine. 5th edition. Philadelphia: Saunders; 2010. p. 1010.

UNITED STATES POSTAL SERVICE®

Statement of Ownership, Management, and Circulation
(All Periodicals Publications Except Requester Publications)

1. Publication Title	2. Publication Number	3. Filing Date
EMERGENCY MEDICINE CLINICS OF NORTH AMERICA	000 – 714	9/18/2019

4. Issue Frequency	5. Number of Issues Published Annually	6. Annual Subscription Price
FEB, MAY, AUG, NOV	4	$349.00

7. Complete Mailing Address of Known Office of Publication (Not printer) (Street, city, county, state, and ZIP+4®)
ELSEVIER INC.
230 Park Avenue, Suite 800
New York, NY 10169

Contact Person: STEPHEN R. BUSHING
Telephone (Include area code): 215-239-3688

8. Complete Mailing Address of Headquarters or General Business Office of Publisher (Not printer)
ELSEVIER INC.
230 Park Avenue, Suite 800
New York, NY 10169

9. Full Names and Complete Mailing Addresses of Publisher, Editor, and Managing Editor (Do not leave blank)

Publisher (Name and complete mailing address)
TAYLOR BALL, ELSEVIER INC.
1600 JOHN F KENNEDY BLVD. SUITE 1800
PHILADELPHIA, PA 19103-2899

Editor (Name and complete mailing address)
Colleen Dietzler, ELSEVIER INC.
1600 JOHN F KENNEDY BLVD. SUITE 1800
PHILADELPHIA, PA 19103-2899

Managing Editor (Name and complete mailing address)
PATRICK MANLEY, ELSEVIER INC.
1600 JOHN F KENNEDY BLVD. SUITE 1800
PHILADELPHIA, PA 19103-2899

10. Owner (Do not leave blank. If the publication is owned by a corporation, give the name and address of the corporation immediately followed by the names and addresses of all stockholders owning or holding 1 percent or more of the total amount of stock. If not owned by a corporation, give the names and addresses of the individual owners. If owned by a partnership or other unincorporated firm, give its name and address as well as those of each individual owner. If the publication is published by a nonprofit organization, give its name and address.)

Full Name	Complete Mailing Address
WHOLLY OWNED SUBSIDIARY OF REED/ELSEVIER, US HOLDINGS	1600 JOHN F KENNEDY BLVD. SUITE 1800 PHILADELPHIA, PA 19103-2899

11. Known Bondholders, Mortgagees, and Other Security Holders Owning or Holding 1 Percent or More of Total Amount of Bonds, Mortgages, or Other Securities. If none, check box ▶ ☐ None

Full Name	Complete Mailing Address
N/A	

12. Tax Status (For completion by nonprofit organizations authorized to mail at nonprofit rates) (Check one)
The purpose, function, and nonprofit status of this organization and the exempt status for federal income tax purposes:
☒ Has Not Changed During Preceding 12 Months
☐ Has Changed During Preceding 12 Months (Publisher must submit explanation of change with this statement)

PS Form 3526, July 2014 (Page 1 of 4 (see instructions page 4)) PSN: 7530-01-000-9931 PRIVACY NOTICE: See our privacy policy on www.usps.com.

---

13. Publication Title	14. Issue Date for Circulation Data Below
EMERGENCY MEDICINE CLINICS OF NORTH AMERICA	AUGUST 2019

15. Extent and Nature of Circulation

		Average No. Copies Each Issue During Preceding 12 Months	No. Copies of Single Issue Published Nearest to Filing Date
a. Total Number of Copies (Net press run)		242	265
b. Paid Circulation (By Mail and Outside the Mail)	(1) Mailed Outside-County Paid Subscriptions Stated on PS Form 3541 (Include paid distribution above nominal rate, advertiser's proof copies, and exchange copies)	137	159
	(2) Mailed In-County Paid Subscriptions Stated on PS Form 3541 (Include paid distribution above nominal rate, advertiser's proof copies, and exchange copies)	0	0
	(3) Paid Distribution Outside the Mails Including Sales Through Dealers and Carriers, Street Vendors, Counter Sales, and Other Paid Distribution Outside USPS®	50	63
	(4) Paid Distribution by Other Classes of Mail Through the USPS (e.g., First-Class Mail®)	0	0
c. Total Paid Distribution (Sum of 15b (1), (2), (3), and (4))		187	222
d. Free or Nominal Rate Distribution (By Mail and Outside the Mail)	(1) Free or Nominal Rate Outside-County Copies included on PS Form 3541	42	26
	(2) Free or Nominal Rate In-County Copies Included on PS Form 3541	0	0
	(3) Free or Nominal Rate Copies Mailed at Other Classes Through the USPS (e.g. First-Class Mail)	0	0
	(4) Free or Nominal Rate Distribution Outside the Mail (Carriers or other means)	0	0
e. Total Free or Nominal Rate Distribution (Sum of 15d (1), (2), (3) and (4))		42	26
f. Total Distribution (Sum of 15c and 15e)		229	248
g. Copies not Distributed (See instructions to Publishers #4 (page #3))		13	17
h. Total (Sum of 15f and g)		242	265
i. Percent Paid (15c divided by 15f times 100)		81.66%	89.52%

* If you are claiming electronic copies, go to line 16 on page 3. If you are not claiming electronic copies, skip to line 17 on page 3.
PS Form 3526, July 2014 (Page 2 of 4)

16. Electronic Copy Circulation

	Average No. Copies Each Issue During Preceding 12 Months	No. Copies of Single Issue Published Nearest to Filing Date
a. Paid Electronic Copies	▶	
b. Total Paid Print Copies (Line 15c) + Paid Electronic Copies (Line 16a)	▶	
c. Total Print Distribution (Line 15f) + Paid Electronic Copies (Line 16a)	▶	
d. Percent Paid (Both Print & Electronic Copies) (16b divided by 16c × 100)	▶	

☒ I certify that 50% of all my distributed copies (electronic and print) are paid above a nominal price.

17. Publication of Statement of Ownership
☒ If the publication is a general publication, publication of this statement is required. Will be printed in the NOVEMBER 2019 issue of this publication.
☐ Publication not required.

18. Signature and Title of Editor, Publisher, Business Manager, or Owner
Stephen R. Bushing
STEPHEN R. BUSHING - INVENTORY DISTRIBUTION CONTROL MANAGER
Date 9/18/2019

I certify that all information furnished on this form is true and complete. I understand that anyone who furnishes false or misleading information on this form or who omits material or information requested on the form may be subject to criminal sanctions (including fines and imprisonment) and/or civil sanctions (including civil penalties).

PS Form 3526, July 2014 (Page 3 of 4) PRIVACY NOTICE: See our privacy policy on www.usps.com.

Printed and bound by CPI Group (UK) Ltd, Croydon, CR0 4YY

08/05/2025

01864747-0002